Soft Tissue Pathology

Editor

ELIZABETH G. DEMICCO

SURGICAL PATHOLOGY CLINICS

www.surgpath.theclinics.com

Consulting Editor
JASON L. HORNICK

March 2019 • Volume 12 • Number 1

ELSEVIER

1600 John F. Kennedy Boulevard • Suite 1800 • Philadelphia, Pennsylvania, 19103-2899

http://www.theclinics.com

SURGICAL PATHOLOGY CLINICS Volume 12, Number 1
March 2019 ISSN 1875-9181, ISBN-13: 978-0-323-66102-7

Editor: Stacy Eastman
Developmental Editor: Donald Mumford

Surgical Pathology Clinics (ISSN 1875-9181) is published quarterly by Elsevier Inc., 360 Park Avenue South, New York, NY 10010. Months of issue are March, June, September, and December. Business and Editorial Office: Elsevier Inc., 1600 John F. Kennedy Blvd., Ste. 1800, Philadelphia, PA 19103-2899. Accounting and Circulation Offices: Elsevier Inc., 3251 Riverport Lane, Maryland Heights, MO 63043. Periodicals postage paid at New York, NY and at additional mailing offices. Subscription prices are $213.00 per year (US individuals), $279.00 per year (US institutions), $100.00 per year (US students/residents), $272.00 per year (Canadian individuals), $318.00 per year (Canadian Institutions), $263.00 per year (foreign individuals), $318.00 per year (foreign institutions), and $120.00 per year (international & Canadian students/residents). Foreign air speed delivery is included in all *Clinics'* subscription prices. All prices are subject to change without notice. **POSTMASTER:** Send address changes to *Surgical Pathology Clinics*, Elsevier, 3251 Riverport Lane, Maryland Heights, MO 63043. **Customer Service: 1-800-654-2452 (US). From outside the United States, call 1-314-447-8871. Fax: 1-314-447-8029. E-mail: JournalsCustomerServiceusa@elsevier.com (for print support) and** JournalsOnlineSupport-usa@elsevier.com **(for online support).**

Reprints. For copies of 100 or more, of articles in this publication, please contact the Commercial Reprints Department, Elsevier Inc., 360 Park Avenue South, New York, NY 10010-1710. Tel. 212-633-3874; Fax: 212-633-3820; E-mail: reprints@elsevier.com.

Surgical Pathology Clinics of North America is covered in *MEDLINE/PubMed (Index Medicus)*.

Contributors

CONSULTING EDITOR

JASON L. HORNICK, MD, PhD
Director of Surgical Pathology and
Immunohistochemistry, Brigham and Women's
Hospital, Professor of Pathology, Harvard
Medical School, Boston, Massachusetts, USA

EDITOR

ELIZABETH G. DEMICCO, MD, PhD
Staff Pathologist, Department of Pathology and
Laboratory Medicine, Mount Sinai Hospital,
Associate Professor, Department of Laboratory
Medicine and Pathobiology, University of
Toronto, Toronto, Ontario, Canada

AUTHORS

ABBAS AGAIMY, MD
Institute of Pathology, Friedrich-Alexander
University Erlangen-Nürnberg (FAU), Erlangen,
Germany

NARASIMHAN P. AGARAM, MBBS
Associate Attending Pathologist, Department
of Pathology, Memorial Sloan Kettering Cancer
Center, New York, New York, USA

CODY S. CARTER, MD
Bone and Soft Tissue Pathology Fellow,
Department of Pathology, Michigan Medicine,
University of Michigan, Ann Arbor, Michigan,
USA

SOFIA DANIELA CARVALHO, MD
Pathologist, Department of Pathology, Hospital
de Braga, Braga, Portugal; Department of
Pathology, Institut Bergonié, Bordeaux, France

JOHN S.A. CHRISINGER, MD
Assistant Professor, Department of Pathology
and Immunology, Washington University
School of Medicine, St Louis, Missouri,
USA

JEAN-MICHEL COINDRE, MD
Professor, Department of Pathology, Institut
Bergonié, University of Bordeaux, Bordeaux,
France

AMANDINE CROMBÉ, MD
Radiologist, Department of Radiology, Institut
Bergonié, Bordeaux, France

**BRENDAN C. DICKSON, BA, BSc, MD, MSc,
FCAP, FRCPC**
Staff Pathologist, Department of Pathology and
Laboratory Medicine, Mount Sinai Hospital,
Associate Professor, Department of
Laboratory Medicine and Pathobiology,
University of Toronto, Toronto, Ontario,
Canada

LEONA A. DOYLE, MD
Associate Pathologist, Department
of Pathology, Brigham and Women's
Hospital, Assistant Professor, Harvard
Medical School, Boston, Massachusetts,
USA

CYRIL FISHER, MD, DSc, FRCPath
Department of Musculoskeletal Pathology,
Royal Orthopaedic Hospital NHS Foundation
Trust, Robert Aitken Institute for Clinical
Research, University of Birmingham,
Birmingham, United Kingdom

KAREN J. FRITCHIE, MD
Associate Professor, Department of
Laboratory Medicine and Pathology, Mayo
Clinic, Rochester, Minnesota, USA

OMAR HABEEB, MD
Fellow, Department of Pathology, NYU
Langone Medical Center, New York University,
New York, New York, USA

VICKIE Y. JO, MD
Assistant Professor, Department of Pathology,
Brigham and Women's Hospital, Boston,
Massachusetts, USA

FRANÇOIS LE LOARER, MD, PhD
Assistant Professor, Department of Pathology,
Institut Bergonié, University of Bordeaux,
Bordeaux, France

ANTHONY P. MARTINEZ, MD
Bone and Soft Tissue Fellow, Department
of Laboratory Medicine and Pathology,
Mayo Clinic, Rochester, Minnesota,
USA

JEFFREY K. MITO, MD, PhD
Clinical Fellow, Department of Pathology,
Brigham and Women's Hospital, Harvard
Medical School, Boston, Massachusetts,
USA

DEVARATI MITRA, MD
Resident, Department of Radiation Oncology,
Brigham and Women's Hospital, Clinical
Fellow, Harvard Medical School, Boston,
Massachusetts, USA

DAVID J. PAPKE Jr, MD, PhD
Department of Pathology, Brigham and
Women's Hospital, Boston, Massachusetts,
USA

RAJIV M. PATEL, MD
Professor, Departments of Pathology and
Dermatology, Sections of Bone and Soft Tissue
Pathology, and Dermatopathology, Michigan
Medicine, University of Michigan, Ann Arbor,
Michigan, USA

DANIEL PISSALOUX, PhD
Molecular Biologist, Department of Pathology,
Centre Leon Berard, Lyon, France

BRIAN P. RUBIN, MD, PhD
Professor and Chair of Pathology, Robert J.
Tomsich Pathology and Laboratory Medicine
Institute, Cleveland Clinic and Lerner Research
Institute, Cleveland, Ohio, USA

KHIN THWAY, MD, FRCPath
Sarcoma Unit, Royal Marsden Hospital, The
Royal Marsden NHS Foundation Trust,
London, United Kingdom

WEI-LIEN WANG, MD
Associate Professor, Departments of
Pathology and Translational Molecular
Pathology, The University of Texas MD
Anderson Cancer Center, Houston, Texas,
USA

Contents

Recent work has revealed SMARCB1/INI1 loss by immunohistochemistry in a subset of epithelioid schwannomas and explored the significance of cytologic atypia and increased mitotic activity in these tumors. Additional studies have evaluated the utility and limitations of histone H3K27 trimethylation in diagnosis of high-grade and low-grade malignant peripheral nerve sheath tumors. New terminology regarding nerve sheath tumors in neurofibromatosis type 1 patients was proposed during a 2016 conference to better define guidelines for classification of this group of tumors. This review highlights novel findings and practical applications relating to these topics in peripheral nerve sheath tumors.

This article reviews the histologic patterns of spindle cell/pleomorphic lipoma, well-differentiated liposarcoma, and dedifferentiated liposarcoma in the context of both usual and atypical anatomic presentation. The utility of molecular and immunohisto-chemical diagnostic modalities to distinguish these entities is described. In addition, more recently described and controversial entities, including atypical spindle cell lipomatous tumor and anisometric cell lipoma, are discussed.

In this review, we provide an update of the recently discovered, diagnostically significant genetic aberrations harbored by a subset of vascular neoplasms. From benign (epithelioid hemangioma, spindle cell hemangioma), to intermediate (pseudomyogenic hemangioendothelioma), to malignant (epithelioid hemangioendothelioma, angiosarcoma), each neoplasm features a mutation or gene fusion that facilitates its diagnosis by immunohistochemistry and/or molecular ancillary testing. The identification of these genetic anomalies not only assists with the objective classification and diagnosis of these neoplasms, but also serves to help recognize potential therapeutic targets.

Myogenic sarcomas include soft tissue sarcomas that show skeletal muscle differentiation (rhabdomyosarcoma) and those with smooth muscle differentiation (leiomyosarcoma). Rhabdomyosarcomas are more common in the pediatric age group and leiomyosarcomas occur more often in the adult population. Based on the clinico-pathologic features and genetic abnormalities identified, the rhabdomyosarcomas are classified into embryonal, alveolar, spindle cell/sclerosing, and pleomorphic subtypes. Each subtype shows distinctive morphology and has characteristic genetic abnormalities. In this update on myogenic sarcomas, each entity is discussed with special emphasis on recent updates in genetic findings and the diagnostic approach to these tumors.

event driving the initiation and/or dedifferentiation of mostly lethal but histogenetically diverse neoplasms in different body organs. This review summarizes and discusses the morphologic and phenotypic diversity of primary soft tissue neoplasms
characterized by SWI/SNF complex deficiency with an emphasis on convergent
and divergent cytoarchitectural patterns.

Among the various genes that can be rearranged in soft tissue neoplasms associated with nonrandom chromosomal translocations, *EWSR1* is the most frequent
one to partner with other genes to generate recurrent fusion genes. This leads to
a spectrum of clinically and pathologically diverse mesenchymal and nonmesenchymal neoplasms, variably manifesting as small round cell, spindle cell, clear cell or
adipocytic tumors, or tumors with distinctive myxoid stroma. This review summarizes the growing list of mesenchymal neoplasms that are associated with *EWSR1*
gene rearrangements.

Round cell sarcomas morphologically similar to Ewing sarcoma, but lacking the
classic immunohistochemical features, *EWSR-ETS* family fusions, and other signs
of differentiation, are classified as Ewing-like sarcomas. Recent molecular advances
led to the discovery and characterization of two recurrent oncogenic fusion rearrangements, *CIC-DUX4* and *BCOR-CCNB3*, in a significant subset of Ewing-like sarcomas. Uncovered alternate fusion partners broadened the proposed classification
of these tumors to *CIC*-rearranged sarcomas and *BCOR*-rearranged sarcomas. This
article summarizes the clinicopathologic and molecular features of these entities,
with particular attention paid to those features that overlap with and distinguish
these sarcomas from other round cell sarcomas.

Prognostication in mesenchymal tumors can be challenging. They exhibit diverse,
and sometimes overlapping, histologic features that are not always predictive of
their true behavior. This article highlights examples of both traditional and emerging
sarcoma biomarkers.

Soft tissue neoplasms are increasingly being sampled by core needle biopsy and
fine-needle aspiration (FNA), and these small biopsy specimens pose unique diagnostic challenges. Many advances in ancillary testing enable detection of characteristic immunophenotypes and molecular alterations, allowing accurate classification
of soft tissue tumors in these small biopsy samples. This review outlines pattern-
based diagnostic approaches to core biopsies and FNAs of soft tissue neoplasms,
including formulation of practical differential diagnoses and relevant application of
ancillary tests.

SURGICAL PATHOLOGY CLINICS

SERIES OF RELATED INTEREST

Clinics in Laboratory Medicine

THE CLINICS ARE AVAILABLE ONLINE!
Access your subscription at:
www.theclinics.com

Preface

A Contemporary Approach to Soft Tissue Tumors

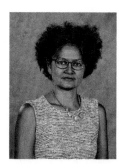

Elizabeth G. Demicco, MD, PhD
Editor

Soft tissue sarcomas are a diverse and diagnostically challenging group of malignancies that may arise at any anatomic site. Classification of these tumors relies on morphology (e.g. spindle cell, round cell, epithelioid, or pleomorphic), line of differentiation (e.g. smooth muscle, vascular, adipocytic, skeletal muscle, nerve sheath, or unrelated to normal tissue lineages), and genomic features (specific gene-fusion, mutation driven, complex karyotype), and the differential diagnosis may vary depending on the tumor site, patient age, and sex. These classification systems overlap and interact in complex ways, such that tumors of myogenic differentiation, for instance, may be classified as mutation associated (a subset of spindle cell/sclerosing rhabdomyosarcoma), translocation driven (alveolar rhabdomyosarcoma, another subset of spindle cell/sclerosing rhabdomyosarcoma), or complex karyotype (pleomorphic rhabdomyosarcoma). Moreover, some sarcomas can behave differently based on site of origin (uterine vs soft tissue leiomyosarcoma), while multiple diverse tumors share *EWSR1*-related gene fusions as common driver event and may display overlapping morphologic features, while showing very different clinical behaviors (e.g., soft tissue myoepithelioma and extraskeletal myxoid chondrosarcoma).

This issue of *Surgical Pathology Clinics* breaks down these complex, interlocking topics into a series of articles focused on tissue lineage of differentiation, predominant morphology, organ of origin, or characteristic molecular event, in order to help readers contextualize these tumors within their histologic, anatomic, or molecular differential diagnosis. These reviews contain state-of-the-art updates on the molecular biology of sarcomas discovered over the past decade, including the identification of specific alterations, contemporary theories on how these alterations drive sarcomagenesis, diagnostic tests derived from these molecular alterations, and in some cases, how changing technologies enabled these discoveries. In addition, the current understanding of the role of prognostic and therapeutic biomarkers in sarcomas is explored, although many proposed biomarkers have yet to reach widespread clinical acceptance. Finally, the diagnosis of mesenchymal tumors in this age of increasingly smaller diagnostic biopsies is reviewed, with a practical focus on what is, and is not, achievable on limited tissue samples.

It is hoped that this issue will serve both as a diagnostic aid and an updated reference for the biology of soft tissue sarcomas.

Elizabeth G. Demicco, MD, PhD
Department of Pathology and Laboratory Medicine
Mount Sinai Hospital
600 University Avenue
Toronto, ON, M5G 1X5, Canada

Department of Laboratory Medicine and Pathobiology
University of Toronto
Toronto, ON M5S 1A1, Canada

E-mail address:
elizabeth.demicco@sinaihealthsystem.ca

Surgical Pathology 12 (2019) ix
https://doi.org/10.1016/j.path.2018.11.003
1875-9181/19/© 2018 Published by Elsevier Inc.

Update on Peripheral Nerve Sheath Tumors

Anthony P. Martinez, MD, Karen J. Fritchie, MD*

KEYWORDS

- SMARCB1/INI1 • H3K27me3 • Epithelioid schwannoma • Nerve sheath tumors

---

Key points

- Approximately 40% of epithelioid schwannomas show loss of SMARCB1/INI1 by immunohistochemistry.

- Loss of Histone H3K27 trimethylation in malignant peripheral nerve sheath tumors ranges from 34% to 73%.

- Low-grade malignant peripheral nerve sheath tumors and other benign peripheral nerve sheath tumors tend to show retained H3K27me3 staining.

- A minority of synovial sarcomas, fibrosarcomatous dermatofibrosarcoma protuberans, and melanoma may show complete loss or mosaic staining for H3K27me3.

- Recent proposed terminology for atypical neurofibromatous tumors in patients with neurofibromatosis type 1 attempts to better define classification of these lesions, including the introduction of the term, *atypical neurofibromatous neoplasm of uncertain biologic potential (ANNUBP)*.

ABSTRACT

Recent work has revealed SMARCB1/INI1 loss by immunohistochemistry in a subset of epithelioid schwannomas and explored the significance of cytologic atypia and increased mitotic activity in these tumors. Additional studies have evaluated the utility and limitations of histone H3K27 trimethylation in diagnosis of high-grade and low-grade malignant peripheral nerve sheath tumors. New terminology regarding nerve sheath tumors in neurofibromatosis type 1 patients was proposed during a 2016 conference to better define guidelines for classification of this group of tumors. This review highlights novel findings and practical applications relating to these topics in peripheral nerve sheath tumors.

EPITHELIOID SCHWANNOMA: WHAT IS NEW

INTRODUCTION

Epithelioid schwannoma, first described by Orosz and colleagues[1] in 1993, is a rare variant of schwannoma composed predominantly of epithelioid Schwann cells. Recently, Hart and colleagues[2] investigated the significance of atypical histologic features in this variant. Additionally, in 2017, Jo and Fletcher[3] studied the rate of SMARCB1/INI loss in a large cohort of these tumors.

CLINICAL

Epithelioid schwannoma usually presents in the fourth and fifth decades of life and occurs equally

---

Disclosure Statement: Nothing to disclose.

Department of Laboratory Medicine and Pathology, Mayo Clinic, 200 First Street Southwest, Rochester, MN 55905, USA

* Corresponding author.

E-mail address: fritchie.karen@mayo.edu

surgpath.theclinics.com

in men and women.[2–5] The majority are dermal and subcutaneous lesions involving the upper and lower extremities, less commonly involving the gastrointestinal tract, back, thorax, and head and neck.[2,3]

PATHOLOGY

Grossly, most cases are unilobulated or multilobulated, well-circumscribed, or encapsulated masses with a median size of 1 cm to 2 cm.[2–5] Microscopic examination reveals cords and clusters of epithelioid cells with a rim of eosinophilic cytoplasm set in a myxoid and/or hyalinized stroma. Although there is no defined percentage of epithelioid cells required for the diagnosis of epithelioid schwannoma, at least 50% of the tumor cells should have epithelioid morphology[2,5] (Fig. 1A–C). Similar to conventional schwannoma, perivascular hyalinization, vascular ectasia, lymphoid aggregates, vague nuclear palisading, and degenerative atypia can be seen in the epithelioid variant. Giant rosettes are present in a subset of cases. The mitotic rate is generally low (1–2/10 high-power fields [HPFs]), without the presence of atypical mitoses or necrosis[2–5] (Fig. 1D).

In 2016 Hart and colleagues[2] examined the impact of atypical histologic features in a series of 58 cases of epithelioid schwannoma. Thirteen tumors (22%) in this study met criteria for atypical as defined by nuclear atypia (nuclear enlargement with hyperchromasia/prominent nucleoli and 3-fold nuclear size variability) and increased mitotic activity (≥3 mitosis/10 HPFs). Only a single tumor recurred and none metastasized, suggesting that even tumors with these features behave in a benign fashion.

Immunohistochemically, epithelioid schwannomas stain like their conventional counterparts, with strong and diffuse S100 protein immunoreactivity (Fig. 1E) and consistent SOX10 positivity. A subset shows glial fibrillary acidic protein (GFAP) staining, and rare cases may stain focally for keratins, but melanocytic-specific markers, such as HMB45 and melan A, are negative.

SMARCB1/INI1 is a tumor suppressor gene located just proximal to NF2 on the long arm of chromosome 22 (22q11.23), and its protein product (SMARCB1/INI1) is part of the human switch/sucrose nonfermentable chromatin-remodeling (SWI/SNF) complex. Molecular studies have confirmed germline mutations in 33% of families with schwannomatosis and a smaller subset of patients with sporadic schwannomatosis.[6] Subsequent work revealed mosaic or partial loss of SMARCB1/INI1 by immunohistochemistry in most familial schwannomatosis cases and up to 50% of schwannomas in sporadic schwannomatosis.[7] Furthermore, up to two-thirds of epithelioid malignant peripheral nerve sheath tumors show loss of this marker. More recently, Jo and Fletcher[3] examined a series of sporadic epithelioid schwannomas and found that 24 of 57 (42%) cases showed complete loss of SMARCB1/INI1 expression (Fig. 1F), suggesting that SMARCB1/INI1 aberrations may play a role in the pathogenesis in a subset of these tumors.

DIFFERENTIAL DIAGNOSIS

Ossifying fibromyxoid tumor, extraskeletal myxoid chondrosarcoma, and myoepithelioma are myxoid mesenchymal neoplasms with epithelioid morphology that should be considered in the differential diagnosis. A peripheral shell of bone favors ossifying fibromyxoid tumor (Fig. 2A), but approximately 25% to 30% of these tumors lack this feature. The lesional cells of extraskeletal myxoid chondrosarcoma are characteristically uniform with deeply eosinophilic cytoplasm (Fig. 2B), and these tumors frequently contain areas of hemorrhage (Fig. 2C). Myoepitheliomas may harbor foci of bone or cartilage with tumor cells arranged in a variety of architectural patterns (Fig. 2D). In contrast to the diffuse pattern of S100 staining seen in epithelioid schwannoma, these other entities typically show only focal S100 staining. A subset of ossifying fibromyxoid tumors shows desmin expression and mosaic loss of SMARCB1/INI1.[8] Complete loss of SMARCB1/INI1 may be seen in malignant myoepithelioma and extraskeletal myxoid chondrosarcoma, but the former typically exhibits coexpression of keratins as well as p63, GFAP, and smooth muscle actin. Molecular testing may be useful in difficult cases or small biopsies because ossifying fibromyxoid tumors harbor PHF1 rearrangements in up to 80% of cases, a majority of extraskeletal myxoid chondrosarcomas show NR4A3 rearrangements, and approximately 50% of myoepitheliomas show fusions involving EWSR1.[9–11]

The most challenging differential diagnosis is epithelioid malignant peripheral nerve sheath tumor because both entities exhibit diffuse S100/SOX10 staining and may show loss of SMARCB1/INI1. Epithelioid malignant peripheral nerve sheath tumors typically harbor more significant nuclear atypia (Fig. 2E) and are less often encapsulated compared with epithelioid schwannoma. Additionally, the presence of atypical

Fig. 1. Low-power examination (*A*) of epithelioid schwannoma frequently reveals circumscription and encapsulation. Higher-power review shows epithelioid cells arranged in cords and clusters in a variably hyalinized (H&E, original magnification ×20) (*B*) and myxoid

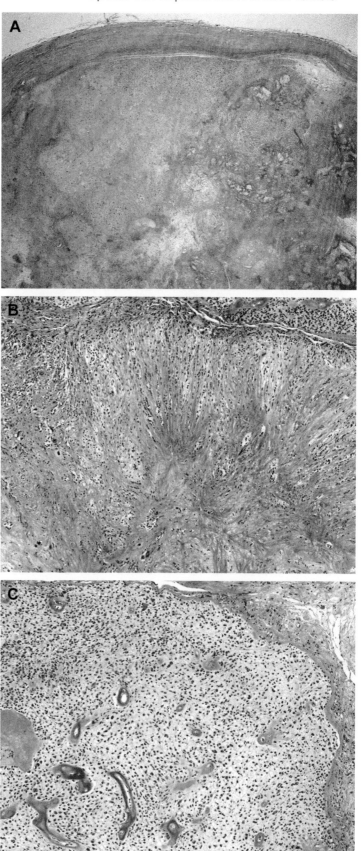

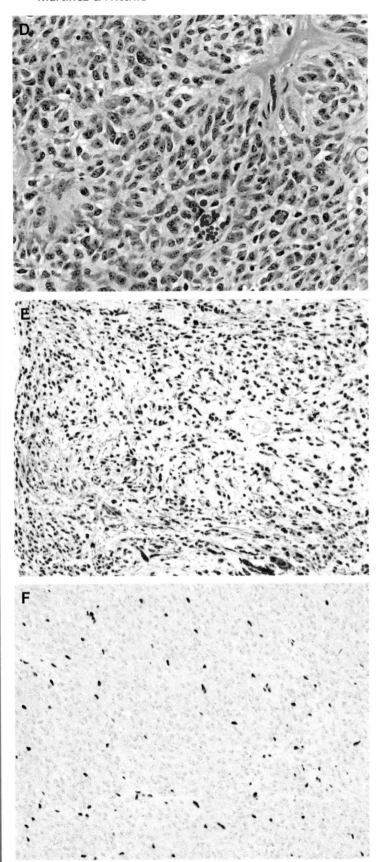

Fig. 1. (*continued*). (H&E, original magnification ×40) (*C*) stroma. Nuclear atypia and mitotic figures (*D*) may be seen, but these features are not associated with adverse prognosis (H&E, original magnification ×400). Tumors show strong and diffuse S100 staining (S100 protein, original magnification) (*E*), and a subset shows loss of SMARCB1/INI1 (*F*) (INI1).

Fig. 2. Ossifying fibromyxoid tumors often show at least a partial rim of peripheral bone (*A*). The lesional cells of extraskeletal myxoid chondrosarcoma show abundant brightly eosinophilic cytoplasm (*B*) (H&E, original magnification ×400), and it is not uncommon to see intralesional hemorrhage (*C*) (H&E, original magnification ×20). Myoepitheliomas may show bone

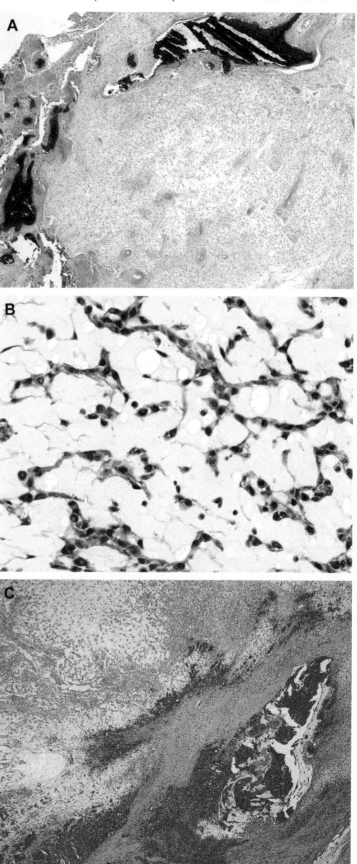

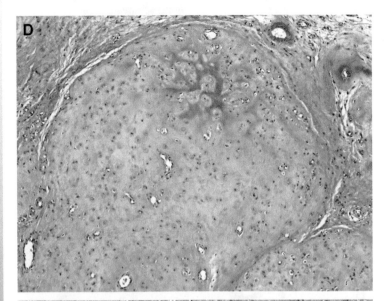

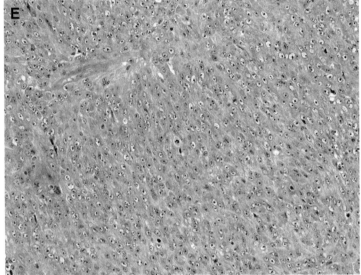

Fig. 2. (continued). (D) (H&E, original magnification ×40) or cartilage matrix. In contrast to epithelioid schwannoma, epithelioid malignant peripheral nerve sheath tumors show more significant cytologic atypia (E) (H&E, original magnification ×100).

mitotic figures and/or necrosis should suggest the diagnosis of epithelioid malignant peripheral nerve sheath tumor.

PROGNOSIS/TREATMENT

The prognosis for epithelioid schwannoma is excellent, with extremely low rates of local recurrence. Complete excision is curative. Rarely, these tumors may undergo malignant transformation to epithelioid malignant peripheral nerve sheath tumor.[3]

Pathologic Key Features

- Well circumscribed or encapsulated
- Cords and clusters of epithelioid cells
- Myxoid or hyalinized stroma
- No atypical mitotic figures or necrosis
- S100/SOX10 positive

Differential Diagnosis

	Helpful Histologic Features	Immunohistochemistry S100/ SOX10	SMARCB1/ INI1 Loss	Genetics
Epithelioid schwannoma	Encapsulation, nuclear palisading, ectatic, and hyalinized vasculature	Diffuse	Subset	
Ossifying fibromyxoid tumor	Peripheral shell of bone	Focal	Subset shows mosaic loss	*PHF1* rearrangements
Extraskeletal myxoid chondrosarcoma	Deep-seated, eosinophilic cytoplasm	Focal	Subset	*NR4A3* rearrangements
Myoepithelioma	Morphologic heterogeneity	Focal	Subset of malignant myoepithelioma	*EWSR1* rearrangements
Epithelioid malignant peripheral nerve sheath tumor	Significant atypia, atypical mitoses, necrosis	Diffuse	Majority	

Pitfall

! Epithelioid schwannoma may show increased mitotic activity or nuclear atypia, and these features do not seem to affect prognosis.

LOSS OF HISTONE H3K27 TRIMETHYLATION IN MALIGNANT PERIPHERAL NERVE SHEATH TUMORS

INTRODUCTION

Malignant peripheral nerve sheath tumors are highly aggressive neoplasms, representing approximately 5% of sarcomas, and can be sporadic, be associated with neurofibromatosis type 1, or arise in the postradiation setting.[12] The morphology of malignant peripheral nerve sheath tumor typically consists of a fascicular/herringbone arrangement of spindle cells, overlapping with monophasic synovial sarcoma and fibrosarcomatous dermatofibrosarcoma protuberans. Because diagnostic criteria for malignant peripheral nerve sheath tumor include peripheral nerve origin, immunohistochemical or ultrastructural support of Schwann cell differentiation, or appropriate clinical history (spindle cell sarcoma in a patient with neurofibromatosis type 1), this diagnosis has traditionally been one of exclusion. Recent studies exploring the loss of histone H3K27 trimethylation in malignant peripheral nerve

sheath tumors have garnered attention in the diagnostic setting.

PATHOPHYSIOLOGY

The polycomb repressive complex 2 (PRC2), which includes associated subunits EZH1/EZH2, SUZ12, and EED, catalyzes the di- and trimethylation of histone H3K27 (H3K27me2 and H3K27me3). Loss of function mutations in *EED* and *SUZ12* results in PRC2 inactivation and subsequent loss of H3K27me3.[13,14] Lee and colleagues[13] showed that functional loss of PRC2 leads to activation of developmentally regulated master regulators and imprinted genes, ultimately driving neoplasia. Additional work has shown that alterations in *EED* and *SUZ12* are present in a majority of malignant peripheral nerve sheath tumors (70%–90%) regardless of clinical setting but not neurofibromas, implicating these genetic changes in the pathogenesis of the former.[13,14] Furthermore, malignant peripheral nerve sheath tumors harboring homozygous loss of *EED* or *SUZ12* show loss of H3K27me3 by immunohistochemistry.[13]

SENSITIVITY AND SPECIFICITY OF HISTONE H3K27 TRIMETHLYATION IMMUNOHISTOCHEMISTRY IN MALIGNANT PERIPHERAL NERVE SHEATH TUMORS

Several groups have explored the diagnostic utility of H3K27me3 in the diagnosis of malignant peripheral nerve sheath tumor and its morphologic mimics (**Table 1**). The frequency of H3K27me3

Table 1
Rates of histone H3k27 trimethylation loss in nerve sheath tumor

	H3K23 Trimethylation Antibody	Definition of Complete Loss	Complete Loss of Histone H3k27 Trimethylation							
			Conventional Malignant Peripheral Nerve Sheath Tumors (All Grades)	Low-Grade Malignant Peripheral Nerve Sheath Tumors	Neurofibroma	Schwannoma	Epithelioid Malignant Peripheral Nerve Sheath Tumors	Melanoma	Synovial Sarcoma	Fibrosarcomatous Dermatofibrosarcoma Protuberans
Rohrich et al,[15] 2016	p	0%—markedly reduced	19/32 (59)	0/3 (0)	0/25 (0)	0/48 (0)	0/1 (0)	—	—	—
Schaefer et al,[16] 2016	p	0%	51/100 (51)	9/31 (29)	0/10 (0)	0/20 (0)	0/10 (0)	0/20 (0)	0/20 (0)	0/10 (0)
Cleven et al,[22] 2016	p	0% or very weak intensity	55/162 (34)	—	0/97 (0)	1/44 (2)	0/2 (0)	1/9 (11)	9/15 (60)	3/8 (38)
Le Guellec et al,[18] 2017	m	<5%	88/122 (72)	4/8 (50)	—	—	—	98/265 (37)	—	—
Asano et al,[20] 2017	m	<5%	30/54 (56)	0/3 (0)	0/43 (0)	0/9 (0)	0/3 (0)	0/8 (0)	0/15 (0)	0/5 (0)
Prieto-Granada et al,[21] 2016	m	<5%	42/68 (62)	1/3 (33)	0/11 (0)	—	0/5 (0)	0/53 (0)	0/113 (0)	—
Pekmezci et al,[19] 2017	m	<5%	7/39 (44)	—	—	—	—	—	7/82 (9)	1/10 (10)
Lee et al,[13] 2014	N/A	N/A	45/62 (73)	—	0/8 (0)	—	0/3 (0)	—	—	—

Abbreviations: m, monoclonal; N/A, not available; p, polyclonal.

Fig. 3. High-grade malignant peripheral nerve sheath tumor (*A*) (H&E, original magnification ×100) with complete loss of H3K27me3 (*B*)

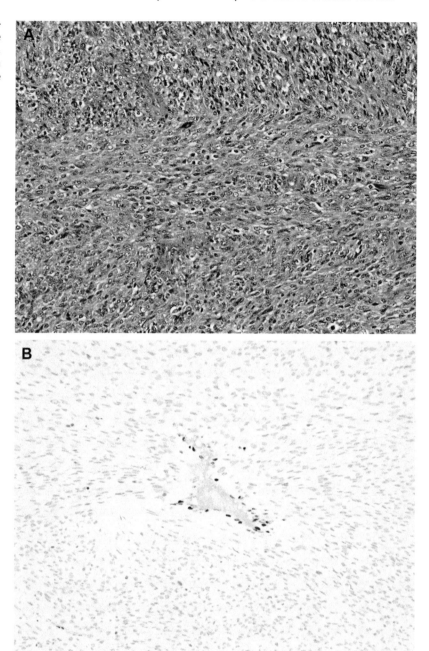

loss (<5% staining) in malignant peripheral nerve sheath tumors, irrespective of grade, in these studies has varied from 34% to 73%, with sporadic and radiation-associated tumors showing higher rates of negative staining than cases arising in patients with neurofibromatosis type 1 (**Fig. 3**).[13,15–19] When specifically evaluating low-grade malignant peripheral nerve sheath tumors, the sensitivity of this marker decreases as rates of loss range from 0% to 50%.[15,16,18,20,21] In contrast, neurofibromas, atypical neurofibromas, epithelioid malignant peripheral nerve sheath tumor, and a vast majority schwannomas have shown intact H3K27me3 staining (**Fig. 4**). Although several studies have found essentially all synovial sarcomas and fibrosarcomatous

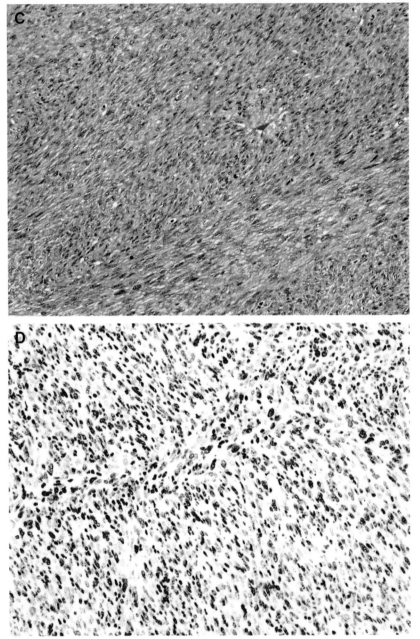

Fig. 3. (*continued*). H&E, original magnification ×100) (*C*) with retained H3K27me3 staining (*D*).

dermatofibrosarcoma protuberans tested to retain H3K27me3, Cleven and colleagues[22] reported H3K27me3 loss in 60% of synovial sarcoma and 38% of fibrosarcomatous dermatofibrosarcoma protuberans.[16,20,21] Because staining with this marker may be heterogeneous, however, especially in synovial sarcoma (**Fig. 5**), the use of tissue microarrays by Cleven and colleagues[22] rather than whole-tissue sections may account for this discrepancy. H3K27me3 loss may also be seen in melanoma (**Fig. 6**)[18,22]; 37% of melanomas, including desmoplastic/spindle cell variant, tested by Le Guellec and colleagues[18] were negative for H3K27me3.

Fig. 4. Examples of low-grade malignant peripheral nerve sheath tumor (*A*, *B*), neurofibroma (H&E, original magnification ×100)

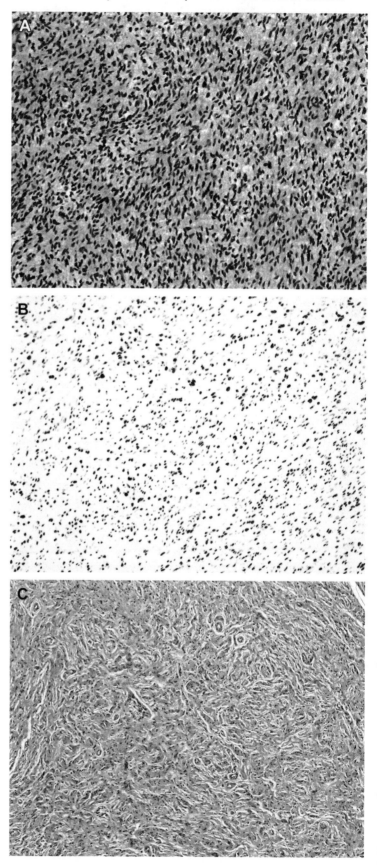

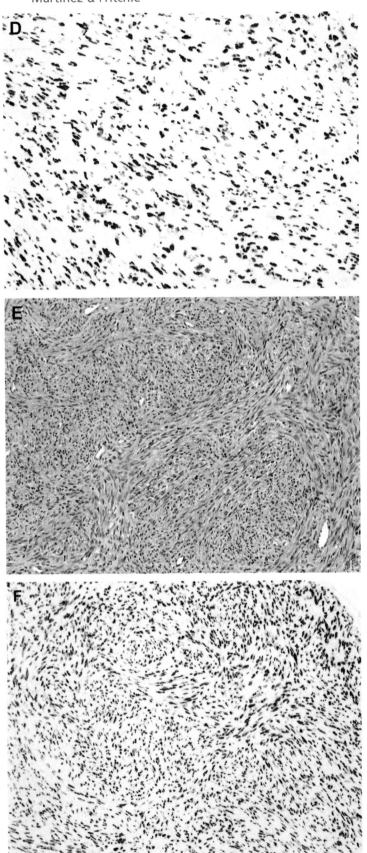

Fig. 4. (continued). (C, D), (H&E, original magnification ×20; H3K27me3) cellular schwannoma (E, F), and epithelioid malignant peripheral nerve sheath tumor (H&E, original magnification ×100; H3K27me3)

Fig. 4. (*continued*). (*G* [H&E, original magnification ×100], *H*) with retained H3K27me3 staining.

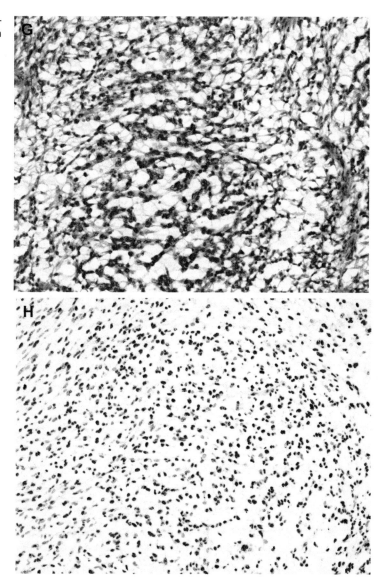

HISTONE H3K27 TRIMETHYLATION LOSS AS A MARKER OF PROGRESSION IN MALIGNANT PERIPHERAL NERVE SHEATH TUMOR

Although aberrations of *NF1* and *CDKN2A* are present in neurofibromas and atypical neurofibromas, there is evidence to suggest that PRC2 inactivation coincides with progression to high-grade malignant peripheral nerve sheath tumor. H3K27me3 is positive in neurofibromas, atypical neurofibromas, and most low-grade malignant peripheral nerve sheath tumors, but this marker is often lost in high-grade malignant peripheral nerve sheath tumors.[16] Furthermore, Cleven and colleagues[22] found loss of H3K27me3 to be an independent prognostic factor for poor survival. Even though subsequent work failed to show correlation between H327me3 status and survival rates, Asano and colleagues[20] did note that H3K27me3-deficient tumors had a higher TNM stage.[19]

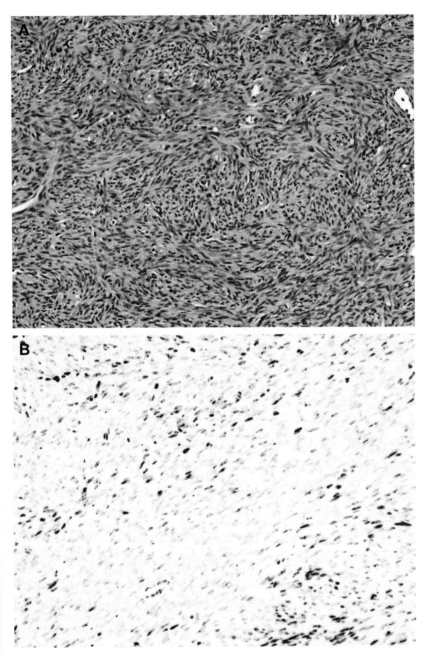

Fig. 5. Synovial sarcoma (A) (H&E, original magnification ×100) with mosaic staining pattern of H3K27me3 (B).

THE SIGNIFICANCE OF HETEROGENEOUS STAINING OF LYSINE 27 OF HISTONE H3 TRIMETHYLATION

Heterogeneous partial loss or mosaic staining (5%–95% staining) may be seen in malignant peripheral nerve sheath tumors as well as a subset of neurofibromas, other sarcomas, and melanomas (see **Figs. 4** and **5**).[16,18–20,23] Although the biological significance of this expression pattern remains uncertain, tumors with this staining pattern may contain a mixture of cells with monoallelic and biallelic mutations in PRC2 subunits. From a practical standpoint, this finding indicates that caution must be exercised when interpreting H3K27me3 staining on biopsies or with limited material. Finally, as with other ancillary testing, H3K27me3 immunohistochemistry is best used within a panel of immunostains in conjunction with assessment of clinical, morphologic, and genetic features (eg, rearrangements of *SYT*, *PDGFB*).

Fig. 6. Malignant melanoma (*A*) (H&E, original magnification ×100) with mosaic staining pattern of H3K27me3 (*B*).

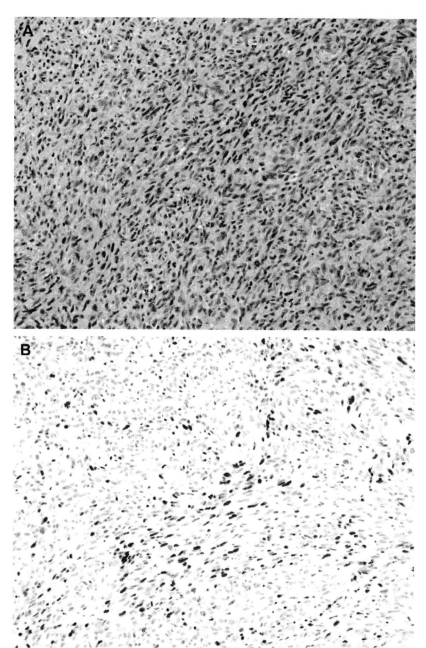

 Pathologic Key Features

- H3K27me3 loss in malignant peripheral nerve sheath tumors ranges from 34% to 73%.

- Low-grade malignant peripheral nerve sheath tumors and other benign peripheral nerve sheath tumors tend to show retained H3K27me3.

- A majority of synovial sarcomas and fibrosarcomatous dermatofibrosarcoma protuberans tested show retained H3K27me3.

 Pitfalls

! H3K27me3 staining can be heterogeneous or mosaic in many tumors.

! Melanomas may show loss of H3K27me3.

PROPOSED TERMINOLOGY FOR NEUROFIBROMATOSIS TYPE 1–ASSOCIATED PERIPHERAL NERVE SHEATH TUMORS

INTRODUCTION

Neurofibromas are benign peripheral nerve sheath tumors consisting of spindled Schwann cells with hyperchromatic wavy nuclei often admixed with fibroblasts and strands of collagen (see **Fig. 4C**). Cytologic atypia in these tumors is considered a degenerative phenomenon and is not a worrisome feature in isolation. High-grade malignant peripheral nerve sheath tumors, representing the opposite end of this histologic spectrum, typically exhibit overtly malignant features including fascicular/herringbone architecture, high mitotic rates, and necrosis (see **Fig. 3A, C**). The diagnosis of low-grade malignant peripheral nerve sheath (see **Fig. 4A**), however, is often problematic because well-defined criteria for this diagnosis are lacking. Furthermore, various terms, such as atypical neurofibroma or neurofibroma with atypical features, have been used to describe tumors with worrisome findings (such as increased cellularity or rare mitotic activity) that fall short of the diagnosis of low-grade malignant peripheral nerve sheath tumor.[24,25]

The utility of cell cycle regulators, such as p16 and p53 as well as Ki-67, and loss of HK27me3 has been explored in this diagnostic setting, but ultimately remains of marginal clinical value. Although malignant peripheral nerve sheath tumors demonstrate loss of the *CDKN2A* gene, which encodes the p16 protein, leading to loss of p16 expression, a majority of neurofibromas retain p16 staining. Beert and colleagues[24] demonstrated, however, that *CDKN2A* can also be lost in atypical neurofibromas. Thus, even though absence of p16 staining may suggest an early stage of malignant transformation, it does not necessarily indicate malignancy. Likewise, malignant peripheral nerve sheath tumors tend to show higher expression of p53 (>10%), but the use of this marker is limited in distinguishing between atypical neurofibroma, neurofibroma with atypical features, and low-grade malignant peripheral nerve tumor because the latter all generally show low expression of p53 (usually <5%).[26–28] Higher Ki-67 rates would be expected in malignant peripheral nerve sheath tumors (>10%) compared with neurofibromas (≤5%), but validated cutoffs are lacking. As discussed previously, H3K27me3 has been shown to be lost in a significant proportion of high-grade malignant peripheral nerve sheath tumors but benign neurofibromas, atypical neurofibromas, and most low-grade malignant peripheral nerve sheath tumors tended to show intact H3K27me3 staining.[15–21] Consequently, differentiating neurofibromas with increased cellularity or rare mitotic activity from low-grade malignant peripheral nerve sheath tumors remains primarily a morphologic distinction.

PROPOSED TERMINOLOGY FOR PERIPHERAL NERVE SHEATH TUMORS IN PATIENTS WITH NEUROFIBROMATOSIS 1

A recent consensus meeting focusing on the pathology of neurofibromatosis 1–associated atypical nerve sheath tumors yielded new terminology for these challenging cases[29] (**Table 2**). The proposed terminology better defines what

Table 2
Proposed terminology for atypical neurofibromatous tumors in patients with neurofibromatosis type 1

Diagnosis	Proposed Definition
Neurofibroma	Schwann cells in a myxoid/collagenous stroma with admixed fibroblasts
Neurofibroma with atypia	Neurofibroma with atypia only
Cellular neurofibroma	Neurofibroma with increased cellularity but lacking fascicular/herringbone architecture and mitotic rate <1/50 HPFs
ANNUBP	Schwann cell neoplasm with ≥2 (of 4) features: • Cytologic atypia • Hypercellularity • Herringbone/fascicular architecture • Mitotic rate >1/50 HPFs but <3/10 HPFs
Low-grade malignant peripheral nerve sheath tumor	Features of ANNUBP with mitotic rate 3–9/10 HPFs and no necrosis
High-grade malignant peripheral nerve sheath tumor	Malignant peripheral nerve sheath tumor with mitotic rate ≥10/10 HPFs or 3–9/10 HPFs and necrosis

Proposed terminology from Miettinen MM, Antonescu CR, Fletcher CDM, et al. Histopathologic evaluation of atypical neurofibromatous tumors and their transformation into malignant peripheral nerve sheath tumor in patients with neurofibromatosis 1-a consensus overview. Hum Pathol 2017;67:1–10.

Fig. 7. An example of ANNUBP showing increased cellularity, loss of neurofibroma architecture (H&E, original magnification ×100) (*A*) and cytologic atypia (*B*) but with a mitotic rate less of than 3/10 HPFs (H&E, original magnification ×200).

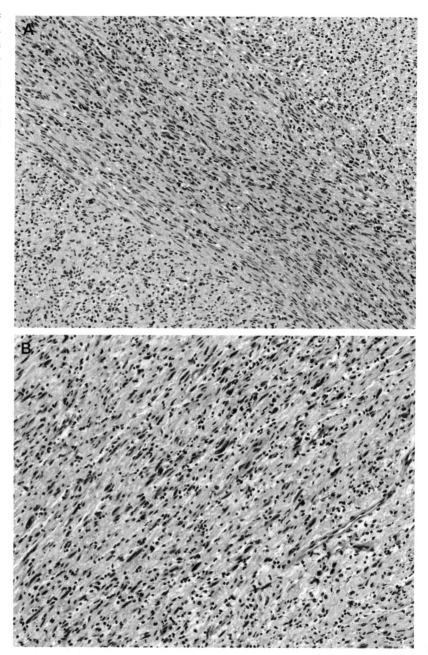

was previously termed, *neurofibroma with atypical features*, and gives specific mitotic count cutoffs to help distinguish between low-grade and high-grade malignant peripheral nerve sheath tumors. Additionally, the term, *atypical neurofibromatous neoplasm of uncertain biologic potential (ANNUBP)*, was introduced for lesions fulfilling at least 2 of the following criteria: cytologic atypia, loss of normal neurofibroma architecture, hypercellularity, and mitoses greater than 1/50 HPF

but less than 3/10 HPFs (**Fig. 7**). Low-grade malignant peripheral nerve sheath tumors harbor features of ANNUBP but have a mitotic count of 3/10 HPFs to 9/10 HPFs, and high-grade malignant peripheral nerve sheath tumors exhibit mitotic rates greater than or equal to 10/10 HPFs or 3/10 HPFs to 9/10 HPFs with necrosis.[29] It seems that tumors that meet criteria for either ANNUBP or low-grade malignant peripheral nerve sheath tumors have relatively low recurrence rates and do not metastasize.[27,30,31] Although these guidelines are intended for lesions arising in the setting neurofibromatosis 1, they likely can be applied to sporadic cases as well.

Because malignant transformation in neurofibromas may be focal, thorough sampling of resections, especially in cases of the plexiform variant, is critical for accurate diagnosis. Painful or rapidly growing lesions or those with worrisome MRI features should trigger tissue sampling, and biopsies in these cases should target the suspicious areas seen on imaging.

REFERENCES

1. Orosz Z, Sapi Z, Szentirmay Z. Unusual benign neurogenic soft tissue tumour. Epithelioid schwannoma or an ossifying fibromyxoid tumour? Pathol Res Pract 1993;189(5):601–5, [discussion: 605–7].

2. Hart J, Gardner JM, Edgar M, et al. Epithelioid schwannomas: an analysis of 58 cases including atypical variants. Am J Surg Pathol 2016;40(5):704–13.

3. Jo VY, Fletcher CDM. SMARCB1/INI1 loss in epithelioid schwannoma: a clinicopathologic and immunohistochemical study of 65 cases. Am J Surg Pathol 2017;41(8):1013–22.

4. Kindblom LG, Meis-Kindblom JM, Havel G, et al. Benign epithelioid schwannoma. Am J Surg Pathol 1998;22(6):762–70.

5. Laskin WB, Fetsch JF, Lasota J, et al. Benign epithelioid peripheral nerve sheath tumors of the soft tissues: clinicopathologic spectrum of 33 cases. Am J Surg Pathol 2005;29(1):39–51.

6. Hadfield KD, Newman WG, Bowers NL, et al. Molecular characterisation of SMARCB1 and NF2 in familial and sporadic schwannomatosis. J Med Genet 2008;45(6):332–9.

7. Patil S, Perry A, Maccollin M, et al. Immunohistochemical analysis supports a role for INI1/SMARCB1 in hereditary forms of schwannomas, but not in solitary, sporadic schwannomas. Brain Pathol 2008; 18(4):517–9.

8. Graham RP, Dry S, Li X, et al. Ossifying fibromyxoid tumor of soft parts: a clinicopathologic, proteomic, and genomic study. Am J Surg Pathol 2011;35(11): 1615–25.

9. Antonescu CR, Sung YS, Chen CL, et al. Novel ZC3H7B-BCOR, MEAF6-PHF1, and EPC1-PHF1 fusions in ossifying fibromyxoid tumors–molecular characterization shows genetic overlap with endometrial stromal sarcoma. Genes Chromosomes Cancer 2014;53(2):183–93.

10. Agaram NP, Zhang L, Sung YS, et al. Extraskeletal myxoid chondrosarcoma with non-EWSR1-NR4A3 variant fusions correlate with rhabdoid phenotype and high-grade morphology. Hum Pathol 2014; 45(5):1084–91.

11. Antonescu CR, Zhang L, Chang NE, et al. EWSR1-POU5F1 fusion in soft tissue myoepithelial tumors. A molecular analysis of sixty-six cases, including soft tissue, bone, and visceral lesions, showing common involvement of the EWSR1 gene. Genes Chromosomes Cancer 2010;49(12): 1114–24.

12. Zou C, Smith KD, Liu J, et al. Clinical, pathological, and molecular variables predictive of malignant peripheral nerve sheath tumor outcome. Ann Surg 2009;249(6):1014–22.

13. Lee W, Teckie S, Wiesner T, et al. PRC2 is recurrently inactivated through EED or SUZ12 loss in malignant peripheral nerve sheath tumors. Nat Genet 2014; 46(11):1227–32.

14. Zhang M, Wang Y, Jones S, et al. Somatic mutations of SUZ12 in malignant peripheral nerve sheath tumors. Nat Genet 2014;46(11):1170–2.

15. Rohrich M, Koelsche C, Schrimpf D, et al. Methylation-based classification of benign and malignant peripheral nerve sheath tumors. Acta Neuropathol 2016;131(6):877–87.

16. Schaefer IM, Fletcher CD, Hornick JL. Loss of H3K27 trimethylation distinguishes malignant peripheral nerve sheath tumors from histologic mimics. Mod Pathol 2016;29(1):4–13.

17. Cleven AH, Sannaa GA, Briaire-de Bruijn I, et al. Loss of H3K27 tri-methylation is a diagnostic marker for malignant peripheral nerve sheath tumors and an indicator for an inferior survival. Mod Pathol 2016; 29(6):582–90.

18. Le Guellec S, Macagno N, Velasco V, et al. Loss of H3K27 trimethylation is not suitable for distinguishing malignant peripheral nerve sheath tumor from melanoma: a study of 387 cases including mimicking lesions. Mod Pathol 2017;30(12): 1677–87.

19. Pekmezci M, Cuevas-Ocampo AK, Perry A, et al. Significance of H3K27me3 loss in the diagnosis of malignant peripheral nerve sheath tumors. Mod Pathol 2017;30(12):1710–9.

20. Asano N, Yoshida A, Ichikawa H, et al. Immunohistochemistry for trimethylated H3K27 in the diagnosis of malignant peripheral nerve sheath tumours. Histopathology 2017;70(3):385–93.

21. Prieto-Granada CN, Wiesner T, Messina JL, et al. Loss of H3K27me3 expression is a highly sensitive marker for sporadic and radiation-induced MPNST. Am J Surg Pathol 2016;40(4):479–89.

22. Cleven AH, Al Sannaa GA, Briaire-de Bruijn I, et al. Loss of H3K27 tri-methylation is a diagnostic marker for malignant peripheral nerve sheath tumors and an indicator for an inferior survival. Mod Pathol 2016; 29(9):1113.

23. Mito JK, Qian X, Doyle LA, et al. Role of histone H3K27 trimethylation loss as a marker for malignant peripheral nerve sheath tumor in fine-needle

aspiration and small biopsy specimens. Am J Clin Pathol 2017;148(2):179–89.

24. Beert E, Brems H, Daniels B, et al. Atypical neurofibromas in neurofibromatosis type 1 are premalignant tumors. Genes Chromosomes Cancer 2011; 50(12):1021–32.

25. Goldblum JR, Folpe AL, Weiss SW, et al. Enzinger and Weiss's soft tissue tumors. 6th edition. Philadelphia: Saunders/Elsevier; 2014.

26. Kindblom LG, Ahlden M, Meis-Kindblom JM, et al. Immunohistochemical and molecular analysis of p53, MDM2, proliferating cell nuclear antigen and Ki67 in benign and malignant peripheral nerve sheath tumours. Virchows Arch 1995;427(1):19–26.

27. Lin BT, Weiss LM, Medeiros LJ. Neurofibroma and cellular neurofibroma with atypia: a report of 14 tumors. Am J Surg Pathol 1997;21(12):1443–9.

28. Zhou H, Coffin CM, Perkins SL, et al. Malignant peripheral nerve sheath tumor: a comparison of grade, immunophenotype, and cell cycle/growth activation marker expression in sporadic and neurofibromatosis 1-related lesions. Am J Surg Pathol 2003; 27(10):1337–45.

29. Miettinen MM, Antonescu CR, Fletcher CDM, et al. Histopathologic evaluation of atypical neurofibromatous tumors and their transformation into malignant peripheral nerve sheath tumor in patients with neurofibromatosis 1-a consensus overview. Hum Pathol 2017;67:1–10.

30. Okada K, Hasegawa T, Tajino T, et al. Clinical relevance of pathological grades of malignant peripheral nerve sheath tumor: a multi-institution TMTS study of 56 cases in Northern Japan. Ann Surg Oncol 2007;14(2):597–604.

31. Bernthal NM, Putnam A, Jones KB, et al. The effect of surgical margins on outcomes for low grade MPNSTs and atypical neurofibroma. J Surg Oncol 2014;110(7):813–6.

Update on Lipomatous Tumors with Emphasis on Emerging Entities, Unusual Anatomic Sites, and Variant Histologic Patterns

John S.A. Chrisinger, MD

KEYWORDS

- Spindle cell lipoma • Pleomorphic lipoma • Liposarcoma • Anisometric cell lipoma
- Dysplastic lipoma • Atypical spindle cell lipomatous tumor
- Fibrosarcoma-like lipomatous neoplasm

Key points

- Spindle cell/pleomorphic lipoma has myriad histologic variants, which can mimic other tumors.

- Seemingly atypical clinical features do not exclude a diagnosis of spindle cell lipoma.

- Anisometric cell/dysplastic lipoma should not be confused with well-differentiated liposarcoma.

- Atypical spindle cell lipomatous tumor and fibrosarcoma-like lipomatous neoplasm are emerging entities, which are distinct from established types of liposarcoma.

- Well-differentiated and dedifferentiated liposarcomas show a very wide range of histologic patterns. Correlation with anatomic site and additional sampling is often very helpful. Molecular analysis can provide support in difficult cases.

ABSTRACT

This article reviews the histologic patterns of spindle cell/pleomorphic lipoma, well-differentiated liposarcoma, and dedifferentiated liposarcoma in the context of both usual and atypical anatomic presentation. The utility of molecular and immunohistochemical diagnostic modalities to distinguish these entities is described. In addition, more recently described and controversial entities, including atypical spindle cell lipomatous tumor and anisometric cell lipoma, are discussed.

and may arise in atypical settings, complicating diagnosis. Moreover, the diagnosis of emerging entities, such as anisometric cell/dysplastic lipoma (ACDL) and atypical spindle cell lipomatous tumor (ASLT), is fraught with many of the same difficulties. Proper classification of established and emerging lipomatous neoplasms is important because prognosis and treatment vary widely.

OVERVIEW

Lipomatous tumors manifest myriad morphologic patterns, substantial areas of histologic overlap,

SPINDLE CELL/PLEOMORPHIC LIPOMA

CLINICAL PRESENTATION

Spindle cell/pleomorphic lipoma (SCPL) is a benign neoplasm that rarely recurs. Tumors show a marked predilection for the subcutis of the shawl area of men greater than 45 years old.

The author has no financial interests to disclose.

Department of Pathology and Immunology, Washington University School of Medicine, 660 South Euclid Avenue, Campus Box 8118, St Louis, MO, USA

E-mail address: jschrisi@wustl.edu

Multiple tumors, some of which are familial, are very rare.

GROSS AND MICROSCOPIC FEATURES

Subcutaneous lesions are well circumscribed, often encapsulated, and usually less than 5 cm. The cut surfaces are variably yellow, gray-white, and myxoid depending on the proportion of mature adipocytes, spindle cells, and myxoid stroma, respectively.

Pure spindle cell lipoma and pleomorphic lipoma represent ends of a histologic spectrum, whereas most lesions show features of both. Spindle cell lipoma is characterized by bipolar cells with scant to moderate cytoplasm, indistinct cytoplasmic borders, and uniform short bland fusiform nuclei with inconspicuous nucleoli. The spindle cells form short bundles, frequently with nuclear palisading, and haphazard arrangements. Admixed mature adipocytes and ropey collagen fibers are typical (**Fig. 1**A). The stroma is variably myxoid, and the vascular network is composed of relatively inconspicuous scattered small- to medium-sized thick-walled vessels, which can be hyalinized. Masts cells are typical, and lipoblasts may be seen. Mitoses are rare. Pleomorphic lipoma additionally shows bizarre pleomorphic cells, which are often multinucleated and floretlike (**Fig. 1**B).

IMMUNOHISTOCHEMICAL AND MOLECULAR FEATURES

SCPL is positive for CD34, whereas typically negative for S100 protein, STAT6, SMA, and desmin. Rb expression is usually lost, which results from deletion of *RB1* at 13q14[1] (**Table 1**).

DIAGNOSIS AND DIFFERENTIAL DIAGNOSIS

SCPL has multifarious histologic patterns, and the differential diagnosis will vary accordingly. First, there is considerable variance in proportion of spindle cells, collagen, fat, and myxoid stroma. Rarely, tumors have extensive areas composed of bundles of collagen,[2] whereas others are predominately myxoid (**Fig. 1**C) and may be mistaken for myxoma. Only rare myxoid SCPL exhibit a plexiform vascular network reminiscent of myxoid liposarcoma (MLS).[3] Cytogenetic analysis for *DDIT3* rearrangement is helpful, if more typical areas cannot be found. Some tumors are mostly composed of mature adipocytes, and resemble lipomas, whereas others have little to no adipocytic component, and thus, the diagnosis relies on recognition of characteristic cytomorphologic features and ropey collagen.[3] Pseudoangiomatous or angiomatous spindle cell lipoma is characterized by villiform projections of tumor into branching cleft-like spaces.[4,5] Dendritic fibromyxolipoma is likely another SCPL variant and is characterized by myxoid stroma, cells with long dendritic processes, a prominent, sometimes plexiform, vascular network,[6] and deletions involving 13q14.3.[7]

SCPL should be distinguished from other neoplasms with spindle cell and adipocytic components (**Table 2**). This distinction can be very difficult, particularly in the case of SCPL, cellular angiofibroma (CAF), and mammary-type myofibroblastoma (MTMFB), which are related neoplasms characterized by the presence of CD34-positive uniform spindle cells, mature adipocytes, myxoid to fibrous stroma with collagen bundles, loss of Rb expression, and deletion of 13q14.[8–10] Although many features overlap, SCPL tends to occur within a shawl distribution, whereas MTMFB and CAF often occur in the genital area. Furthermore, cellular fascicular growth with course hyalinized collagen and prominent small- to medium-sized hyalinized vessels supporting a uniformly cellular spindle cell proliferation are characteristic of MTMFB and CAF, respectively. Rarely, SCPL displays a hemangiopericytomatous vascular pattern[3] simulating fat-forming solitary fibrous tumor (SFT). However, ropey collagen is not a typical feature of SFT, and STAT6 is negative in SCPL.[11,12]

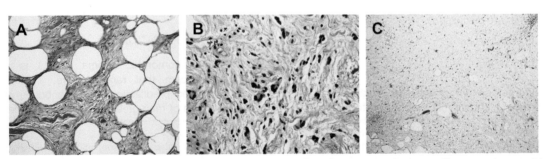

Fig. 1. (*A*) Spindle cell lipoma with admixed bland spindle cells, adipocytes, and ropey collagen set in myxoid stroma (H&E, original magnification ×100). (*B*) Pleomorphic lipoma with multiple floretlike cells (H&E, original magnification ×400). (*C*) Spindle cell lipoma with extensive myxoid stroma (H&E, original magnification ×40).

Table 1
Key features: molecular genetics in select adipocytic neoplasms and mimics

Tumor Type	Cytogenetic Alteration	Molecular Alteration
Lipoma	Rearrangement of 12q13–15, deletion of 13q, rearrangement of 6p21–23	HMGA2 rearrangement most common
ACDL	Variable loss of 13q14	Variable loss of RB1
SCPL	Loss of 13q14 ± loss of 16q	Loss of RB1, ± low-level MDM2 copy gain
ASLT	Variable loss of 13q and monosomy 7	Variable loss of RB1
CAF	Loss of 13q14	Loss of RB1
MTMFB	Loss of 13q14	Loss of RB1
SFT	Inv(12)(q13q13)	NAB2-STAT6 fusion
Myolipoma	t(9;12)(p22;q14) (limited data)	HMGA2-C9orf92 fusion (limited data)
Angiomyolipoma	Mutations in 9q34 or 16p13.3	Mutations in TSC1 or TSC2
Well-differentiated/ DDLS	Supernumerary ring and giant chromosomes (12q13–15)	Amplification of MDM2, CDK4, FRS2, HMGA2, and others
Pleomorphic liposarcoma	Complex karyotype	Alterations involving TP53 and NF1
MLS	t(12;16)(q13;p11) or t(12;22)(q13;q12)	FUS-DDIT3 or EWSR1-DDIT3 fusion (rare)

UNUSUAL ANATOMIC LOCATIONS

The stereotypical presentation of SCPL in the subcutis of the shawl area of middle-aged men can make recognition outside this context challenging. However, SCPL can arise over a wide anatomic distribution, including the buttock, perineum, inguinal region, and distal extremities, including digits.[13] Moreover, most SCPL in women affect sites outside the shawl area and are more frequently dermal.[14] Adding to the potential confusion, most dermal lesions exhibit infiltrative borders,[15] and SCPL may rarely involve muscle, particularly when arising on the face.[16]

ANISOMETRIC CELL/DYSPLASTIC LIPOMA

CLINICAL PRESENTATION

ACDL is a recently described entity that occurs in the subcutis of adults (usually middle aged) and shows a marked male predominance. There is a strong predilection for the head and neck or cephalad trunk, particularly the posterior neck, upper back, and shoulders. The arms, inguinal/genital area, and scrotum may also be affected; lower extremity or superficial skeletal muscle involvement is exceptional. ACDL is benign and infrequently recurs. Most ACDLs are solitary, but approximately 20% are multifocal. Rare tumors arise in patients with a history of retinoblastoma.[17–19]

GROSS FEATURES

Tumors are well circumscribed, are lobulated, may be encapsulated, and appear as unremarkable adipose or fibroadipose tissue. Tumors are often small but may grow to more than 10 cm.

MICROSCOPIC FEATURES

Anisometric cell lipomas are composed of adipocytes with significant variation in size and only minimal nuclear atypia, and scattered foci of fat necrosis frequently involving single adipocytes. Fibrous or fibromyxoid areas without atypical cells may make up a minor component. Scattered lipoblast-like cells can be seen. Some tumors, termed dysplastic lipoma, show scattered atypical hyperchromatic adipocyte nuclei with course chromatin, nuclear enlargement, and Lochkern change[19] (**Fig. 2**).

IMMUNOHISTOCHEMICAL AND MOLECULAR FEATURES

Immunohistochemical (IHC) studies are of limited utility. S100 protein and CD163 highlight adipocytes and histiocytes, respectively; scattered

Table 2
Differential diagnosis: neoplasms with adipocytic and uniform spindle cell components

Features	Spindle Cell Lipoma	CAF	MTMFB	Fat-Forming SFT	ASLT	Myolipoma	Angiomyolipoma
Clinical	Adults; M > F; subcutis; shawl distribution or extremities particularly in women; rare in deep sites	Adults; M = F; subcutis; typically vulvovaginal or inguinoscrotal area but can involve extragenital sites	Adults; M > F; subcutis; inguinal, scrotal, and vulvovaginal areas most common but wide anatomic distribution; rare in deep sites	Adults; M > F; deep; retroperitoneum and thigh most common but wide anatomic distribution	Adults; M > F; superficial or deep; often limb girdles and extremities (including distal) but wide anatomic distribution	Adults; F > M; deep; retroperitoneum and abdominopelvic region	Adults; F > M (sporadic), F = M (TSC); kidney (most common), also retroperitoneum, pelvis, liver, and lung
Histologic	Typically well-circumscribed and often encapsulated; broad histologic range; variable mixture of short bland spindle cells, ropey collagen, myxoid stroma, and mature uniform adipocytes; mitoses rare, scattered atypical mononuclear or multinucleated cells; mast cells; lipoblasts may be present; staghorn vessels usually absent or focal	Well-circumscribed; uniformly cellular; short fascicles or haphazard arrangement; bland ovoid cells; prominent small- to medium-caliber vessels often with hyalinization; fibrous to myxoid stroma; wispy collagen; mitoses rare, mast cells; often with small mature adipocytic component	Well-circumscribed; prominent short fascicles of bland spindle cells; prominent course hyalinized collagen bundles; typically inconspicuous vasculature without hyalinization or staghorn configuration; mitoses rare; masts cells; often with mature uniform adipocytic component	"Patternless" proliferation of bland spindle cells, alternating hypercellular and hypocellular areas or diffusely cellular, branching thick-walled vessels, collagenous stroma, admixed mature adipocytes, may have floretlike cells	Infiltrative or well-circumscribed but unencapsulated; broad histologic range; hyperchromatic atypical spindle cells; adipocytic component with variation in size; myxoid to fibrous stroma; lipoblasts variably present; scattered bizarre cells; ropey collagen rare	Well-circumscribed; intermixed mature bland smooth muscle and adipocytes; thick-walled vessels absent	May be infiltrative; variable proportion of mature adipose, smooth muscle and thick-walled dystrophic vessels

IHC	CD34+, Rb lost, STAT6−, desmin and S100− (rarely +), ER+ (subset)	CD34+, Rb lost, STAT6−, ER+, PR+, focal SMA or desmin+ (subset), S100−	CD34+, Rb lost, STAT6−, desmin+, SMA+ (subset)	CD34+, Rb retained, STAT6+, desmin−, focal SMA and S100+ (subset)	CD34+ (majority), Rb lost (about 50%), S100+ (variable), desmin+ (subset), MDM2 and CDK4− (weak+ in rare tumors)	Desmin+, SMA+, caldesmon+, ER+, CD34−, S100−, HMB-45−, melan A−	SMA+, desmin+ (subset), HMB-45+, melan A+, ER+, CD34−(rarely+), STAT6−
Molecular	Loss of 13q14 (RB1)	Loss of 13q14 (RB1)	Loss of 13q14 (RB1)	NAB2-STAT6 fusion	Variable loss of 13q14 (RB1)	HMGA2 rearrangement (limited data)	Alterations in TSC1 or TSC2

Abbreviations: M, male; F, female; TSC, tuberous sclerosis complex.

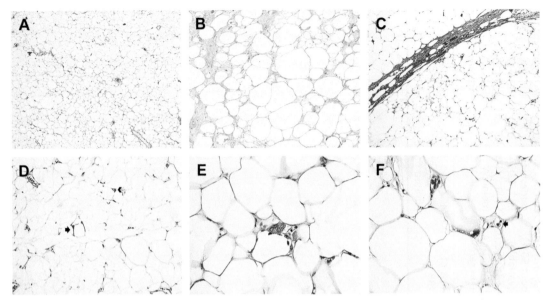

Fig. 2. ACDL. (*A*) There is marked variation in adipocyte size (H&E, original magnification ×20). (*B*) Tumors may have a minor fibrous component (H&E, original magnification ×40) (photomicrograph courtesy of Dr Wei-Lien Wang, Houston, TX). (*C*) A capsule separates the tumor from the subcutis (*upper left*) (H&E, 20× magnification). (*D*) Foci of fat necrosis (*arrow*) and enlarged adipocyte nuclei with Lochkern change (*arrowhead*) are present (H&E, 200× magnification). (*E*) Fat necrosis often involves single adipocytes (H&E, original magnification ×400). (*F*) Adipocyte nuclei may show chromatin coarsening and enlargement. Note adjacent fat necrosis (*arrow*) (H&E, original magnification ×400).

spindle cells are positive for CD34.[18,19] Expression of p53 is seen in 2% to 20% of tumor nuclei, particularly those with atypia.[19] A significant subset of dysplastic lipomas shows focal staining with MDM2, but CDK4 expression is absent (weak staining may be seen in histiocytes).[18,19] Rb expression is completely or partially lost, and some cases show deletion of *RB1*, whereas *MDM2* amplification is not detected[18,19] (see **Table 1**).

DIAGNOSIS AND DIFFERENTIAL DIAGNOSIS

Marked variation in adipocyte size and nuclear atypia rightly raise concern for well-differentiated liposarcoma (WDL). However, ACDL is subcutaneous and lacks large fibrous areas, and atypia is restricted to adipocytes, whereas WDL is only very rarely superficial and usually contains fibrous septa with increased cellularity and atypical stromal cells. ACDL can be separated from traumatized lipomas by the presence of larger areas of fat necrosis with associated reactive myofibroblastic proliferation and hemorrhage in the latter. Furthermore, atypical-appearing cells in traumatized lipomas are generally macrophages, whereas hyperchromatic mononucleated or multinucleated adipocytes are absent. SCPL and ACDL display very similar clinical features, loss of Rb expression, and *RB1* deletion. However, ACDL does not show ropey collagen; striking variation

in adipocyte size and fat necrosis are not features of SCPL, and lesions with hybrid features have not been reported.

ATYPICAL SPINDLE CELL LIPOMATOUS TUMOR

ASLT[20,21] is a controversial designation that encompasses tumors with a wide range of clinical presentations and histomorphologies. Tumors present over a broad age range but are most common in middle-aged adults with a slight male predominance. Tumors present in both subcutis and subfascial tissue, and the extremities (particularly distal), limb girdles, and head and neck are most frequently affected. Involvement of body cavities is rare. The recurrence rate is approximately 12%, and there is minimal metastatic risk.[21]

GROSS AND MICROSCOPIC FEATURES

The median tumor size is 5 cm (0.5 cm to 28 cm).[21] Tumors are infiltrative, or less frequently well circumscribed, and are characterized by a low- to moderately cellular proliferation of uniform hyperchromatic spindle cells, atypical adipocytes with marked variation in size, and a collagenous to myxoid stroma (**Fig. 3**). The relative proportion of each component varies considerably. There are often scattered pleomorphic hyperchromatic

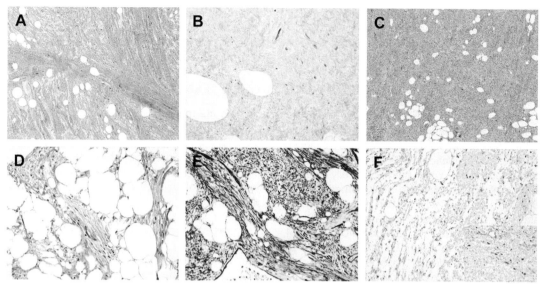

Fig. 3. ASLT. (*A*) Hyperchromatic spindle cells and admixed adipocytes are set in a collagenous to myxoid stroma (H&E, original magnification ×20). (*B, C*) Cellularity varies greatly between tumors (H&E, original magnification ×200, ×20). (*D*) Spindle cells are intimately associated with adipocytes and lipoblasts with significant variation in morphology (H&E, original magnification ×200). CD34 is frequently positive (*E*) (H&E, original magnification ×200), loss of Rb1 (*F*) (H&E, original magnification ×40) and S100 protein expression may be seen (*inset*) (H&E, original magnification ×40). (*Courtesy of* Dr Elizabeth G. Demicco, Toronto, Ontario, Canada.)

mononucleated and multinucleated cells. The mitotic rate is low, and necrosis is absent. Lipoblasts may be present, whereas ropey collagen is rare.[21]

IMMUNOHISTOCHEMICAL AND MOLECULAR FEATURES

The IHC profile is variable. CD34 is positive in most cases, and S100 protein and desmin are expressed in a significant subset. Rb staining is lost in approximately half of tumors.[21] Focal weak MDM2 or CDK4 expression may be noted. There is variable loss of *RB1* and monosomy 7[20–22] (see **Table 1**). Amplification of *MDM2* and *CDK4* is absent.[20,21]

DIAGNOSIS AND DIFFERENTIAL DIAGNOSIS

Atypical adipocytic tumors with a predominant spindle cell component, originally described as spindle cell liposarcoma,[23] represent a heterogenous group of neoplasms, including cases that can now be confirmed as morphologic variants of WDL, dedifferentiated liposarcoma (DDLS), or MLS. However, tumors remain that are difficult to classify. The designation ASLT has been proposed for a subset of such tumors, as described above; however, the broad morphologic spectrum and lack of specific IHC or molecular features make the diagnosis of ASLT challenging.

Low cellularity tumors, which often have mild atypia, can manifest extensive morphologic overlap with spindle cell lipoma. In fact, the designation atypical spindle cell lipoma has also been proposed for such lesions, and it is hypothesized that atypical spindle cell lipoma represents progression from spindle cell lipoma in at least some cases.[20,24] In addition to tumors with spindle cell lipoma-like morphology, lesions with atypical pleomorphic lipoma-like features characterized by wide anatomic distribution, ill-defined periphery, floret-like cells, frequent presence of ropey collagen, variably cellular proliferation of hyperchromatic spindle cells, bizarre (often multinucleated) cells, admixed atypical adipocytic component with significant variation in size, pleomorphic lipoblasts, and variably collagenous to myxoid stroma have been termed atypical pleomorphic lipomatous tumors (APLT).[25] Given overlapping histologic and molecular features, ASLT (including atypical spindle cell lipoma) and APLT may be part of the same spectrum (atypical spindle cell/pleomorphic lipomatous tumor)[25,26] and can be difficult to distinguish from SCPL. Distal extremity location, spindle cell atypia, marked variation in adipocyte size, infiltrative growth, and lack of ropey collagen favor ASLT[21]; however, criteria for separating SCPL from ASLT/APLT are evolving.[27–29] Other Rb loss family tumors, especially MTMFB, can also mimic ASLT (see **Table 2**).

Furthermore, ASLT should be distinguished from WDL and DDLS. Both WDL and DDLS tend to occur in the retroperitoneum and are rare above the fascia, whereas the reverse is true of ASLT. Most

DDLS show clearly high-grade features and an abrupt transition, which is exceptional in ASLT.[21] Less frequently, DDLS produces a morphologically low-grade spindle cell appearance similar to ASLT. The intimate association spindle cells and adipocytes favor ASLT, although a similar (comingling) pattern is rarely observed DDLS.

A more uniform group of tumors designated fibrosarcoma-like lipomatous neoplasms are also in the differential. They are characterized by vaguely nodular growth, bland spindle cell component with parallel orientation, which morphologically recapitulates embryonic adipocyte development, a fine branching capillary network, and a variably myxoid stroma.[30] There is variable expression of S100 protein, CD34, and desmin, whereas MDM2, CDK4, SMA, myogenin, and MyoD1 are negative.[30] By definition, tumors do not show loss of 13q, rearrangement of *DDIT3*, or amplification of *MDM2*.[30] Whether fibrosarcoma-like lipomatous neoplasm lies at the cellular end of the ASLT spectrum or represents a distinct entity is debated.

ATYPICAL LIPOMATOUS TUMOR/WELL-DIFFERENTIATED LIPOSARCOMA

CLINICAL PRESENTATION

WDL is a locally aggressive neoplasm, which most commonly occurs in middle-aged to elderly adults. Tumors are typically deep and involve the retroperitoneum, extremities, abdominopelvic cavity, spermatic cord, and mediastinum. Superficial tumors are rare. WDL is known as atypical lipomatous tumor (ALT) when it occurs in the extremities or superficial locations.

GROSS FEATURES

Tumors are multilobular and appear well circumscribed. Predominately, adipocytic areas are yellow; fibrous areas are firm and tan-white and often take the form of broad bands. Areas with a significant inflammatory infiltrate are fleshy. Dedifferentiation often appears fibrous or fleshy and may be focal.

MICROSCOPIC FEATURES AND HISTOLOGIC VARIANTS

WDL can be divided into 3 types: lipoma-like, sclerosing, and inflammatory, although many tumors are mixed. Lipoma-like tumors are predominately composed of mature variably sized adipocytes with scattered, markedly enlarged, hyperchromatic stromal cells. Broad bands and sheets of collagen, which range from finely fibrillary to sclerotic, divide variable amounts of adipose tissue in the sclerosing type. Scattered pleomorphic stromal cells and floretlike cells are often prominent, especially within fibrous areas. The inflammatory type is characterized by adipose tissue and paucicellular fibrous stroma with scattered atypical stromal cells and a dense inflammatory infiltrate (**Fig. 4**).

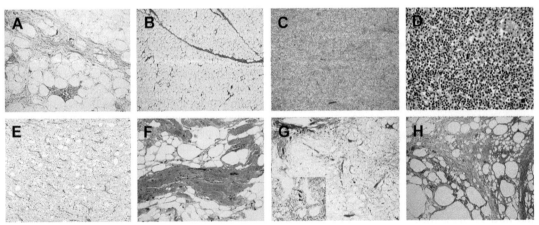

Fig. 4. WDL and mimics. (*A*) Fibrous bands with atypical stromal cells divide sheets of adipocytes with variation in size; lymphoid aggregates are frequently present (H&E, original magnification ×40). WDL shows many patterns including lipoma-like (*B*) (H&E, original magnification ×20) and sclerotic (*C*) (H&E, original magnification ×20). (*D*) Marked mixed inflammation can partly obscure scattered atypical stromal cells (H&E, original magnification ×200). (*E*) Some WDL have areas composed of small bland spindle cells and a branching capillary network reminiscent of MLS (H&E, original magnification ×20). (*F*) Skeletal muscle atrophy in an intramuscular lipoma can mimic atypical stromal cells or floretlike cells. Furthermore, associated fat necrosis produces variably sized adipocytes (H&E, original magnification ×200). (*G*) Fibrous bands and floretlike cells (*inset*) are also seen in herniated orbital fat (H&E, original magnification ×100). (*H*) Fibrosis and foreign body giant cell reaction to silicone should not be confused with WDL (H&E, original magnification ×40).

IMMUNOHISTOCHEMICAL AND MOLECULAR FEATURES

WDL and DDLS are characterized by giant marker and ring chromosomes composed of an amplified region (12q13~15) most commonly including *MDM2*, *CDK4*, *FRS2*, and *HMGA2*, among others[31] (see **Table 1**). Amplification is usually high level (>10 copies), and low-level copy number gains (3–4 copies) or polysomy, should prompt alternative diagnoses. IHC for MDM2 and CDK4 are of limited utility in the diagnosis of WDL because they tend to highlight atypical nuclei, which are rare to absent in ambiguous cases.[32] Moreover, MDM2 IHC is positive in histiocytes,[33] which may be prominent in lipomas with fat necrosis potentially leading to overdiagnosis of malignancy. However, MDM2 and CDK4 IHC may be useful screening tools in the diagnosis of DDLS, pending confirmatory fluorescence in situ hybridization (FISH) or molecular testing to confirm expression is due to gene amplification.

DIAGNOSIS AND DIFFERENTIAL DIAGNOSIS

Atypia in lipoma-like WDL can be focal, particularly in extremity tumors, and thus these tumors can be mistaken for lipoma. Inversely, deep location, large size, and entrapped atrophic skeletal muscle mimicking atypical stromal and floretlike cells (see **Fig. 4**F) can cause intramuscular lipoma to be confused with WDL. Most large retroperitoneal neoplasms with mature adipocytic differentiation are WDL. However, in retroperitoneal tumors without atypia, particularly smaller lesions, other cell types, such as are present in fat-dominant angiomyolipoma, myolipoma, and fat-forming SFT, should be sought. Furthermore, if WDL is excluded after thorough histologic examination and molecular analysis, retroperitoneal lipoma can also be cautiously considered.[34]

Dense lymphocytic, lymphoplasmacytic, or mixed inflammation in the inflammatory type of WDL can mask the underlying tumor. This morphology may lead to a mistaken impression of lymphoma, sclerosing mesenteritis, retroperitoneal fibrosis, Castleman disease, or inflammatory myofibroblastic tumor.[35–38] Diagnosis largely relies on a high index of suspicion and identifying atypical stromal cells in the background.

WDL can also exhibit prominent myxoid stroma. When combined with short uniform spindle cells, small lipoblasts, microcystic pattern, and a plexiform vascular network, there is a close resemblance to MLS.[39–41] Significant pleomorphism strongly favors WDL over MLS. Furthermore, although rare primary MLS of the retroperitoneum

have been described,[42] the vast majority of retroperitoneal MLS-like tumors are WDL or DDLS with MLS-like features.[41] As a caveat, MLS metastases have a predilection for deep soft tissue sites, including the retroperitoneum, so a distant primary (usually the thigh) should also be considered. Interestingly, WDL and DDLS with amplification of *DDIT3* along with *MDM2* may be more likely to show MLS-like features.[43]

Several other usual histologic patterns can cause diagnostic problems, particularly on biopsy. WDL may show bland smooth muscle differentiation. This finding should not be taken for evidence of dedifferentiation or confused with low-grade leiomyosarcoma, angiomyolipoma, leiomyoma, or myolipoma.[44,45] Rarely, hibernoma-like areas are present, and additional sampling may be necessary to identify recognizable areas of liposarcoma.[39,46] Identifying atypia is particularly important because hibernomas may be predominately composed of multivacuolated lipoblast-like cells, causing concern for liposarcoma.[47] WDL may have proliferations of small mild to moderately atypical spindle cells. Such tumors should be separated from ASLT, which, at the cellular end of the spectrum, may be morphologically indistinguishable from cellular ALT.[21]

UNUSUAL ANATOMIC LOCATIONS

Involvement of unusual locations can present site-specific challenges. For example, herniated orbital fat should not be overinterpreted as a rare orbital WDL. Herniated orbital fat is likely a reactive condition characterized by mature adipose tissue, fibrous septa, Lochkern change, and multinucleated floretlike cells (see **Fig. 4**G). Atypical stromal cells characteristic of WDL are absent.[48,49] In addition, the face, genitals, and breast may be sites of silicone injection or leakage. The resulting tissue reaction may somewhat mimic WDL (**Fig. 4**H).

DEDIFFERENTIATED LIPOSARCOMA

CLINICAL PRESENTATION

DDLS is generally characterized by transition from WDL to a pleomorphic and spindle cell sarcoma either in the primary tumor (90%) or in a recurrence (10%). Tumors afflict middle-aged to elderly adults and arise in the retroperitoneum, abdominopelvic cavity, spermatic cord, and deep soft tissues of the extremities and head and neck. DDLS carries a better prognosis than most pleomorphic sarcomas. The metastatic rate is approximately 20%, although mortality is more often attributable to local recurrence.

GROSS FEATURES

DDLSs are multinodular and large. The character of the cut surfaces depends on the distribution of well-differentiated and dedifferentiated areas as well as the composition of each. The dedifferentiated component often manifests as a discrete fibrous or fleshy area. Necrosis and hemorrhage may be present. The well-differentiated component can exhibit a range of gross features; however, it is often recognizable as adipocytic. In fact, clinically, the presence of the well-differentiated component may not be recognized, leading to resection aimed at only the dedifferentiated element. Thus, it is important to sample peripheral fat.

IMMUNOHISTOCHEMICAL AND MOLECULAR FEATURES

See WDL section for more information on immuno-histochemical and molecular features.

MICROSCOPIC FEATURES AND HISTOLOGIC VARIANTS

Microscopically, there is an abrupt or gradual transition from the well-differentiated component to a typically nonlipogenic sarcoma. Rarely, the 2 components are comingled.[50] Dedifferentiated areas are most often composed of undifferentiated markedly atypical polygonal and spindle cells growing in sheets, fascicles, and loose storiform arrays (**Fig. 5**). However, DDLS has myriad histologic patterns that may present a diagnostic dilemma (**Boxes 1 and 2**,

---

Box 1
Pitfalls: dedifferentiated liposarcoma

The well-differentiated component is not always sampled (biopsy or resection without removal of surrounding "normal fat")

DDLS shows an incredible histologic range mimicking numerous neoplasms, including lymphoma, carcinoma, pleomorphic, myxoid, round cell and spindle cell sarcomas, inflammatory myofibroblastic tumor, paraganglioma, and others

Heterologous differentiation is not uncommon and includes leiomyosarcomatous, rhabdomyosarcomatous, osteosarcomatous, chondrosarcomatous, and angiosarcomatous components

The vast majority of myxofibrosarcoma-like and primary MLS-like tumors of the retroperitoneum are DDLS; however, MLS may metastasize to the retroperitoneum

Neural or meningioma-like morphology can mimic follicular dendritic cell sarcoma, which can show staining with MDM2 and harbor amplification of MDM2. CD21 and CD35 are negative in DDLS.

Solitary fibrous tumorlike histology may be seen in DDLS, which can also express STAT6

---

see **Fig. 5**). The myxofibrosarcoma-like pattern can be particularly challenging to distinguish from true myxofibrosarcoma in deep extremity tumors; however, nearly all cases with this appearance in the retroperitoneum and abdominopelvic cavity are ultimately found to be DDLS.[40] Low-grade

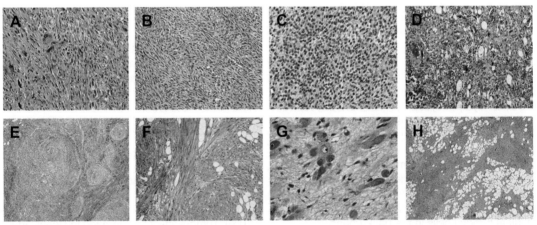

Fig. 5. DDLS. (*A*) The dedifferentiated component is most often histologically indistinguishable from undifferentiated pleomorphic sarcoma (H&E, original magnification ×200). However, numerous other patterns may be seen, including fibrosarcomatous (*B*) (H&E, original magnification ×100), round cell (*C*), inflammatory (also note lipoblasts and emperipolesis) (*D*) (H&E, original magnification ×40), neural or meningioma-like whorling (*E*) (H&E, original magnification ×20), leiomyosarcomatous (*F*) (H&E, original magnification ×40), and rhabdomyosarcomatous (*G*) (H&E, original magnification ×400) among many others. Although an abrupt transition often separates dedifferentiated and well-differentiated components, rare tumors show a comingling pattern (*H*) (H&E, original magnification ×20).

Box 2
Morphologic patterns of DDLS including pitfalls
Undifferentiated pleomorphic sarcoma-like (most common)
Fibrosarcomatous
Round cell
Epithelioid
Inflammatory
Neural/meningioma-like whorls +/- metaplastic bone
Myxoid
Myxoid liposarcoma-like
Myxofibrosarcoma-like
Pleomorphic liposarcoma-like ("homologus" lipoblastic differentiation)
Inflammatory myofibroblastic tumor-like
Solitary fibrous tumor-like
Paraganglioma-like
Leiomyosarcomatous
Rhabdomyosarcomatous
Osteosarcomatous
Chondrosarcomatous
Angiosarcomatous

dedifferentiation in DDLS may also mimic fibromatosis,[51] which can be a particular challenge in intra-abdominal tumors. Furthermore, heterologous differentiation is present in approximately 10% of DDLS, and although dedifferentiation usually takes the form of a nonadipocytic sarcoma, pleomorphic liposarcoma-like ("homologous" lipoblastic differentiation) may also occur.[52,53]

DDLS displays impressive mimicry, but most cases can still be correctly diagnosed histologically through identification of a WDL component and consideration of tumor site. Further correlation with imaging is extremely helpful if the adipocytic component is not sampled, particularly in biopsies. In difficult cases, detection of amplification of MDM2 can provide strong support for DDLS; however, care must be taken because MDM2 amplification is not specific for WDL and DDLS. Extranodal follicular dendritic cell sarcoma can histologically resemble DDLS with neural or meningothelial-like whorling,[54,55] express MDM2,[56] and demonstrate MDM2 amplification by FISH.[57] Furthermore, intimal sarcoma,

rhabdomyosarcoma, and well-differentiated osteosarcoma (intramedullary and parosteal) can also harbor MDM2 amplification.

DDLS can show little or no well-differentiated component and most (Undifferentiated pleomorphic sarcoma) UPS-like tumors of the retroperitoneum are DDLS.[58] It may be that similar tumors in the periphery are underdiagnosed. It has been suggested that peripheral pure UPS or undifferentiated sarcomas with divergent differentiation should be screened with an IHC study for MDM2 followed by confirmatory FISH testing if positive.[59] Peripheral UPS-like tumors with MDM2 amplification appear to be more similar to peripheral DDLS than to UPS.[59]

SUMMARY

Established and emerging lipomatous neoplasms are histologically diverse. Familiarity with typical features as well as variant morphologies and atypical presentations allows for accurate diagnosis in most cases. However, in difficult cases, limited ancillary testing (ie, FISH for MDM2 amplification, DDIT3 rearrangement, or 13q14 deletion) can be informative. Proper classification is important because prognosis and treatment can vary considerably.

REFERENCES

1. Dal Cin P, Sciot R, Polito P, et al. Lesions of 13q may occur independently of deletion of 16q in spindle cell/pleomorphic lipomas. Histopathology 1997; 31(3):222–5.
2. Diaz-Cascajo C, Borghi S, Weyers W. Fibrous spindle cell lipoma: report of a new variant. Am J Dermatopathol 2001;23(2):112–5.
3. Billings SD, Folpe AL. Diagnostically challenging spindle cell lipomas: a report of 34 "low-fat" and "fat-free" variants. Am J Dermatopathol 2007;29(5):437–42.
4. Hawley IC, Krausz T, Evans DJ, et al. Spindle cell lipoma–a pseudoangiomatous variant. Histopathology 1994;24(6):565–9.
5. Zamecnik M, Michal M. Angiomatous spindle cell lipoma: report of three cases with immunohistochemical and ultrastructural study and reappraisal of former 'pseudoangiomatous' variant. Pathol Int 2007;57(1):26–31.
6. Karim RZ, McCarthy SW, Palmer AA, et al. Intramuscular dendritic fibromyxolipoma: myxoid variant of spindle cell lipoma? Pathol Int 2003;53(4):252–8.
7. Wong YP, Chia WK, Low SF, et al. Dendritic fibromyxolipoma: a variant of spindle cell lipoma with extensive myxoid change, with cytogenetic evidence. Pathol Int 2014;64(7):346–51.
8. Howitt BE, Fletcher CD. Mammary-type myofibroblastoma: clinicopathologic characterization in a

series of 143 cases. Am J Surg Pathol 2016;40(3):361–7.

9. Flucke U, van Krieken JH, Mentzel T. Cellular angiofibroma: analysis of 25 cases emphasizing its relationship to spindle cell lipoma and mammary-type myofibroblastoma. Mod Pathol 2011;24(1):82–9.

10. Chen BJ, Marino-Enriquez A, Fletcher CD, et al. Loss of retinoblastoma protein expression in spindle cell/pleomorphic lipomas and cytogenetically related tumors: an immunohistochemical study with diagnostic implications. Am J Surg Pathol 2012;36(8):1119–28.

11. Cheah AL, Billings SD, Goldblum JR, et al. STAT6 rabbit monoclonal antibody is a robust diagnostic tool for the distinction of solitary fibrous tumour from its mimics. Pathology 2014;46(5):389–95.

12. Doyle LA, Vivero M, Fletcher CD, et al. Nuclear expression of STAT6 distinguishes solitary fibrous tumor from histologic mimics. Mod Pathol 2014;27(3):390–5.

13. Ud Din N, Zhang P, Sukov WR, et al. Spindle cell lipomas arising at atypical locations. Am J Clin Pathol 2016;146(4):487–95.

14. Ko JS, Daniels B, Emanuel PO, et al. Spindle cell lipomas in women: a report of 53 cases. Am J Surg Pathol 2017;41(9):1267–74.

15. French CA, Mentzel T, Kutzner H, et al. Intradermal spindle cell/pleomorphic lipoma: a distinct subset. Am J Dermatopathol 2000;22(6):496–502.

16. Cheah A, Billings S, Goldblum J, et al. Spindle cell/pleomorphic lipomas of the face: an under-recognized diagnosis. Histopathology 2015;66(3):430–7.

17. Evans HL. Anisometric cell lipoma: a predominantly subcutaneous fatty tumor with notable variation in fat cell size but not more than slight nuclear enlargement and atypia. Ajsp: Rev Rep 2016;21:195–9.

18. Agaimy A. Anisometric cell lipoma: Insight from a case series and review of the literature on adipocytic neoplasms in survivors of retinoblastoma suggest a role for RB1 loss and possible relationship to fat-predominant ("fat-only") spindle cell lipoma. Ann Diagn Pathol 2017;29:52–6.

19. Michal M, Agaimy A, Contreras AL, et al. Dysplastic lipoma: a distinctive atypical lipomatous neoplasm with anisocytosis, focal nuclear atypia, p53 overexpression, and a lack of MDM2 gene amplification by FISH: a report of 66 cases demonstrating occasional multifocality and a rare association with retinoblastoma. Am J Surg Pathol 2018;42(11):1530–40.

20. Mentzel T, Palmedo G, Kuhnen C. Well-differentiated spindle cell liposarcoma ('atypical spindle cell lipomatous tumor') does not belong to the spectrum of atypical lipomatous tumor but has a close relationship to spindle cell lipoma: clinicopathologic, immunohistochemical, and molecular analysis of six cases. Mod Pathol 2010;23(5):729–36.

21. Marino-Enriquez A, Nascimento AF, Ligon AH, et al. Atypical spindle cell lipomatous tumor: clinicopathologic characterization of 232 cases demonstrating a morphologic spectrum. Am J Surg Pathol 2017;41(2):234–44.

22. Italiano A, Chambonniere ML, Attias R, et al. Monosomy 7 and absence of 12q amplification in two cases of spindle cell liposarcomas. Cancer Genet Cytogenet 2008;184(2):99–104.

23. Dei Tos AP, Mentzel T, Newman PL, et al. Spindle cell liposarcoma, a hitherto unrecognized variant of liposarcoma. Analysis of six cases. Am J Surg Pathol 1994;18(9):913–21.

24. Creytens D, van Gorp J, Savola S, et al. Atypical spindle cell lipoma: a clinicopathologic, immunohistochemical, and molecular study emphasizing its relationship to classical spindle cell lipoma. Virchows Archiv 2014;465(1):97–108.

25. Creytens D, Mentzel T, Ferdinande L, et al. "Atypical" pleomorphic lipomatous tumor: a clinicopathologic, immunohistochemical and molecular study of 21 cases, emphasizing its relationship to atypical spindle cell lipomatous tumor and suggesting a morphologic spectrum (atypical spindle cell/pleomorphic lipomatous tumor). Am J Surg Pathol 2017;41(11):1443–55.

26. Creytens D, Mentzel T, Ferdinande L, et al. Atypical multivacuolated lipoblasts and atypical mitoses are not compatible with the diagnosis of spindle cell/pleomorphic lipoma. Hum Pathol 2018;74:188–9.

27. Michal M, Kazakov DV, Hadravsky L, et al. Lipoblasts in spindle cell and pleomorphic lipomas: a close scrutiny. Hum Pathol 2017;65:140–6.

28. Michal M, Babaoglu B, Kazakov DV, et al. Atypical mitoses in pleomorphic lipomas. Hum Pathol 2017;70:143.

29. Michal M, Kazakov DV, Michalova K, et al. Atypical multivacuolated lipoblasts and atypical mitoses are not compatible with the diagnosis of spindle cell/pleomorphic lipoma-reply. Hum Pathol 2018;74:189.

30. Deyrup AT, Chibon F, Guillou L, et al. Fibrosarcoma-like lipomatous neoplasm: a reappraisal of so-called spindle cell liposarcoma defining a unique lipomatous tumor unrelated to other liposarcomas. Am J Surg Pathol 2013;37(9):1373–8.

31. Comprehensive and integrated genomic characterization of adult soft tissue sarcomas. Cell 2017;171(4):950–65.e28.

32. Clay MR, Martinez AP, Weiss SW, et al. MDM2 and CDK4 immunohistochemistry: should it be used in problematic differentiated lipomatous tumors?: A new perspective. Am J Surg Pathol 2016;40(12):1647–52.

33. Dei Tos AP. Liposarcomas: diagnostic pitfalls and new insights. Histopathology 2014;64(1):38–52.

34. Macarenco RS, Erickson-Johnson M, Wang X, et al. Retroperitoneal lipomatous tumors without cytologic atypia: are they lipomas? A clinicopathologic and molecular study of 19 cases. Am J Surg Pathol 2009;33(10):1470–6.

35. Kraus MD, Guillou L, Fletcher CD. Well-differentiated inflammatory liposarcoma: an uncommon and easily

overlooked variant of a common sarcoma. Am J Surg Pathol 1997;21(5):518–27.

36. Argani P, Facchetti F, Inghirami G, et al. Lymphocyte-rich well-differentiated liposarcoma: report of nine cases. Am J Surg Pathol 1997;21(8):884–95.

37. Snover DC, Sumner HW, Dehner LP. Variability of histologic pattern in recurrent soft tissue sarcomas originally diagnosed as liposarcoma. Cancer 1982; 49(5):1005–15.

38. Weaver J, Goldblum JR, Turner S, et al. Detection of MDM2 gene amplification or protein expression distinguishes sclerosing mesenteritis and retroperitoneal fibrosis from inflammatory well-differentiated liposarcoma. Mod Pathol 2009;22(1):66–70.

39. Evans HL. Atypical lipomatous tumor, its variants, and its combined forms: a study of 61 cases, with a minimum follow-up of 10 years. Am J Surg Pathol 2007;31(1):1–14.

40. Sioletic S, Dal Cin P, Fletcher CD, et al. Well-differentiated and dedifferentiated liposarcomas with prominent myxoid stroma: analysis of 56 cases. Histopathology 2013;62(2):287–93.

41. de Vreeze RS, de Jong D, Tielen IH, et al. Primary retroperitoneal myxoid/round cell liposarcoma is a nonexisting disease: an immunohistochemical and molecular biological analysis. Mod Pathol 2009; 22(2):223–31.

42. Setsu N, Miyake M, Wakai S, et al. Primary retroperitoneal myxoid liposarcomas. Am J Surg Pathol 2016;40(9):1286–90.

43. Mantilla JG, Ricciotti RW, Chen EY, et al. Amplification of DNA damage-inducible transcript 3 (DDIT3) is associated with myxoid liposarcoma-like morphology and homologous lipoblastic differentiation in dedifferentiated liposarcoma. Mod Pathol 2018. [Epub ahead of print].

44. Folpe AL, Weiss SW. Lipoleiomyosarcoma (well-differentiated liposarcoma with leiomyosarcomatous differentiation): a clinicopathologic study of nine cases including one with dedifferentiation. Am J Surg Pathol 2002;26(6):742–9.

45. Evans HL. Smooth muscle in atypical lipomatous tumors. A report of three cases. Am J Surg Pathol 1990;14(8):714–8.

46. Hallin M, Schneider N, Thway K. Well-differentiated liposarcoma with hibernoma-like morphology. Int J Surg Pathol 2016;24(7):620–2.

47. Al Hmada Y, Schaefer IM, Fletcher CDM. Hibernoma mimicking atypical lipomatous tumor: 64 cases of a morphologically distinct subset. Am J Surg Pathol 2018;42(7):951–7.

48. Schmack I, Patel RM, Folpe AL, et al. Subconjunctival herniated orbital fat: a benign adipocytic lesion that may mimic pleomorphic lipoma and atypical lipomatous tumor. Am J Surg Pathol 2007;31(2): 193–8.

49. Stacy RC, Bernardo LA, Nielsen GP. Absence of chromosomal abnormalities in herniated orbital fat. Histopathology 2014;65(2):273–7.

50. Iwasa Y, Nakashima Y. Dedifferentiated liposarcoma with lipoma-like well-differentiated liposarcoma: clinicopathological study of 30 cases, with particular attention to the comingling pattern of well- and dedifferentiated components: a proposal for regrouping of the present subclassification of well-differentiated liposarcoma and dedifferentiated liposarcoma. Int J Surg Pathol 2013;21(1):15–21.

51. Henricks WH, Chu YC, Goldblum JR, et al. Dedifferentiated liposarcoma: a clinicopathological analysis of 155 cases with a proposal for an expanded definition of dedifferentiation. Am J Surg Pathol 1997; 21(3):271–81.

52. Marino-Enriquez A, Fletcher CD, Dal Cin P, et al. Dedifferentiated liposarcoma with "homologous" lipoblastic (pleomorphic liposarcoma-like) differentiation: clinicopathologic and molecular analysis of a series suggesting revised diagnostic criteria. Am J Surg Pathol 2010;34(8):1122–31.

53. Boland JM, Weiss SW, Oliveira AM, et al. Liposarcomas with mixed well-differentiated and pleomorphic features: a clinicopathologic study of 12 cases. Am J Surg Pathol 2010;34(6):837–43.

54. Fanburg-Smith JC, Miettinen M. Liposarcoma with meningothelial-like whorls: a study of 17 cases of a distinctive histological pattern associated with dedifferentiated liposarcoma. Histopathology 1998;33(5): 414–24.

55. Nascimento AG, Kurtin PJ, Guillou L, et al. Dedifferentiated liposarcoma: a report of nine cases with a peculiar neurallike whorling pattern associated with metaplastic bone formation. Am J Surg Pathol 1998;22(8):945–55.

56. Creytens D. MDM2 expression in extranodal abdominal and retroperitoneal follicular dendritic cell sarcomas, mimicking dedifferentiated liposarcomas. Appl Immunohistochem Mol Morphol 2016;24(4): e25–7.

57. Agaimy A, Michal M, Hadravsky L, et al. Follicular dendritic cell sarcoma: clinicopathologic study of 15 cases with emphasis on novel expression of MDM2, somatostatin receptor 2A, and PD-L1. Ann Diagn Pathol 2016;23:21–8.

58. Coindre JM, Mariani O, Chibon F, et al. Most malignant fibrous histiocytomas developed in the retroperitoneum are dedifferentiated liposarcomas: a review of 25 cases initially diagnosed as malignant fibrous histiocytoma. Mod Pathol 2003;16(3): 256–62.

59. Le Guellec S, Chibon F, Ouali M, et al. Are peripheral purely undifferentiated pleomorphic sarcomas with MDM2 amplification dedifferentiated liposarcomas? Am J Surg Pathol 2014;38(3):293–304.

The Molecular Diagnostics of Vascular Neoplasms

Omar Habeeb, MD[a], Brian P. Rubin, MD, PhD[b],*

KEYWORDS

- Molecular diagnostics • Vascular neoplasms • Review

Key points

- Epithelioid hemangioma: *FOS* rearrangements (including *ZFP36-FOSB* gene fusion)
- Spindle cell hemangioma: mutation of *IDH1* or *IDH2*
- Pseudomyogenic hemangioendothelioma: *SERPINE1-FOSB* gene fusion
- Epithelioid hemangioendothelioma: *WWTR1-CAMTA1* gene fusion
- *YAP1-TFE3* fused hemangioendothelioma: *YAP1-TFE3* gene fusion
- Angiosarcoma: multiple aberrations (eg, *MYC* amplification; *CIC* abnormalities; recurrent *PTPRB* and *PLCG1* mutations)

ABSTRACT

In this review, we provide an update of the recently discovered, diagnostically significant genetic aberrations harbored by a subset of vascular neoplasms. From benign (epithelioid hemangioma, spindle cell hemangioma), to intermediate (pseudomyogenic hemangioendothelioma), to malignant (epithelioid hemangioendothelioma, angiosarcoma), each neoplasm features a mutation or gene fusion that facilitates its diagnosis by immunohistochemistry and/or molecular ancillary testing. The identification of these genetic anomalies not only assists with the objective classification and diagnosis of these neoplasms, but also serves to help recognize potential therapeutic targets.

characteristic genetic alterations of vascular neoplasms. However, some of them are now recognized by their specific genetic aberrations, including epithelioid hemangioma (*FOS* rearrangements, including *ZFP36-FOSB*)[3,4]; spindle cell hemangioma (*IDH1* or *IDH2* mutation)[5–7]; pseudomyogenic hemangioendothelioma (*SERPINE1-FOSB*)[8]; epithelioid hemangioendothelioma (*WWTR1-CAMTA1*)[9,10]; *YAP1-TFE3* fused hemangioendothelioma[11]; and angiosarcoma (eg, *MYC* amplification in secondary angiosarcoma; *CIC* mutation and/or rearrangement; recurrent mutations of *PTPRB* and *PLCG1*).[12–14] The recent discovery of most of these findings is indicative of the impact that molecular diagnostics have had on our current understanding of vascular neoplasia.

OVERVIEW

Neoplasms of vascular origin encompass a complex array of pathologic entities.[1,2] For many years, there was little information regarding the

METHODS

The International Society for the Study of Vascular Anomalies (ISSVA)[1] and World Health Organization (WHO)[2] have each issued their own

Disclosure Statement: This research did not receive any specific grant from funding agencies in the public, commercial, or not-for-profit sectors.

[a] Department of Pathology, Langone Medical Center, New York University, 160 East 34th Street, New York, NY 10016, USA; [b] Robert J. Tomsich Pathology & Laboratory Medicine Institute, Cleveland Clinic and Lerner Research Institute, Department of Pathology, 9500 Euclid Avenue L25, Cleveland, OH 44195, USA
* Corresponding author.
E-mail address: rubinb2@ccf.org

Surgical Pathology 12 (2019) 35–49
https://doi.org/10.1016/j.path.2018.10.002

classification of vascular neoplasms. Those neoplasms that harbor diagnostically significant genetic aberrations across both classifications have been selected for review; however, items beyond the scope of this review include the vascular malformations (and their causal genes)[1]; vascular neoplasms whose mutations do not specifically facilitate their diagnosis or classification, for example, *KRAS2, TP53* rearrangements in Kaposi sarcoma (KS)[2]; and a comprehensive review of the genetic alterations linked to angiosarcoma.

SELECTED VASCULAR NEOPLASMS

EPITHELIOID HEMANGIOMA

Overview

Classified as benign,[1] epithelial hematioma (EH) has a low recurrence rate (8/67, 12%), but can rarely metastasize to regional lymph nodes (2/67, 3%).[15,16] Known for its multifocal growth pattern in bone,[15] EH histologically consists of epithelioid endothelial cells; intravascular growth; florid stromal inflammation (eg, eosinophils, lymphocytes); and a cellular/solid growth pattern (**Fig. 1**).[3] EH presents in a variety of anatomic locations, including soft tissue (54%), intraosseous (29%), and cutaneous sites (17%).[2,3]

Associated Genetic Changes/Alterations

The main genetic alteration found in EH is rearrangement of *FOS* (26/104, 25%).[3,4] Most *FOS*-rearranged cases occur in either bone or soft tissue (each 12/26, 46%), are not multifocal (17/20, 85%), and are the cellular/mostly solid subtype (15/26, 58%).[3,4] *ZFP36-FOSB* is the most common gene fusion identified in EH (7/26, 27%), and most cases with this fusion (4/7, 57%) display atypical features (ie, necrosis and/or mild-moderate nuclear pleomorphism).[4] Rare cases of *WWTR1-FOSB* (1), *FOS-LMNA* (1), and *FOS-VIM* (2) fusions have also been reported in EH.[3,4] However, in most cases (15/26, 58%), the gene partner of *FOS* remains unknown.[3,4]

EH cases with the morphology of angiolymphoid hyperplasia with eosinophilia do not harbor *FOS* abnormalities (0/12).[3] However, by immunohistochemistry (IHC), FOS-B overexpression occurs consistently in angiolymphoid hyperplasia with eosinophilia (15/15).[17] And although neither FOS-B expression nor rearrangement of *FOSB* is unique to EH (see the section Pseudomyogenic Hemangioendothelioma), its immunophenotype (FOS-B+; negative for cytokeratin, TFE-3, CAMTA-1, MYC) is a consistently diagnostic immunophenotype.[17]

Molecular Pathology

FOS (Finkel-Biskis-Jinkins murine osteosarcoma viral oncogene homolog) belongs to the *Fos* gene family, including *FOSB, FOSL1,* and *FOSL2*. Normally, *FOS* encodes a transcription factor that leads to overexpression of vascular endothelial growth factor-D (VEGF-D) via its role in forming the activating protein-1 (AP-1) complex with the Jun family (c-Jun, JunB, JunD). In human umbilical cord vein endothelial cells, VEGF-D binds to its corresponding receptors (VEGFR-2, VEGFR-3) producing an extensive network of capillary-like cords.[3] In contrast, *FOS* rearrangement in EH produces a shortened gene that truncates FOS protein (resulting in loss of a C-terminal sequence required for proteasomal degradation of FOS).[18] As a result, FOS degradation becomes impaired, allowing FOS to stimulate abnormal vessel growth.[19]

ZFP36 (zinc finger protein 36) regulates the stability of adenosine/uridine-rich element mRNAs by removing the poly(A) tail and increasing mRNA turnover.[4] In doing so, ZFP36 helps control cytokine and chemokine production, including tumor necrosis factor-α.[4] *LMNA* encodes for lamins A and C, which not only support the architecture of the nucleus, but also DNA replication, transcription, and nuclear organization.[3] *VIM* encodes for vimentin, the well-known intermediate filament that helps support the cytoskeleton.[3] A discussion of the molecular pathology of *WWTR1* follows (see section Epithelioid Hemangioendothelioma). The specific role of each of these partner genes in EH, however, remains unclear.

Techniques

Rearrangements of *FOS* in EH were detected using RNA sequencing (with bioinformatics analysis by FusionSeq to identify gene fusions); fluorescence in situ hybridization (FISH); reverse transcriptase polymerase chain reaction (RT-PCR); and/or DNA-based PCR.[3,4]

SPINDLE CELL HEMANGIOMA

Overview

Now regarded as a benign neoplasm that lacks metastatic potential,[1,20] spindle cell hemangioma (SCH) was first reported as a variant of hemangioendothelioma in its original, 1986 case series (n = 26). In that series, 1 patient developed (what was regarded as) a regional lymph node metastasis following radiotherapy, despite a long follow-up (40 years), and multiple recurrences (19). Hence, the term "spindle cell hemangioendothelioma" (spindle cell HE) was proposed to describe this "low-grade angiosarcoma."[21]

Fig. 1. EH. (*A*) Low-power hematoxylin-eosin (H&E) showing rounded blood vessels with occasional lumina admixed with hemorrhage and chronic inflammatory cells (H&E, original magnification ×200). (*B*) Higher power H&E view showing endothelial cells lining vessels with epithelioid morphology (H&E, original magnification ×400). (*C*) CD31 immunostain highlights epithelioid morphology (H&E, original magnification ×400).

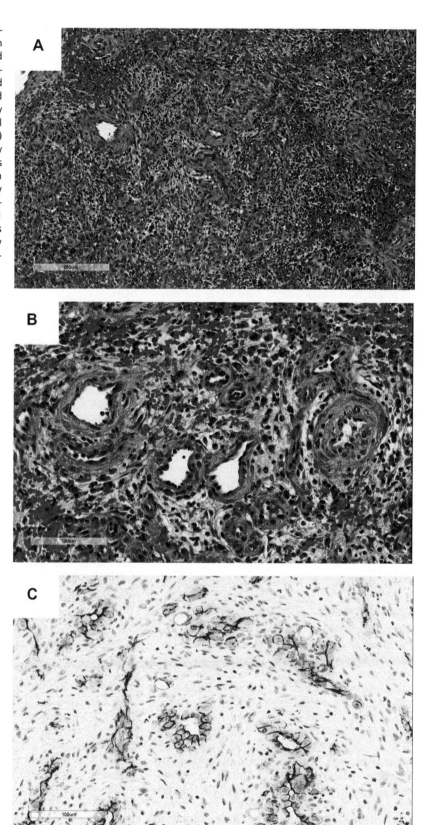

However, ensuing studies could not confirm another case with metastasis (0/7),[22] and instead suggested that the neoplasm could actually represent a reactive, vascular proliferation.[23] The largest case series to date in 1996 (n = 78) confirmed the benign clinical behavior of "spindle cell HE," and thus, it was renamed SCH.[20]

The 1986 case series described "spindle cell HE" as resembling the combination of cavernous hemangioma and KS.[21] The 1996 case series refined the description of the KS-like areas by highlighting the collapsed blood spaces, often lined by epithelioid endothelial cells with cytoplasmic vacuolation, along with the bland, spindled fibroblastic cells, which separated the cavernous and collapsed vessels (Fig. 2).[20]

In the 1996 case series, SCH "recurred" in 58% of patients (29/40). However, because 58% (45/78) of the SCH cases overall were either partially or completely intravascular, and accompanied by similar intimal changes within nearby vessels, these "recurrences" were deemed to likely represent contiguous spread along or multifocal involvement of a vessel. However, no metastases were reported, nor did any patients die directly due to the neoplasm itself. Thus, the lymph node "metastasis" from the 1986 case series most likely reflected the spread of a radiation-induced sarcoma.[20,21]

With an anatomic predilection for the distal extremities,[5–7] SCH occurs either in the setting of Maffucci syndrome (characterized by its associated enchondromatosis),[5] or sporadically.[6,7] The first case series of SCH (ie, "spindle cell HE") in patients with Maffucci syndrome was reported in 1995 (n = 6).[24] The next year, the 1996 case series confirmed that a subset of SCH cases was also found in patients with Maffucci syndrome (4/78, 5%).[20]

Associated Genetic Changes/Alterations

The principal genetic alteration that characterizes the development of SCH is a mutation of IDH1 or IDH2.[5–7] In 2011, a somatic heterozygous mutation in exon 4 of IDH1 (c.394C > T encoding an R132C substitution) was first identified in patients with Maffucci syndrome with SCH (7/10, 70%), and in their associated cartilaginous neoplasms (ie, enchondroma, chondrosarcoma) (total: 13/17, 76%).[5] This R132C substitution was also noted in synchronous SCH cases, as well as a metachronous presentation of an SCH and an enchondroma (over 6 years).[5] However, the R132H IDH1 mutation (c.395G > A) was not detected in a separate series of SCH cases from patients with Maffucci syndrome (0/14),[5] nor in a series of sporadic SCH cases (0/28).[6]

In contrast, the presence of the R132C IDH1 mutation has been confirmed in 3 separate series of sporadic SCH cases, in 2013 (18/28, 64%), and December 2017 (13/17, 76%).[6,7] Both series also established mutations in exon 4 of IDH2 in SCH, as substitutions of R172M (c.515G > T), R172T, P167S, R172G (c.514A > G), and R172S (c.516G > T).[6,7] In contrast, a variant R172S IDH2 mutation (c.516G > C) was not found in the SCH cases from Maffucci syndrome patients in the 2011 case series (0/10).[5]

Across all 3 series, 78% of cases with SCH (43/55) harbored a mutation of IDH1 (38) or IDH2 (5). The mutation of IDH1 or IDH2 is also specific for SCH, in comparison with other vascular neoplasms/proliferations (0/386). Hence, the mutation of IDH1 or IDH2 in a vascular neoplasm constitutes a diagnostically significant finding in support of SCH.[5–7]

Molecular Pathology

The mutation of IDH1 or IDH2 corresponds to altered forms of isocitrate dehydrogenase (IDH). The altered form not only retains the ability to convert isocitrate to α-ketoglutarate (α-KG) in the cytoplasm (IDH1) and mitochondria (IDH2), but also becomes capable of converting α-KG to the structurally similar D-2-hydroxyglutarate (D2HG). D2HG reduces α-KG production, and competitively inhibits enzymes that are dependent on α-KG, thereby blocking histone and DNA demethylation.[5–7]

The ensuing hypermethylation and inhibition of gene expression also stabilizes hypoxia-inducible factor-1α (HIF-1α), a known inducer of angiogenesis; however, a subset of SCH cases in the 2013 series was negative for HIF-1α (0/16). Therefore, the exact mechanism by which SCH develops remains elusive.[6]

Techniques

In the 2011 series, a separate series of SCH cases (collected by tissue microarray) was evaluated by IHC for the mutant R132H IDH1 protein.[5] In the 2013 series, a subset of the sporadic SCH cases was evaluated by IHC for HIF-1α expression.[6] Both were negative (0/14, 0/16).[5,6]

In patients with Maffucci syndrome with SCH, PCR amplification detected the R132C IDH1 mutation (7/10, 70%), but not a variant R172S IDH2 mutation (c.516G > C) (0/10).[5]

In the series of sporadic SCH cases, the R132C IDH1 mutation was confirmed by the combination of Sanger sequencing; multiplex ligation-dependent probe amplification; conventional next generation sequencing (NGS); and/or NGS using

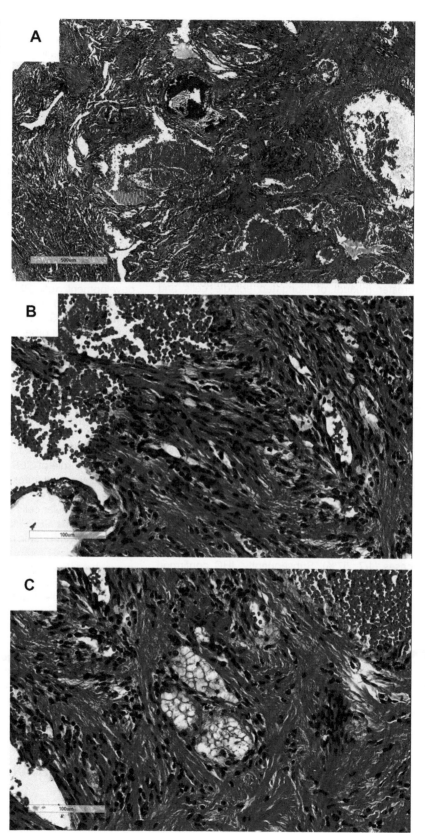

Fig. 2. SCH. (*A*) Low-power H&E view showing multiple dilated vascular spaces with occasional intraluminal calcification (H&E, original magnification ×100). (*B*) Higher power H&E view showing benign appearing spindle cell component in SCH (H&E, original magnification ×400). (*C*) Prominent endothelial vacuolization (H&E) in a case of SCH (H&E, original magnification ×400).

a single molecule, molecular inversion probes (smMIP)-based library preparation (31/45, 69%).[6,7] Sanger sequencing or NGS techniques also identified the *IDH2* mutations (5/45, 11%),[6,7] as described in the section Associated Genetic Changes/Alterations . However, the R132H *IDH1* mutation was not identified in sporadic SCH cases by Sanger sequencing (0/28).[6]

PSEUDOMYOGENIC HEMANGIOENDOTHELIOMA

Overview

Pseudomyogenic hemangioendothelioma (PMHE) was first described as the "fibroma-like variant of epithelioid sarcoma" in a 1992 case series (n = 5). Initially, it was noted to have a desmoid/fibroblastic appearance, whereas recurrences featured a greater mixture of elongated spindle cells and plump rhabdoid/myoid cells. By IHC, the neoplastic cells expressed cytokeratin and vimentin (5/5), but were negative for S-100, desmin, and myoglobin. These findings led to the conclusion that the tumor represented a variant of epithelioid sarcoma (which lacked the usual necrobiosis).[25]

The tumor's nomenclature was revisited in a 2003 case series (n = 7). For each case in which the referring diagnosis was available (6/7, 86%), the tumor had been (at least partially) misclassified as an epithelioid sarcoma due to morphologic similarity (ie, sheets/nodules/fascicles of epithelioid to spindled cells set in a desmoplastic stroma), lack of vascular channel formation and/or hemorrhage, and diffuse keratin expression by IHC. However, the 2003 series detected intracytoplasmic vacuolation (and thus, the possibility of vascular lumen formation) in rare tumor cells within a subset of cases (4/7, 57%). Subsequently, IHC confirmed the findings from the 1992 series: the neoplastic cells were positive for cytokeratin and vimentin (6/6), but negative for S-100 and desmin. IHC also established the vascular lineage of the tumor: its cells were positive for CD31 (5/6, 83%) and FLI-1 (6/6), but negative for CD34. Therefore, the tumor became designated as "epithelioid sarcoma-like hemangioendothelioma," a vascular tumor of intermediate malignancy.[26]

The term "PMHE" then emerged into the literature through a 2011 case series (n = 50), the largest to date. Histologically, this series emphasized the brightly eosinophilic cytoplasm and rhabdomyoblastic appearance of the spindle cells; the prominent neutrophilic infiltrate (27/50, 54%), plus occasional foci of necrosis and vascular invasion (each 7/50, 14%) (**Fig. 3**). All cases in this series confirmed the pertinent IHC findings from the 2003 series: the tumor cells were positive for cytokeratin

and FLI-1, but were negative for CD34, S-100, and desmin. This series also noted that INI1 expression by IHC was intact in all cases, thereby distinguishing PMHE from epithelioid sarcoma.[27]

Across all 3 series,[25–27] the extremities were the most common anatomic site (49/62, 79%). In addition, 65% of cases (40/62) were multifocal, whereas 60% (26/43) recurred, either locally or via satellite-like spread. Intraosseous involvement varied (13/62, 21%), whereas lymph node metastasis (1/43, 2%), distant metastasis (3/43, 7%), and death due to the neoplasm itself (2/43, 5%) were all rare events. Consequently, PMHE is still regarded as an intermediate malignant vascular tumor in the WHO classification.[2]

Associated Genetic Changes/Alterations

The main genetic anomaly responsible for the development of PMHE is a translocation, t(7;19)(q22;q13), resulting in the fusion of *SERPINE1* and *FOSB*. Because *FOSB* is part of the pathogenesis of other tumors (eg, EH: see section Epithelioid Hemangioma), its expression by IHC is not restricted to PMHE (48/50, 96%)[28]; however, the *SERPINE1-FOSB* fusion is unique: to date, it has been reported only in PMHE, and was identified in all cases from the series that described the gene fusion (n = 10).[8]

Molecular Pathology

The normal role of *SERPINE1* (ie, *PAI-1*, plasminogen activator inhibitor type 1) is to inhibit fibrinolysis by blocking the conversion of plasminogen to plasmin. Vascular cells express high levels of *SERPINE1*, but the *SERPINE1-FOSB* fusion does not produce an oncogenic protein. Instead, *SERPINE1* functions as a promoter, thereby facilitating the overexpression of *FOSB* mRNA.[8] The molecular pathology of *FOSB* has been described earlier (see section Molecular Pathology under Epithelioid Hemangioma).

Techniques

The *SERPINE1-FOSB* gene fusion was identified using a variety of genetic methods: cytogenetics (cell culture); FISH; mRNA sequencing; and RT-PCR. Quantitative real-time PCR also identified the overexpression of *FOSB* mRNA in 2 cases of PMHE, relative to a control series of soft tissue neoplasms.[8]

EPITHELIOID HEMANGIOENDOTHELIOMA

Overview

Designated as a "borderline" malignancy in its first series of soft tissue cases (n = 41),[29] epithelioid hemangioendothelioma (EHE) is now classified

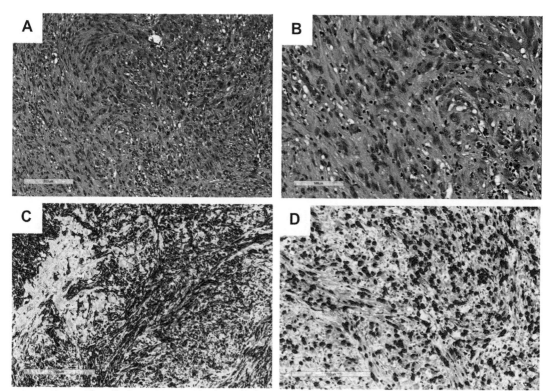

Fig. 3. PMHE. (*A*) Low-power H&E showing sheets of plump spindle cells with abundant eosinophilic cytoplasm (H&E, original magnification ×200). (*B*) High power H&E demonstrating round to oval shaped cells with nuclei showing variably prominent nucleoli and extensive a moderate degree of cytoplasmic vacuolization. Note the scattered neutrophils, which are frequently seen in dermal-based lesions (H&E, original magnification ×400). (*C*) PMHEs are diffusely and strongly positive for cytokeratins such as is seen in this case with extensive AE1/ AE3 immunoreactivity (H&E, original magnification ×200). (*D*) Pseudomyogenic hemangiomas are also diffusely and strongly positive for ERG (shown here) and other vascular markers (CD31), supporting their classification as neoplasms showing endothelial differentiation. Interestingly, CD34 is usually negative in these neoplasms (H&E, original magnification ×200).

as malignant.[1] EHE has a relatively consistent histologic appearance: epithelioid endothelial cells; evident intracytoplasmic vacuolation; glassy, eosinophilic cytoplasm; and a stroma ranging from myxoid to myxochondroid to densely hyalinized/sclerotic (**Fig. 4**).[12,29] Typical anatomic sites affected by EHE include skin/soft tissue, as well as bone, liver, and lung (which commonly reveals multifocal involvement).[2] The reported rates of recurrence (up to 15%),[29] metastasis (up to 31%),[30] and tumor-related deaths (up to 18%)[31] have stayed consistent across multiple case series of skin/soft tissue EHE. In contrast, survival in skeletal EHE (92% at 10 years)[32] is excellent, and surpasses its pulmonary (60% at 5 years)[33] and hepatic (41% at 5 years) counterparts.[34]

Associated Genetic Changes/Alterations

The main genetic alteration that leads to the development of EHE is *WWTR1-CAMTA1*. Heralded by the report of a translocation, t(1;3)(p36.3;q25), in 2

EHE cases,[35] the gene fusion was identified in 2 separate case series in 2011.[9,10] Across both series, 90% of EHE cases (56/62) showed rearrangements of *WWTR1* and *CAMTA1*,[9,10] and although rearrangement of *WWTR1* or *CAMTA1* was not identified in a wide range of other vascular tumors/proliferations (0/140),[9,10] EH does rarely harbor a *WWTR1-FOSB* fusion (see section Associated Genetic Changes/Alterations).

Based on these findings, an investigation of CAMTA1 expression by IHC in EHE was performed in a 2016 series, which demonstrated that 86% (51/59) were CAMTA1+. In contrast, only one epithelioid angiosarcoma was CAMTA1+ in the control group (1/145, 0.7%), which included vascular and mesenchymal/nonendothelial tumors. Therefore, a vascular neoplasm that expresses cytokeratin (25%–40%),[2] endothelial lineage markers (eg, CD31), and CAMTA1 by IHC is indicative of EHE.[36]

In 2013, a case series reported the rearrangement of *TFE3* (10/10) and *YAP1* (8/10, 80%) in a subset of

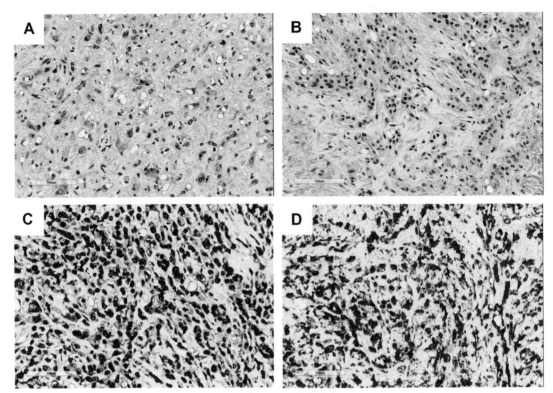

Fig. 4. EHE. (*A*) H&E showing liver lesion with scattered epithelioid cells embedded in a myxohyaline background with prominent cytoplasmic vacuolization. (*B*) Pleural lesion showing cords and sheets of epithelioid cells in a myxohyaline and fibrotic stroma (H&E). (*C*) ERG immunohistochemistry is diffuse and strong in a nuclear pattern in a pulmonary EHE. (*D*) Diffuse and strong nuclear CAMTA1 immunoreactivity is highly sensitive and specific for the diagnosis of EHE and is a surrogate for *WWTR1(TAZ)-CAMTA1* gene fusion. This case of pleural EHE is positive in a nuclear and cytoplasmic pattern (H&E, original magnification [*A–D*] ×400).

cases deemed to represent a distinct subset of EHE. The rearrangement was first identified via a combination of findings in the index case: pseudoalveolar (luminal) growth; lack of *WWTR1-CAMTA1*; and diffuse TFE3+ expression by IHC (Fig. 5). In contrast, the control cases (of epithelioid vascular tumors) revealed no genetic anomalies of *TFE3*. Both *YAP1*-negative cases were also negative for *WWTR1* fusion,[11] and in the 2016 series, 75% (6/8) of the CAMTA1- EHE cases were TFE3+.[36]

However, we contend that the *YAP1-TFE3* neoplasms represent a unique entity, characterized by epithelioid cytomorphology, vascular lumen formation, and *YAP1-TFE3* gene fusions. Two cases in the original, 2013 series were also described as having "abundant stromal chronic inflammation and scattered eosinophils," findings that better replicate the stroma of EH (see section Epithelioid Hemangioma: Overview). And although at least one case did contain a myxoid matrix, this finding appears to be the exception in the 2013 series, as a solid growth pattern with minimal intervening stroma was the most consistent finding.[11] Thus,

the characteristic myxoid to myxochondroid to densely hyalinized/sclerotic stroma of EHE[12,29] does not seem to be a consistent finding in the *YAP1-TFE3* neoplasms. Consequently, they are better regarded as a distinct entity, which we provisionally term *YAP1-TFE3* fused hemangioendothelioma.

Molecular Pathology

The process by which the *WWTR1* (WW domain-containing transcription regulator 1)- *CAMTA1* (Calmodulin binding transcription activator 1) gene fusion exerts its oncogenic effect in EHE has been reported in detail.[37] Briefly, the phosphorylation of *WWTR1* (ie, TAZ: *t*ranscriptional co*a*ctivator with PD*Z* binding motif) normally leads to its translocation from the nucleus to the cytoplasm, where it undergoes degradation via ubiquitination. However, the *WWTR1-CAMTA1* gene fusion facilitates constitutive nuclear localization (and thus, activation) of the *WWTR1* portion. The resulting gene fusion protein becomes insensitive

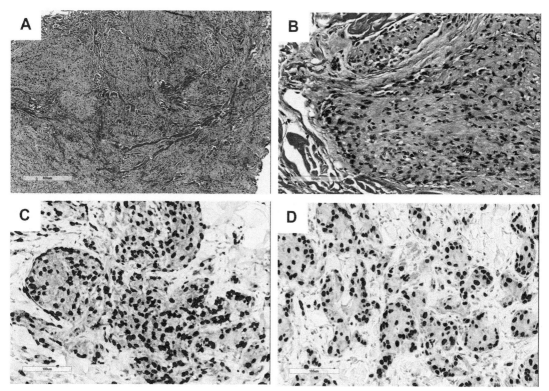

Fig. 5. YAP1-TFE3 fused hemangioendothelioma. (*A*) Low-power H&E of YAP1-TFE3 fused hemangioendothelioma showing sheetlike growth pattern (dermal case) (H&E, original magnification ×100). (*B*) Higher power H&E demonstrating sheets of epithelioid cells with focal vascular lumina at periphery. (*C*) The lesions are diffusely and strongly positive for ERG (nuclear), supporting vascular differentiation. (*D*) The lesions are also diffusely and strongly positive for TFE3 (nuclear pattern), which is an immunohistochemical surrogate for *YAP1-TFE3* gene fusion (H&E, original magnification [*B–D*] ×400).

to its regulatory pathway (Hippo), which normally functions as a tumor suppressor by negatively regulating tissue growth. This loss of inhibition is the basis on which *WWTR1-CAMTA1* EHE tumorigenesis occurs.[37]

In *WWTR1-CAMTA1* EHE, most cases are driven by the fusion of *WWTR1* exon 3 with *CAMTA1* exons 8 or 9 (9/13, 69%).[38] However, variant in-frame gene fusions of *WWTR1-CAMTA1* have now been described: *WWTR1* exon 3/*CAMTA1* within exon 9; *WWTR1* within exon 3/*CAMTA1* within exon 9; and *WWTR1* exon 2/*CAMTA1* within exon 9.[10,38] Nevertheless, the mechanism of action of the *WWTR1-CAMTA1* gene fusion transcript (as described previously) remains preserved.

As a paralogue of *WWTR1*, *YAP1* (Yes-associated protein 1) functions similarly, and thus, its fusion with *TFE3* (Transcription Factor E3) also likely produces constitutive nuclear localization. *TFE3* is part of the MiT family of transcription factors (*MITF, TFEB, TFEC, TFE3*). The role that *TFE3* plays in the oncogenesis of other neoplasms (eg, alveolar soft part sarcoma; translocation-

associated renal cell carcinoma) is well recognized.[11]

Techniques

IHC established the diffuse/nuclear expression of CAMTA1 and TFE3 in *WWTR1-CAMTA1* EHE and in *YAP1-TFE3* fused hemangioendothelioma, respectively.[11,36] The gene fusions were identified by using complementary DNA (cDNA) library construction, followed by paired-end whole-transcriptome sequencing (and FusionSeq analysis); along with FISH and RT-PCR confirmation.[9–11] RT-PCR studies also show that the gene fusions are independent of each other.[37]

ANGIOSARCOMA

Overview

A malignancy demonstrating endothelial differentiation, angiosarcoma (AS) has the most clinically aggressive behavior of all the vascular neoplasms, highlighted by its high rate of recurrence (76/108, 70%) and tumor-related death (50/108, 46%).[13] Known for involving the skin (especially the head and neck region), breast, soft tissue, bone, and viscera,[13] AS arises either as a primary neoplasm or as a secondary neoplasm due to radiotherapy, chronic lymphedema, or vinyl chloride exposure.[12,13] Histologically, AS displays a wide range of appearances, ranging from well-formed vascular spaces with minimal cytologic atypia, to solid sheets of poorly differentiated epithelioid/spindled cells that lack evident vascular structures (Fig. 6).[12] Multifocal spread is well known in AS,[2] which not only demonstrates consistent expression of vascular markers (eg, CD31, CD34, ERG), but can also stain for podoplanin (D2-40) or epithelial markers (eg, epithelial membrane antigen, cytokeratin) by IHC.[12]

Associated Genetic Changes/Alterations

Although a comprehensive discussion of the genetic changes associated with AS is beyond the scope of this review, secondary AS (that is, radiation-induced AS, most often in the setting of breast cancer; lymphedema-associated AS [Stewart-Treves syndrome]) is frequently driven by *MYC*. A 2010 series first revealed how *MYC* amplification was the exclusive genetic anomaly

present in most secondary AS cases (18/33, 55%).[39] *MYC* amplification in secondary AS was then confirmed in a 2011 series (22/22),[40] and recently, in a 2016 series (34/43, 79%).[13] Consequently, secondary AS illustrates consistent MYC expression by IHC, as noted in a 2012 case series (21/22, 95%).[41] And although primary AS also rarely harbors *MYC* amplification (8/75, 11%),[13,42] *MYC* amplification has not been found in atypical vascular lesions (0/12), or radiation-induced sarcomas unrelated to AS (0/8).[40]

In the 2010 and 2011 series, co-amplification of *FLT4* was identified in a subset of secondary AS cases (8/36, 22%),[39,40] but not in atypical vascular lesions (0/12).[40] And although the 2016 series confirmed the co-amplification of *FLT4* in *MYC*-amplified AS (5/39, 13%), 1 case of primary AS also harbored *FLT4* amplification, in which it occurred as an independent event.[13]

The 2016 series also identified a subset of AS cases (9/98, 9%) in which alterations of *CIC* were described. Representing mostly primary AS cases (8/9, 89%), this subset consisted of: a mutation of *CIC*, without an associated translocation (6/9, 67%); both a mutation and rearrangement of *CIC* (2/9, 22%); and a rearrangement of wild-type *CIC*

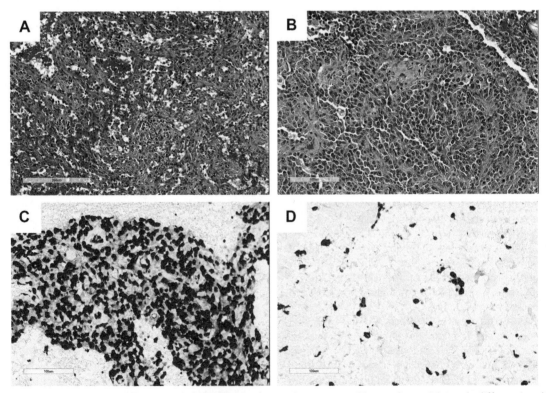

Fig. 6. AS. (*A*) H&E of AS of soft tissue showing pseudovascular spaces and hemorrhage. (*B*) Poorly differentiated epithelioid AS demonstrating subtle "cracking," a clue to the diagnosis. (*C*) ERG is sensitive for the diagnosis of AS (nuclear stain). (*D*) MYC immunohistochemistry is strongly positive in a nuclear pattern in radiation-associated AS.

(1/9, 11%). Regardless of the *CIC* alteration, these AS cases consistently displayed (at least a partially) round/epithelioid cell morphology (6/9, 67%), and presented, on average, in patients younger than expected (41 years).[13]

Finally, a 2014 series described recurrent mutations of *PTPRB* and *PLCG1* in association with AS. Driven by truncating/missense mutations (10/39, 26%), alterations of *PTPRB* involved either known cases of secondary AS (9/19, 47%), or whose

Table 1
Summary of genetic alterations

Tumor	Genetic Alteration	Details	References
EH	*FOS* rearrangements (n = 26)	*FOS*-unknown (15, 58%) *ZFP-FOSB* (7, 27%) *FOS-VIM* (2), *WWTR1-FOSB* (1), *FOS-LMNA* (1) (4, 15%)	Huang et al,[3] 2015; Antonescu et al,[4] 2014
SCH	Mutation of *IDH1* or *IDH2* (43/55 = 78%)	*IDH1* R132C (38, 88%) *IDH2* R172T, R172G, R172M (1 each), R172S (2) (5, 12%)	Pansuriya et al,[5] 2011; Kurek et al,[6] 2013; Ten Broek et al,[7] 2017
PMHE	*SERPINE1-FOSB* (n = 10)	Original series: 100% (10)	Walther et al,[8] 2014
EHE	*WWTR1-CAMTA1* (n = 62)	First 2 series: 90% (56)	Errani et al,[9] 2011; Tanas et al,[10] 2011
YAP1-TFE3 fused HE	*YAP1-TFE3* (n = 10)	Original series: *TFE3* (10), *YAP1* (8, 80%) rearranged	Antonescu et al,[11] 2013
Primary AS	*MYC* amplification (n = 90)	*MYC* (9, 10%)	Huang et al,[13] 2016; Behjati et al,[14] 2014; Italiano et al,[42] 2012
	FLT4 amplification (n = 110)	*FLT4* (1, 0.9%)	Huang et al,[13] 2016
	CIC anomalies (8/98 = 8%)	*CIC* mutation (5, 62.5%) *CIC* rearranged (37.5%): mutated (2), wild-type (1)	Huang et al,[13] 2016
	PLCG1 mutation (n = 129)	*PLCG1* (6, 4.7%)	Huang et al,[13] 2016; Behjati et al,[14] 2014
	PLCG1 mutation with... (n = 6)	*CIC* mutation (1, 17%)	Huang et al,[13] 2016
Secondary AS	*MYC* amplification (n = 117)	*MYC* (85, 73%)	Huang et al,[13] 2016; Behjati et al,[14] 2014; Manner et al,[39] 2010; Guo et al,[40] 2011
	MYC/FLT4 co-amplification (n = 74)	*MYC/FLT4* (13, 18%)	Huang et al,[13] 2016; Manner et al,[39] 2010; Guo et al,[40] 2011
	CIC mutation (1/98 = 1%)	No *CIC* rearrangement	Huang et al,[13] 2016
	PTPRB mutation (n = 19)	Truncating/missense (9, 47%)	Behjati et al,[14] 2014
	PTPRB mutation with... (n = 9)	*MYC* amplification (7, 78%)	Behjati et al,[14] 2014
	PTPRB mutation with... (n = 6)	*PLCG1* mutation (2, 33%)	Behjati et al,[14] 2014
	PLCG1 mutation (n = 132)	Missense (7, 5.3%)	Huang et al,[13] 2016; Behjati et al,[14] 2014
	PLCG1 mutation with... (n = 7)	*MYC* amplification (5, 71%)	Huang et al,[13] 2016; Behjati et al,[14] 2014

Abbreviations: AS, angiosarcoma; EH, epithelial hematioma; EHE, epithelioid hemangioendothelioma; PMHE, pseudomyogenic hemangioendothelioma; SCH, spindle cell hemangioma.

primary/secondary status was unknown (1/5, 20%). Concomitant *MYC* amplification consistently occurred in AS cases with *PTPRB* mutation (8/10, 80%), composed again of secondary AS (7/9, 78%), and the lone case of unknown status (1/1). No mutations of *PTPRB* were found in any of the primary AS cases (0/15), or in the control group (EH, KS, EHE) (0/19).[14]

In contrast, primary AS (6/129, 4.7%) and secondary AS (7/132, 5.3%),[13,14] as well as cases of unknown primary/secondary status (1/5, 20%),[14] can show mutated *PLCG1*. Featuring missense mutations, *PLCG1* changes and *MYC* amplification occur together in secondary AS (5/7, 71%),[13,14] and in AS cases of unknown status (1/1),[14] but not in primary AS (0/6).[13,14] And in the 2014 series, all of the AS cases with a *PLCG1*

mutation harbored mutations of *PTPRB* (2 secondary, 1 unknown status), but only half of AS cases with *PTPRB* mutations had a mutation of *PLCG1* (3/6, 50%).[14] No mutation of *PLCG1* was noted in the control group (EH, KS, EHE) (0/18).[14]

Molecular Pathology

Amplification of MYC (v-myc myelocytomatosis viral oncogene homolog) exerts its oncogenic effect in AS by upregulating the miR-17 to 92 microRNA cluster, which then lowers the half-life of THBS1 (thrombospondin-1) mRNA. Normally, THBS1 inhibits angiogenesis and mediates apoptosis of endothelial cells via the Fas/Fas ligand pathway. However, downregulation of THBS1 leads to a loss of this inhibition, thereby

Table 2
Tumor profile by immunohistochemistry (IHC)

Tumor	Pertinent IHC Positive	Pertinent IHC Negative	Comments	References
EH	FOSB	Keratin, CAMTA1, TFE3, MYC	Exclude other tumors	Llamas-Velasco et al,[17] 2017
SCH	None	None	Mutation of *IDH1* or *IDH2*	Pansuriya et al,[5] 2011; Kurek et al,[6] 2013; Ten Broek et al,[7] 2017
PMHE	Keratin, FOSB	S-100, desmin, myoglobin, CD34, CAMTA1, TFE3	INI1 expression retained No *MYC* amplification	Llamas-Velasco et al,[17] 2017; Mirra et al,[25] 1992; Billings et al,[26] 2003; Hornick et al,[27] 2011; Hung et al,[28] 2017
EHE	Keratin, CAMTA1	None reported	Keratin+ in 25%–40% Rarely FOSB+	[2]; Hung et al,[28] 2017; Doyle et al,[36] 2016
YAP1-TFE3 fused HE	TFE3	None reported	Currently classified in literature as EHE variant	Antonescu et al,[11] 2013
Primary AS	D2-40, epithelial membrane antigen, Keratin	MYC	Rarely *MYC* amplified; Rarely *FLT4* amplified; Rarely FOSB+, CAMTA1+	Antonescu,[12] 2014; Huang et al,[13] 2016; Hung et al,[28] 2017; Doyle et al,[36] 2016; Mentzel et al,[41] 2012
Secondary AS	MYC	None reported	FLT4 by IHC may be indicative of for *FLT4* amplification by FISH	Huang et al,[13] 2016; Mentzel et al,[41] 2012

Abbreviations: AS, angiosarcoma; EH, epithelial hematioma; EHE, epithelioid hemangioendothelioma; PMHE, pseudomyogenic hemangioendothelioma; SCH, spindle cell hemangioma.

permitting unregulated angiogenesis.[12,42] Co-amplification of *FLT4* (FMS-like tyrosine kinase 4, VEGFR3) likely augments this angiogenesis, but does not connote (partial) lymphatic differentiation, as these tumors were negative for D2-40 by IHC.[40]

The mechanism by which alterations of *CIC* (capicua transcriptional repressor) promote oncogenesis in AS is not well understood, but a loss of inhibition may play a role. Of note, the only gene partner in *CIC*-rearranged AS identified so far is *LEUTX*, which belongs to the same class of paired homeobox genes as *DUX4*, whose role in *EWSR1*-negative small round blue cell tumors is well established.[13]

Expressed in vascular endothelium, PTPRB (Protein Tyrosine Phosphatase, Receptor Type B) normally blocks angiogenesis by inhibiting vascular endothelial growth factor receptor 2 (VEGFR2), vascular endothelial cadherin, and angiopoietin. Subsequently, the truncating/missense mutations of *PTPRB* produce disinhibited angiogenesis.[14] On the other hand, *PLCG1* (Phospholipase C, gamma 1) is expressed in all normal tissue, but its missense mutations (p.R707Q, p.S345F) activate phospholipase Cγ1 (PLCγ1), which then produces uncontrolled angiogenesis due to unregulated signaling.[13,14]

Techniques

In the 2010 series, the presence of *MYC* amplification in secondary AS was identified by using array-comparative genomic hybridization and FISH.[39] In the 2011 series, *MYC* amplification and *FLT4* co-amplification were confirmed via gene expression profiling and FISH.[40] IHC then confirmed the consistent expression of MYC in secondary AS in the 2012 series.[41] The *CIC* alterations were discovered via a combination of RNA sequencing (including FusionSeq, for results analysis), RT-PCR, FISH, and Sanger sequencing.[13] Molecular techniques that identified the recurrent mutations of *PTPRB* and *PLCG1* included whole genome, exome, and targeted gene sequencing.[13,14]

SUMMARY

Our review has highlighted the characteristic genetic aberrations in EH, SCH, PMHE, EHE, *YAP1-TFE3* fused hemangioendothelioma, and AS (**Table 1**). Despite their range in biological behavior, these vascular neoplasms share common features, which include an epithelioid morphology (in at least a subset of cases), a predisposition for multifocality, and a consistent immunophenotype (**Table 2**). Molecular methods

have improved the reproducible evaluation of these diagnostically challenging neoplasms, whose more accurate classification makes it possible to help find potential targets for therapeutic intervention.

REFERENCES

1. International Society for the Study of Vascular Anomalies. Classification. 2014. Available at: http://www.issva.org/UserFiles/file/Classifications-2014-Final.pdf. Accessed January 20, 2018.
2. Vascular tumours, [Chapter: 8]. In: Fletcher CDM, Bridge JA, Hogendoorn P, et al, editors. WHO classification of tumours of soft tissue and bone. 4th edition. Lyon (France): IARC Press; 2013.
3. Huang SC, Zhang L, Sung YS, et al. Frequent FOS gene rearrangements in epithelioid hemangioma: a molecular study of 58 cases with morphologic reappraisal. Am J Surg Pathol 2015;39(10):1313–21.
4. Antonescu CR, Chen HW, Zhang L, et al. ZFP36-FOSB fusion defines a subset of epithelioid hemangioma with atypical features. Genes Chromosomes Cancer 2014;53(11):951–9.
5. Pansuriya TC, van Eijk R, d'Adamo P, et al. Somatic mosaic IDH1 and IDH2 mutations are associated with enchondroma and spindle cell hemangioma in Ollier disease and Maffucci syndrome. Nat Genet 2011;43(12):1256–61.
6. Kurek KC, Pansuriya TC, van Ruler MA, et al. R132C IDH1 mutations are found in spindle cell hemangiomas and not in other vascular tumors or malformations. Am J Pathol 2013;182(5):1494–500.
7. Ten Broek RW, Bekers EM, de Leng WWJ, et al. Mutational analysis using Sanger and next generation sequencing in sporadic spindle cell hemangiomas: a study of 19 cases. Genes Chromosomes Cancer 2017;56(12):855–60.
8. Walther C, Tayebwa J, Lilljebjörn H, et al. A novel SERPINE1-FOSB fusion gene results in transcriptional up-regulation of FOSB in pseudomyogenic haemangio-endothelioma. J Pathol 2014;232(5):534–40.
9. Errani C, Zhang L, Sung YS, et al. A novel WWTR1-CAMTA1 gene fusion is a consistent abnormality in epithelioid hemangioendothelioma of different anatomic sites. Genes Chromosomes Cancer 2011;50(8):644–53.
10. Tanas MR, Sboner A, Oliveira AM, et al. Identification of a disease-defining gene fusion in epithelioid hemangioendothelioma. Sci Transl Med 2011;3(98):98ra82.
11. Antonescu CR, Le Loarer F, Mosquera JM, et al. Novel YAP1-TFE3 fusion defines a distinct subset of epithelioid hemangioendothelioma. Genes Chromosomes Cancer 2013;52(8):775–84.

12. Antonescu C. Malignant vascular tumors—an update. Mod Pathol 2014;27(Suppl 1):S30–8.

13. Huang SC, Zhang L, Sung YS, et al. Recurrent CIC gene abnormalities in angiosarcomas: a molecular study of 120 cases with concurrent investigation of PLCG1, KDR, MYC, and FLT4 gene alterations. Am J Surg Pathol 2016;40(5):645–55.

14. Behjati S, Tarpey PS, Sheldon H, et al. Recurrent PTPRB and PLCG1 mutations in angiosarcoma. Nat Genet 2014;46(4):376–9.

15. Nielsen GP, Srivastava A, Kattapuram S, et al. Epithelioid hemangioma of bone revisited: a study of 50 cases. Am J Surg Pathol 2009;33:270–7.

16. Errani C, Zhang L, Panicek DM, et al. Epithelioid hemangioma of bone and soft tissue: a reappraisal of a controversial entity. Clin Orthop Relat Res 2012;470:1498–506.

17. Llamas-Velasco M, Kempf W, Cota C, et al. Multiple eruptive epithelioid hemangiomas: a subset of cutaneous cellular epithelioid hemangioma with expression of FOS-B. Am J Surg Pathol 2017. https://doi.org/10.1097/PAS.0000000000001003.

18. van IJzendoorn DG, de Jong D, Romagosa C, et al. Fusion events lead to truncation of FOS in epithelioid hemangioma of bone. Genes Chromosomes Cancer 2015;54(9):565–74.

19. van IJzendoorn DGP, Forghany Z, Liebelt F, et al. Functional analyses of a human vascular tumor FOS variant identify a novel degradation mechanism and a link to tumorigenesis. J Biol Chem 2017 29;292(52):21282–90.

20. Perkins P, Weiss SW. Spindle cell hemangioendothelioma. An analysis of 78 cases with reassessment of its pathogenesis and biologic behavior. Am J Surg Pathol 1996;20(10):1196–204.

21. Weiss SW, Enzinger FM. Spindle cell hemangioendothelioma. A low-grade angiosarcoma resembling a cavernous hemangioma and Kaposi's sarcoma. Am J Surg Pathol 1986;10(8):521–30.

22. Scott GA, Rosai J. Spindle cell hemangioendothelioma. Report of seven additional cases of a recently described vascular neoplasm. Am J Dermatopathol 1988;10(4):281–8.

23. Imayama S, Murakamai Y, Hashimoto H, et al. Spindle cell hemangioendo-thelioma exhibits the ultrastructural features of reactive vascular proliferation rather than of angiosarcoma. Am J Clin Pathol 1992;97(2):279–87.

24. Fanburg JC, Meis-Kindblom JM, Rosenberg AE. Multiple enchondromas associated with spindle-cell hemangioendotheliomas. An overlooked variant of Maffucci's syndrome. Am J Surg Pathol 1995;19(9):1029–38.

25. Mirra JM, Kessler S, Bhuta S, et al. The fibroma-like variant of epithelioid sarcoma. A fibrohistiocytic/myoid cell lesion often confused with benign and malignant spindle cell tumors. Cancer 1992;69(6):1382–95.

26. Billings SD, Folpe AL, Weiss SW. Epithelioid sarcoma-like hemangioendothelioma. Am J Surg Pathol 2003;27(1):48–57.

27. Hornick JL, Fletcher CD. Pseudomyogenic hemangioendothelioma: a distinctive, often multicentric tumor with indolent behavior. Am J Surg Pathol 2011;35(2):190–201.

28. Hung YP, Fletcher CD, Hornick JL. FOSB is a useful diagnostic marker for pseudomyogenic hemangioendothelioma. Am J Surg Pathol 2017;41(5):596–606.

29. Weiss SW, Enzinger FM. Epithelioid hemangioendothelioma: a vascular tumor often mistaken for a carcinoma. Cancer 1982;50(5):970–81.

30. Weiss SW, Ishak KG, Dail DH, et al. Epithelioid hemangioendothelioma and related lesions. Semin Diagn Pathol 1986;3(4):259–87.

31. Deyrup AT, Tighiouart M, Montag AG, et al. Epithelioid hemangioendothelioma of soft tissue: a proposal for risk stratification based on 49 cases. Am J Surg Pathol 2008;32(6):924–7.

32. Angelini A, Mavrogenis AF, Gambarotti M, et al. Surgical treatment and results of 62 patients with epithelioid hemangioendothelioma of bone. J Surg Oncol 2014;109(8):791–7.

33. Bagan P, Hassan M, Le Pimpec Barthes F, et al. Prognostic factors and surgical indications of pulmonary epithelioid hemangioendothelioma: a review of the literature. Ann Thorac Surg 2006;82(6):2010–3.

34. Mehrabi A, Kashfi A, Fonouni H, et al. Primary malignant hepatic epithelioid hemangioendothelioma: a comprehensive review of the literature with emphasis on the surgical therapy. Cancer 2006;107(9):2108–21.

35. Mendlick MR, Nelson M, Pickering D, et al. Translocation t(1;3)(p36.3;q25) is a nonrandom aberration in epithelioid hemangioendothelioma. Am J Surg Pathol 2001;25(5):684–7.

36. Doyle LA, Fletcher CD, Hornick JL. Nuclear expression of CAMTA1 distinguishes epithelioid hemangioendothelioma from histologic mimics. Am J Surg Pathol 2016;40(1):94–102.

37. Tanas MR, Ma S, Jadaan FO, et al. Mechanism of action of a WWTR1(TAZ)-CAMTA1 fusion oncoprotein. Oncogene 2016;35(7):929–38.

38. Patel NR, Salim AA, Sayeed H, et al. Molecular characterization of epithelioid haemangioendotheliomas identifies novel WWTR1-CAMTA1 fusion variants. Histopathology 2015;67(5):699–708.

39. Manner J, Radlwimmer B, Hohenberger P, et al. MYC high level gene amplification is a distinctive feature of angiosarcomas after irradiation or chronic lymphedema. Am J Pathol 2010;176(1):34–9.

40. Guo T, Zhang L, Chang NE, et al. Consistent MYC and FLT4 gene amplification in radiation-induced angiosarcoma but not in other radiation-associated atypical vascular lesions. Genes Chromosomes Cancer 2011;50(1):25–33.

41. Mentzel T, Schildhaus HU, Palmedo G, et al. Post-radiation cutaneous angiosarcoma after treatment of breast carcinoma is characterized by MYC amplification in contrast to atypical vascular lesions after radiotherapy and control cases: clinicopathological, immunohistochemical and molecular analysis of 66 cases. Mod Pathol 2012;25(1): 75–85.

42. Italiano A, Thomas R, Breen M, et al. The miR-17-92 cluster and its target THBS1 are differentially expressed in angiosarcomas dependent on MYC amplification. Genes Chromosomes Cancer 2012; 51(6):569–78.

Update on Myogenic Sarcomas

Narasimhan P. Agaram, MBBS

KEYWORDS

- Rhabdomyosarcoma • Embryonal • Alveolar • Spindle cell/Sclerosing • Pleomorphic
- Leiomyosarcoma • *MYOD1* • *FOXO1*

Key points

- Clinico-pathologic and molecular analysis classify rhabdomyosarcomas into different histologic and prognostic subtypes.

- Embryonal rhabdomyosarcomas and infantile *VGLL2* gene fusion-positive rhabdomyosarcoma have favorable prognosis.

- Alveolar rhabdomyosarcoma and *MYOD1*-mutant spindle cell/sclerosing rhabdomyosarcomas are aggressive tumors and have poor prognosis.

- Leiomyosarcoma should be diagnosed only if the morphologic and immunohistochemical features correlate and not based on the immunohistochemical features alone.

- Tumor size (>10 cm) and histologic grade are the most important prognostic factors of leiomyosarcoma.

ABSTRACT

Myogenic sarcomas include soft tissue sarcomas that show skeletal muscle differentiation (rhabdomyosarcoma) and those with smooth muscle differentiation (leiomyosarcoma). Rhabdomyosarcomas are more common in the pediatric age group and leiomyosarcomas occur more often in the adult population. Based on the clinico-pathologic features and genetic abnormalities identified, the rhabdomyosarcomas are classified into embryonal, alveolar, spindle cell/sclerosing, and pleomorphic subtypes. Each subtype shows distinctive morphology and has characteristic genetic abnormalities. In this update on myogenic sarcomas, each entity is discussed with special emphasis on recent updates in genetic findings and the diagnostic approach to these tumors.

RHABDOMYOSARCOMA

Rhabdomyosarcomas (RMSs) comprise the single largest category of soft tissue sarcomas in children and adolescents in the United States, occurring in 4.5 million persons younger than 20 years. Currently, RMS is classified based on histology into 4 different subtypes: embryonal rhabdomyosarcoma (ERMS), alveolar rhabdomyosarcoma (ARMS), pleomorphic rhabdomyosarcoma (PRMS) and spindle cell/sclerosing rhabdomyosarcoma (SRMS). The key features of each subtype are listed in **Table 1**.

EMBRYONAL RHABDOMYOSARCOMA

ERMS is a primitive, malignant soft tissue tumor that recapitulates the phenotypic and biological features of embryonic skeletal muscle. It is the most common subtype, occurring in 2.6 per million children younger than 15 years in the United States, with children younger than 5 years being most commonly affected. They are more common in boys than girls with a ratio of 1.4:1.0.[1,2]

The tumors occur in equal proportion in the head and neck and the genitourinary system.[3] Common locations in the genitourinary tract include the urinary bladder, prostate, vulva/vagina, cervix, and

Disclosure Statement: No disclosures.
Department of Pathology, Memorial Sloan Kettering Cancer Center, 1275 York Avenue, New York, NY 10065, USA
E-mail address: agaramn@mskcc.org

Surgical Pathology 12 (2019) 51–62
https://doi.org/10.1016/j.path.2018.10.003

Table 1
Comparison of rhabdomyosarcoma subtypes with respect to clinico-pathologic and genetic features

Clinico-pathologic Features	Embryonal RMS	Alveolar RMS	Spindle Cell/Sclerosing RMS	Pleomorphic RMS
Age at presentation (most common)	Pediatric (0–5)	Pediatric (10–20)	Infantile, pediatric, and adults	Adults
Location	H&N, GU, GYN tract	Extremities	H&N, paratesticular, extremities	Extremities
Morphology	Primitive to small blue round cells, scattered rhabdomyoblasts, botryoid pattern	Alveolar pattern, sheets of medium-sized cells, scattered giant cells	Spindle cells in fascicles; sclerosing "pseudovascular" pattern	Pleomorphic rhabdomyoblasts
Immunohistochemistry	Desmin-pos; Myogenin - focal	Desmin-pos; Myogenin-diffuse	Desmin-pos; Myogenin-focal; MYOD1-diffuse	Desmin-pos; Myogenin-focal
Genetic alterations	Aneuploidy with chromosomal gains and losses; alterations of the RAS family genes (HRAS, NRAS, KRAS), FGFR4, PIK3CA, NF1, and FBXW7	PAX3-FOXO1 gene fusion; PAX7-FOXO1 gene fusion	VGLL2 gene fusions (infantile); MYOD1 gene mutation	Complex genetic alterations
Prognosis	Favorable	Poor	Infantile-favorable; MYOD1 mutant-poor	Poor

Abbreviations: GU, genitourinary; GYN, gynecologic; H&N, head and neck; pos, positive; RMS, rhabdomyosarcoma.

paratesticular soft tissues. Besides these 2 general regions, ERMS occurs in the biliary tract, retroperitoneum, pelvis, perineum, and abdomen and has been reported in various visceral organs, such as the liver, kidney, heart, and lungs. The botryoid variant of ERMS arises beneath a mucosal epithelial surface, limiting it to organs such as the urinary bladder, biliary tract, vulva/vagina, cervix, pharynx, conjunctiva, or auditory canal.

Clinically, ERMS presents as a rapidly growing soft tissue mass. The head and neck lesions can cause proptosis, diplopia, sinusitis, or unilateral deafness, depending on their location. Tumors in the genitourinary tract present as a scrotal mass or urinary retention, and biliary tumors may cause jaundice. ERMS forms poorly circumscribed, fleshy, pale tan masses that directly impinge on neighboring structures. Botryoid tumors have a characteristic polypoid appearance with clusters

of small, sessile, or pedunculated nodules that abut an epithelial surface.[4]

Histologically, ERMS shows primitive oval to spindle cells with minimal cytoplasm. Some areas show small, blue, round cell morphology. As these cells differentiate, they progressively acquire more cytoplasmic eosinophilia and elongate shapes, varyingly described as "tadpole," "strap," and "spider" cells and deemed to be evidence of rhabdomyoblastic differentiation (Fig. 1A, B). Differentiation tends to be more evident after chemotherapy, as differentiated elements become the predominant cell population, separated by therapy-induced necrosis and fibrosis. The botryoid variant of ERMS contains linear aggregates of tumor cells (cambium layer) that tightly abut an epithelial surface. This variant also shows variable numbers of polypoid nodules, often with an abundant, loose, myxoid stroma.[4] The anaplastic variant of ERMS is characterized by

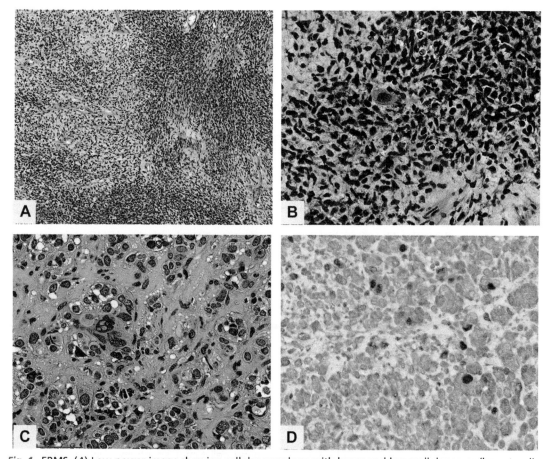

Fig. 1. ERMS. (A) Low-power image showing cellular neoplasm with hyper and hypocellular areas (hematoxylin-eosin stain [H&E], original magnification ×200). (B) High-power image showing primitive spindle cells with scattered rhabdomyoblasts (H&E, original magnification ×400). (C) High-power image of ERMS with scattered large anaplastic cells. (H&E, original magnification ×400). (D) Immunohistochemical stain for myogenin showing scattered nuclear positivity.

the presence of enlarged, atypical cells with hyperchromatic nuclei.[5] Anaplastic features can be focal or diffuse and bizarre, multipolar, mitoses are also often present (**Fig. 1**).

Immunohistochemically, markers of skeletal muscle differentiation are positive in ERMS. Desmin is the most frequently used diagnostic marker and shows diffuse staining. Antibodies against MyoD1 and myogenin, highly specific and sensitive for rhabdomyosarcoma, are routinely used for diagnosis.[6,7] ERMS typically shows patchy positivity for myogenin (see **Fig. 1**D).

DIFFERENTIAL DIAGNOSIS

The morphologic differential diagnoses include other subtypes of rhabdomyosarcoma (alveolar and spindle cell/sclerosing) and other tumors in the small, blue, round cell tumor spectrum such as Ewing sarcoma and desmoplastic small round cell tumors. Immunohistochemical and ancillary cytogenetic and molecular studies are helpful to arrive at the correct diagnosis.

GENETICS

ERMS does not show any gene fusions. Molecular analyses typically show aneuploidy with multiple copy number gains and losses noted. Whole chromosome gains with polysomy of chromosome 8 are common. Whole chromosome losses of 10 and 15 are noted.[8] The specific genes associated with ERMS include RAS family genes (*HRAS, NRAS, KRAS*), *FGFR4, PIK3CA, NF1,* and *FBXW7*.[9,10]

PROGNOSIS

Prognosis can be determined by stage, histologic classification, age, and site of origin. Staging, in children, is accomplished by clinical evaluation (Intergroup Rhabdomyosarcoma Study Group [IRSG] stage) and/or surgicopathological evaluation (IRSG group).[11] The IRSG subdivides RMS into low-risk, intermediate-risk, and high-risk groups for purposes of protocol-based therapy. Younger patients (1–9 years) tend to have a more favorable prognosis than infants and adolescents.[12] ERMS has a better prognosis than ARMS, and botryoid variants have a superior outcome as a group.[13] ERMS with diffuse anaplasia may have a worse outcome than the other subsets of ERMS.[5]

In adults, the reported range of ERMS is from 21% to 54%. Although historical data indicate that ERMS in adults fares poorly and has a higher relapse rate, recent studies have shown that using IRSG groups and staging for adult ERMS and treating them with pediatric protocols significantly improves the survival of adult patients.[14,15]

ALVEOLAR RHABDOMYOSARCOMA

ARMS is a cellular malignant neoplasm composed of a monomorphous population of primitive cells with round nuclei and features of arrested myogenesis. ARMS occurs at all ages, more often in adolescents and young adults than in younger children. The median ages of occurrence is between 6.8 and 9.0 years.[3] ARMS occurs less frequently than ERMS and comprises approximately 20% of all pediatric RMS. The male: female ratio is approximately even, and no geographic or racial predilection is reported.

ARMS commonly arises in the extremities. Additional sites of involvement include the paraspinal and the perineal regions and the paranasal sinuses. Clinically, ARMS typically presents as rapidly growing extremity masses. Tumors at other sites, such as paranasal, perirectal, and paraspinal, mainly cause symptoms of compression of the surrounding structures. ARMS tends to be high-stage lesions at presentation and forms expansile, rapidly growing soft tissue tumors.[16]

Histologically, they are highly cellular neoplasms and composed of primitive cells with round nuclei, with fibrovascular septa that separate the tumor cells into discrete nests. These nests contain central clusters of cells with loss of cohesion around the periphery, giving an "alveolar" appearance (**Fig. 2**A, B). Giant cells with rhabdomyoblastic differentiation are common. Solid variants of ARMS lack the fibrovascular stroma and form sheets of round cells with variable rhabdomyoblastic differentiation.[17]

Immunohistochemically, ARMS stains strongly for desmin. Myogenin and MyoD1 typically show a diffuse, strong nuclear staining pattern[18] (**Fig. 2**C, D). The diffuse positivity for myogenin is unlike the focal patchy staining seen in ERMS and can provide a clue to the subtype on small biopsy material. Approximately one-third to one-half of ARMSs in the head and neck have been reported to show positivity for epithelial markers.[19]

DIFFERENTIAL DIAGNOSIS

The morphologic differential diagnoses include other subtypes of rhabdomyosarcoma (embryonal and sclerosing) and other tumors in the small, blue, round cell tumor spectrum, such as Ewing sarcoma and desmoplastic small round cell tumors. Immunohistochemical and ancillary cytogenetic and molecular studies are helpful to arrive at the correct diagnosis.

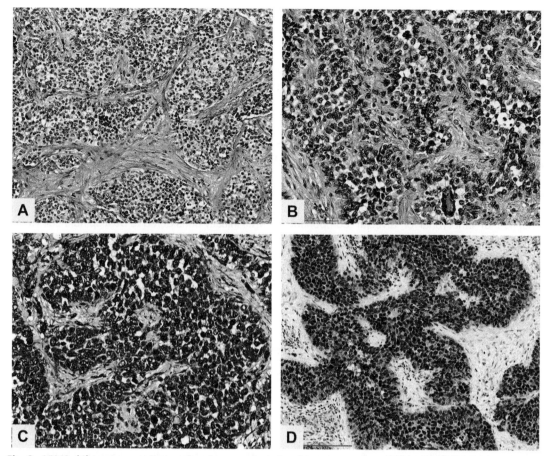

Fig. 2. ARMS. (*A*) Low-power image showing a nested alveolar pattern of arrangement of the tumor cells with the nests separated by fibrous septae (H&E, original magnification ×100). (*B*) High-power image showing medium-sized tumor cells with scattered giant cells (H&E, original magnification ×400) Immunohistochemical stains for Desmin (*C*) and myogenin (*D*) showing diffuse positivity.

GENETICS

ARMS is characterized by recurrent translocations. A t(2;13)(q35;q14) is found in most cases and a t(1;13)(p36;q14) is seen in a smaller subset of cases.[20] These translocations juxtapose the *PAX3* or *PAX7* genes on chromosomes 2 and 1, respectively, with the *FOXO1* gene on chromosome 13, to generate fusion genes that encode PAX3-FOXO1 and PAX7-FOXO1 fusion proteins.[21,22] *PAX3* and *PAX7* are related members of the paired box family of transcription factors, whereas *FOXO1* is a member of the forkhead transcription factor family. The *PAX3-FOXO1* and *PAX7-FOXO1* fusion products contain the *PAX3/PAX7* DNA binding domain and the *FOXO1* transcriptional activation domain, and function as potent transcriptional activators.[23] In addition to this functional change, the translocations generate high levels of these chimeric proteins, which activate downstream transcriptional targets, and are

postulated to exert oncogenic effects by altering control of proliferation, apoptosis, and differentiation.[1] The most frequent amplifications seen in ARMS involve chromosomal regions 12q13–15 and 2p24,[24] regions that contains many growth-related genes, such as the *GLI*, *CDK4*, *MDM2*, and *MYCN* genes. The *PAX7-FOXO1* fusion gene is amplified in most ARMS cases with the t(1;13) translocation.[25]

PROGNOSIS

ARMSs are high-grade neoplasms that are more aggressive than ERMS.[26] IRSG grouping is predictive of outcome. Although some studies postulate that *PAX7-FOXO1* positive tumors behave in a more benign fashion than *PAX3-FOXO1* tumors,[27] the prognostic value of the different type of gene fusion is uncertain. Unlike ERMS, ARMS is one of the few sarcomas that can metastasize to the regional lymph nodes. Imaging of the regional lymph nodes should be part of the workup for these patients. In some institutions, sentinel lymph node mapping is used. In adults, the reported proportion of ARMS relative to other RMS types is 18% to 33%. Similar to the pediatric population, ARMS in adults seems to have a worse prognosis when compared with ERMS.[14,15]

PLEOMORPHIC RHABDOMYOSARCOMA

PRMS is a high-grade sarcoma occurring almost exclusively in adults and consisting of bizarre polygonal, round, and spindle cells that display evidence of skeletal muscle differentiation with no evidence of embryonal or alveolar component. These lesions are more common in men and present at a median age in the sixth to seventh decade.[28] These tumors usually occur in the deep soft tissues of the lower extremities but have been reported in a wide variety of other locations.[29,30]

Clinically, most patients present with a rapidly growing painful swelling. Tumors are usually large (5–15 cm), well circumscribed, and often surrounded by a pseudocapsule. The cut surface is tan and fleshy with variable hemorrhage and necrosis. Morphologically, these are pleomorphic sarcomas composed of undifferentiated round to spindle cells and an admixture of polygonal cells with densely eosinophilic cytoplasm in spindle, tadpole, and racquetlike contours. Cross striations are not usually seen (**Fig. 3**). Immunohistochemically, PRMS, like other rhabdomyosarcoma subtypes, expresses desmin, MyoD1, and myogenin, with MyoD1 and myogenin showing focal positivity. Genetically, PRMS shows a complex karyotype with copy number alterations and unbalanced structural alterations.[31] The prognosis for these tumors is poor.[30]

The morphologic differential diagnoses include other high-grade tumors in adults, including dedifferentiated liposarcoma and high-grade undifferentiated pleomorphic sarcoma. Immunohistochemical stains and ancillary studies help to make the right diagnosis.

SPINDLE CELL/SCLEROSING RHABDOMYOSARCOMA

Spindle cell/sclerosing rhabdomyosarcoma (SpRMS) is an uncommon subtype of RMS that was initially considered to be a spindle cell variant of ERMS. Given the characteristic morphology of the tumor, it was recently classified as a separate subtype of RMS in the most recent World Health Organization classification (2013).[1] SpRMS has been reported in a wide age range from infants to elderly with most cases occurring in children and adolescents. The tumor occurs predominantly in the head and neck location with other sites of presentation being extremities and paratesticular.[32–35] Tumors can occur as painless masses or can have symptoms due to compression. Grossly they are usually well circumscribed with sections showing a gray-white whorled cut surface. Microscopically, SpRMS can show a varying morphology. Some tumors show a bland spindle cell proliferation, with eosinophilic, fibrillary cytoplasm, resembling true smooth muscle differentiation. The cells are typically arranged in intersecting long fascicles, reminiscent of the "herring bone" pattern of adult-type fibrosarcoma (**Fig. 4**A). Evidence of rhabdomyoblasts with cross-striations can be seen in some tumors. Other patterns that

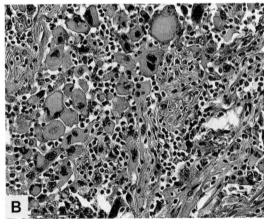

Fig. 3. PRMS. (*A*) Low-power image showing sheets of tumor cells (H&E, original magnification ×100). (*B*) High-power image showing large cells with rhabdoid morphology and large pleomorphic nuclei (H&E, original magnification ×400).

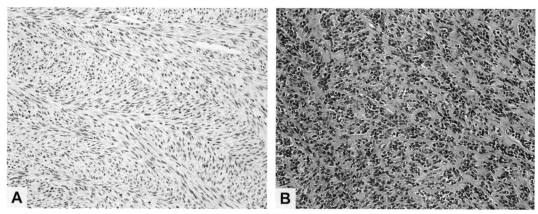

Fig. 4. SpRMS. (*A*) Spindle cell morphology showing uniform spindle cells in fascicles, in a herring bone pattern (H&E, original magnification ×200). (*B*) Sclerosing "pseudovascular" morphology composed of small nests of tumor cells with central clearing, in a sclerosing collagenous background (H&E, original magnification ×200).

can be seen in SpRMS are those of a cellular proliferation of spindle cells with morphology closely resembling fibrosarcoma, leiomyosarcoma, or malignant peripheral nerve sheath tumor. The sclerosing variant of SpRMS shows tumor cells in an extensive hyalinized matrix with focal alveolar architecture giving a pseudovascular appearance (**Fig. 4**B). Some sclerotic areas may mimic osteosarcoma. Immunohistochemically, SpRMS shows diffuse positivity for desmin. Myogenin usually shows rare focal positivity with some cases being negative. MyoD1 stain is positive in the tumor cells.[36]

GENETICS

Recent molecular studies on SpRMS have shed light on the genetic alterations of this entity and molecularly classify it into 3 categories: (1) SpRMS occurring in the infantile/congenital setting that shows recurrent *NCOA2* and *VGLL2* associated gene fusions, including *VGLL2-CITED2*, *VGLL2-NCOA2*, *TEAD1-NCOA2*, and *SRF-NCOA2*.[37,38] (2) *MYOD1* p.L122R gene mutations have been identified as a frequent event in adult and pediatric spindle cell RMS.[39,40] A subset (up to one-third) of the *MYOD1*-mutant SpRMS has coexistent mutations in the *PIK3CA* gene mutations.[36,41] (3) SpRMS with no known recurrent abnormalities. Recent studies note that *MYOD1*-mutated SpRMS tumors are aggressive and show a worse prognosis in both pediatric and adult patients.[36,41]

PROGNOSIS

The recent genetic findings in SpRMS have significantly increased our understanding of the biology of SpRMS. The infantile SpRMS with the *VGLL2* associated gene fusions appear to have a favorable prognosis.[37] In contrast, the *MYOD1*-mutated SpRMS tumors seem to be aggressive and have a significantly worse prognosis, despite aggressive chemoradiation therapy, in both the pediatric and adult age groups[36] (**Fig. 5**).

DIAGNOSTIC APPROACH TO RHABDOMYOSARCOMA

RMSs that occur in the pediatric age group include embryonal, alveolar, and spindle cell/sclerosing subtypes. In adults, PRMS should also be included as part of the differential diagnosis. Based on the clinical presentation and imaging findings, the initial approach for a tissue diagnosis is to get a surgical core biopsy. A core biopsy is preferable to fine needle aspiration biopsy to assess the morphologic architecture as well as to obtain adequate tissue for cytogenetic and molecular analysis. The immunohistochemical panel used for diagnosis depends on the morphology of the tumor. If the tumor shows morphology of a small, blue, round cell tumor with no hint of rhabdomyoblastic differentiation, immunohistochemical stains for desmin, myogenin, and MyoD1 should be included in the panel of stains performed. If the tumor shows distinctive rhabdomyoblastic differentiation, immunohistochemical stains for desmin, myogenin, and MyoD1 should be performed. Although the morphology and immunohistochemical stains suggest a subtype of RMS, it is standard practice to perform ancillary fluorescence in situ hybridization (FISH) or molecular studies for the detection of *FOXO1* gene rearrangement on all newly diagnosed cases to exclude the possibility of fusion-positive ARMS. If the morphology is suggestive of SpRMS, recent studies[36,37,41] suggest the utility of performing

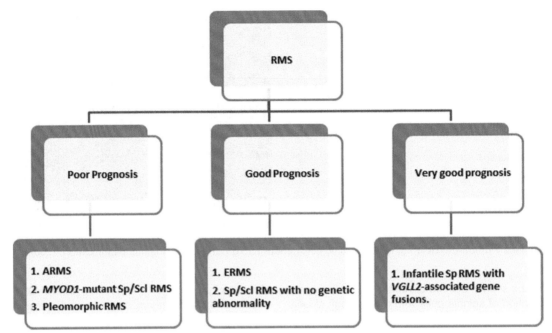

Fig. 5. Schematic showing the prognostic classification of RMS based on the current prognostic information. Sp/Scl RMS, spindle cell/sclerosing RMS.

molecular studies to detect presence of *MYOD1* mutation, a finding that predicts aggressive behavior of the disease.

LEIOMYOSARCOMA

Leiomyosarcoma is a malignant tumor composed of cells showing distinct smooth muscle features. Soft tissue leiomyosarcoma usually occurs in middle-aged or older persons, although it may develop in young adults and even in children.[42] The tumor occurs more frequently in women in the retroperitoneal and inferior vena cava locations, but leiomyosarcomas in other soft tissue sites occur in both men and women.

The common locations of soft tissue leiomyosarcoma include the retroperitoneum, including the pelvis, and the extremities.[43,44] A subset of leiomyosarcomas arise in large blood vessels, most commonly the inferior vena cava and the large veins of the lower extremity.[45] Intramuscular and subcutaneous localizations occur in approximately equal proportion, and some of these tumors show evidence of origin from a small to medium-sized vein. Leiomyosarcomas also develop in the dermis and have been termed cutaneous leiomyosarcoma or atypical intradermal smooth muscle neoplasm.

Soft tissue leiomyosarcoma generally presents as a mass lesion. It typically forms a fleshy tan mass with a characteristic whorled cut surface.

Hemorrhage, necrosis, or cystic changes are often noted in large tumors. The typical histologic pattern of leiomyosarcoma is that of intersecting fascicles of sharply marginated groups of spindle cells (**Fig. 6**A). Myxoid change may be seen. The tumor cell nuclei are characteristically elongated and blunt-ended and may be indented or lobated. Nuclear hyperchromasia and pleomorphism are generally noted (**Fig. 6**B). Mitotic figures can usually be found readily and atypical mitoses are often seen. The cytoplasm varies from typically eosinophilic to pale. Cytoplasmic vacuolation is frequently apparent, particularly in cells cut transversely. Epithelioid cytomorphology, multinucleated osteoclastlike giant cells, very prominent chronic inflammatory cells, and granular cytoplasmic change are rare findings.[1] Occasional soft tissue leiomyosarcomas contain areas with a nonspecific, poorly differentiated, pleomorphic appearance in addition to typical areas.[46] Rarely dedifferentiated liposarcomas can show divergent differentiation to leiomyosarcoma.

Immunohistochemical stains for smooth muscle actin (SMA), desmin, and h-caldesmon are positive in a great majority of soft tissue leiomyosarcomas. Generally, diffuse cytoplasmic positivity for 2 of these markers is needed to diagnose a leiomyosarcoma (**Fig. 6**C, D). It must be emphasized that the diagnosis of soft tissue leiomyosarcoma should be made only in the presence of appropriate morphologic

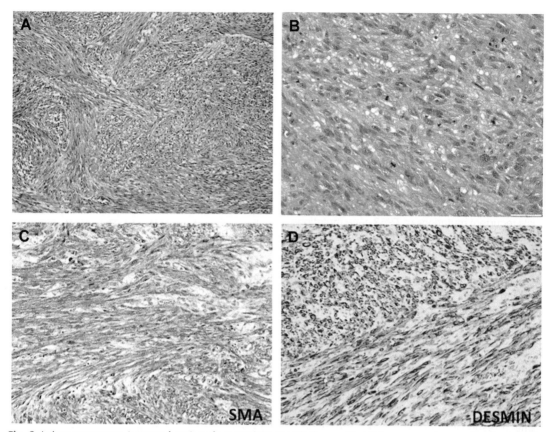

Fig. 6. Leiomyosarcoma. Images showing characteristic morphology with (*A*) low-power image showing cellular spindle cell neoplasm with spindle cells in intersecting fascicles (H&E, original magnification ×100) and (*B*) high-power image showing characteristic "plump" elongated nucleoli (H&E, original magnification × 400). Immuno-histochemical stains for SMA (*C*) and Desmin (*D*) showing diffuse cytoplasmic positivity.

features and not based on immunohistochemical findings alone.

Uterine leiomyosarcoma arises from the uterus and is the most common subtype of uterine sarcoma. They are most common in the perimeno-pausal age group (fifth to sixth decades). The histologic criteria used for the diagnosis of uterine leiomyosarcomas (Stanford criteria) include the presence of cytologic atypia, elevated mitotic activity, and presence of coagulative tumor cell necrosis.[47] This varies slightly from the criteria for soft tissue leiomyosarcoma in that the presence of tumor necrosis is essential for the diagnosis of uterine leiomyosarcoma.

DIFFERENTIAL DIAGNOSIS

The differential diagnoses of leiomyosarcoma are based on the location of the tumor. In extremities, the differential includes undifferentiated pleomorphic sarcoma. Immunohistochemical stains for SMA, desmin, and h-caldesmon help to distinguish leiomyosarcomas from these tumors.

In retroperitoneal locations, the differential includes undifferentiated pleomorphic liposarcoma, dedifferentiated liposarcoma with divergent leiomyosarcomatous differentiation, and malignant perivascular epithelioid cell neoplasms (PEComa). Immunohistochemical stains and/or FISH studies for *CDK4* and *MDM2* gene amplifications help to distinguish dedifferentiated liposarcoma with divergent leiomyosarcomatous differentiation from leiomyosarcoma. Immunohistochemical stains for HMB45, Melan A, and Cathepsin-K help in differentiating malignant PEComa from leiomyosarcoma.

GENETICS

Leiomyosarcomas belong to the class of sarcomas with complex genomic alterations characterized by nonrecurrent structural and copy number alterations.[48] Cytogenetic studies have shown that the loss of 1p12, 2p, 13q, 10q, and 16q are most frequent, and gains are seen in chromosomes 17p, 8q, and 5p. The 5p region is frequently amplified in leiomyosarcoma. The 10q and 13q region losses most likely affect the tumor suppressor genes PTEN and Rb.[48,49]

Chromosome 17p amplification is one of the most frequent amplifications seen in leiomyosarcoma.[50,51] The target of this amplification is a gene encoding myocardin (MYOCD), a transcriptional cofactor of serum response factor (SRF) regulating smooth muscle development and differentiation. Myocardin (MYOCD) gene is highly amplified and overexpressed in a subset of retroperitoneal leiomyosarcoma. MYOCD induces smooth muscle differentiation and promotes cell migration.[50,52] Deep-sequencing methodology reveals recurrent mutations of TP53 gene mutations, seen in more than one-third of the cases. The low mutation frequency in these tumors suggests that leiomyosarcoma genesis is driven primarily by copy number alterations. Chromosomal losses involving tumor suppressor genes PTEN, RB1, and TP53 are common events and emerge as the hallmark genetic abnormalities in these tumors.[50,53]

Uterine leiomyosarcomas have genetic copy number alterations similar to other soft tissue leiomyosarcomas. However, they may have distinct methylation and messenger RNA signatures, with uterine leiomyosarcoma showing a higher DNA damage response score and hypomethylation of ESR1 target genes.[53]

DIAGNOSTIC APPROACH TO ABDOMINAL SMOOTH MUSCLE TUMORS

Smooth muscle tumors of the abdomen and retroperitoneum can be of different types, including leiomyoma and leiomyosarcoma. If the patient is male, then pure soft tissue criteria can be used for differentiating benign leiomyomas from the malignant leiomyosarcomas, similar to extremity tumors. In female patients, benign smooth muscle tumors similar to uterine leiomyoma can occur in the pelvis, parametria, and other abdominal sites not contiguous with the uterus. These tumors are characterized by sharp circumscription, lack of cytologic atypia, lack of increased mitotic activity (<5 per 50 high-power fields), absent necrosis, and consistent diffuse positivity for SMA, desmin, estrogen receptors (ERs), and progesterone receptors (PRs) by immunohistochemistry. These tumors have been termed "parasitic leiomyoma," "GYN-type leiomyoma," or "ER-positive leiomyoma."

When tissue is limited, as in a biopsy setting, and the tumor does not show all the features of malignancy (increased cellularity, cytologic atypia, or increased mitoses) the terminology of "smooth muscle tumor of uncertain malignant potential" could be used. It is advisable not to use this terminology when a complete resection of the tumor is performed.

Leiomyosarcomas of the retroperitoneum and abdomen can occur as de novo lesions or as recurrent/metastatic uterine leiomyosarcoma. Stains for ER and PR are not helpful to distinguish leiomyosarcomas of soft tissue from tumors of uterine origin.

PROGNOSIS

Soft tissue leiomyosarcomas can locally recur and show distant metastasis. The most important prognostic factors by far are tumor grade and size.[43] Retroperitoneal leiomyosarcomas are fatal in the great majority of cases; they are typically large (larger than 10 cm), often difficult or impossible to excise with clear margins, and prone to both local recurrence and metastasis. Leiomyosarcomas of large vessels also tend to have a poor prognosis, although local control rates are higher except for those in the upper inferior vena cava, and very small examples (1–2 cm) may be less prone to metastasize. Nonretroperitoneal soft tissue leiomyosarcomas are generally smaller than those in the retroperitoneum, more amenable to local control, and more favorable in outlook overall. Local recurrences and metastases of soft tissue leiomyosarcoma usually become manifest within the first few years after diagnosis, but may appear as many as 10 years later in 6% to 9% of cases.[43] For retroperitoneal leiomyosarcomas, the most common sites of metastases are the lungs and liver, whereas the lungs are the dominant location when the primary tumor is nonretroperitoneal. Metastases frequently occur in skin, soft tissue, and bone.

Uterine leiomyosarcomas are staged by using the Federation of Gynecology and Obstetrics (FIGO) 2009 staging system, as opposed to the American Joint Committee of Cancer Staging System. The FIGO staging system does not use tumor grade as a criterion. Five-year survival estimates of uterine leiomyosarcoma by FIGO stage are 76%, 60%, 45%, and 29% for stages I, II, III and IV respectively.[54] The modality of treatment includes hysterectomy for patients with disease limited to the uterus and adjuvant chemotherapy in cases of recurrence/metastasis.[54]

REFERENCES

1. Fletcher C, Bridge JA, Hogendoorn PC, et al. WHO classification of tumours of soft tissue and bone. Lyon (France): IARC; 2013.

2. Ognjanovic S, Linabery AM, Charbonneau B, et al. Trends in childhood rhabdomyosarcoma incidence and survival in the United States, 1975-2005. Cancer 2009;115(18):4218–26.

3. Newton WA Jr, Soule EH, Hamoudi AB, et al. Histopathology of childhood sarcomas, intergroup rhabdomyosarcoma studies I and II: clinicopathologic correlation. J Clin Oncol 1988;6(1):67–75.

4. Newton WA Jr, Gehan EA, Webber BL, et al. Classification of rhabdomyosarcomas and related sarcomas. Pathologic aspects and proposal for a new classification—an Intergroup Rhabdomyosarcoma Study. Cancer 1995;76(6):1073–85.

5. Kodet R, Newton WA Jr, Hamoudi AB, et al. Childhood rhabdomyosarcoma with anaplastic (pleomorphic) features. A report of the Intergroup Rhabdomyosarcoma Study. Am J Surg Pathol 1993;17(5):443–53.

6. Cessna MH, Zhou H, Perkins SL, et al. Are myogenin and myoD1 expression specific for rhabdomyosarcoma? A study of 150 cases, with emphasis on spindle cell mimics. Am J Surg Pathol 2001;25(9):1150–7.

7. Wang NP, Marx J, McNutt MA, et al. Expression of myogenic regulatory proteins (myogenin and MyoD1) in small blue round cell tumors of childhood. Am J Pathol 1995;147(6):1799–810.

8. Weber-Hall S, Anderson J, McManus A, et al. Gains, losses, and amplification of genomic material in rhabdomyosarcoma analyzed by comparative genomic hybridization. Cancer Res 1996;56(14):3220–4.

9. Paulson V, Chandler G, Rakheja D, et al. High-resolution array CGH identifies common mechanisms that drive embryonal rhabdomyosarcoma pathogenesis. Genes Chromosomes Cancer 2011;50(6):397–408.

10. Shern JF, Chen L, Chmielecki J, et al. Comprehensive genomic analysis of rhabdomyosarcoma reveals a landscape of alterations affecting a common genetic axis in fusion-positive and fusion-negative tumors. Cancer Discov 2014;4(2):216–31.

11. Meyer WH, Spunt SL. Soft tissue sarcomas of childhood. Cancer Treat Rev 2004;30(3):269–80.

12. Sultan I, Qaddoumi I, Yaser S, et al. Comparing adult and pediatric rhabdomyosarcoma in the surveillance, epidemiology and end results program, 1973 to 2005: an analysis of 2,600 patients. J Clin Oncol 2009;27(20):3391–7.

13. Wexler LH, Ladanyi M. Diagnosing alveolar rhabdomyosarcoma: morphology must be coupled with fusion confirmation. J Clin Oncol 2010;28(13):2126–8.

14. Bompas E, Campion L, Italiano A, et al. Outcome of 449 adult patients with rhabdomyosarcoma: an observational ambispective nationwide study. Cancer Med 2018;7(8):4023–35.

15. Gerber NK, Wexler LH, Singer S, et al. Adult rhabdomyosarcoma survival improved with treatment on multimodality protocols. Int J Radiat Oncol Biol Phys 2013;86(1):58–63.

16. Raney RB Jr, Tefft M, Maurer HM, et al. Disease patterns and survival rate in children with metastatic soft-tissue sarcoma. A report from the Intergroup Rhabdomyosarcoma Study (IRS)-I. Cancer 1988;62(7):1257–66.

17. Tsokos M, Webber BL, Parham DM, et al. Rhabdomyosarcoma. A new classification scheme related to prognosis. Arch Pathol Lab Med 1992;116(8):847–55.

18. Dias P, Chen B, Dilday B, et al. Strong immunostaining for myogenin in rhabdomyosarcoma is significantly associated with tumors of the alveolar subclass. Am J Pathol 2000;156(2):399–408.

19. Thompson LDR, Jo VY, Agaimy A, et al. Sinonasal tract alveolar rhabdomyosarcoma in adults: a clinicopathologic and immunophenotypic study of fifty-two cases with emphasis on epithelial immunoreactivity. Head Neck Pathol 2018;12(2):181–92.

20. Barr FG. Molecular genetics and pathogenesis of rhabdomyosarcoma. J Pediatr Hematol Oncol 1997;19(6):483–91.

21. Barr FG, Chatten J, D'Cruz CM, et al. Molecular assays for chromosomal translocations in the diagnosis of pediatric soft tissue sarcomas. JAMA 1995;273(7):553–7.

22. Davis RJ, D'Cruz CM, Lovell MA, et al. Fusion of PAX7 to FKHR by the variant t(1;13)(p36;q14) translocation in alveolar rhabdomyosarcoma. Cancer Res 1994;54(11):2869–72.

23. Bennicelli JL, Advani S, Schafer BW, et al. PAX3 and PAX7 exhibit conserved cis-acting transcription repression domains and utilize a common gain of function mechanism in alveolar rhabdomyosarcoma. Oncogene 1999;18(30):4348–56.

24. Gordon AT, Brinkschmidt C, Anderson J, et al. A novel and consistent amplicon at 13q31 associated with alveolar rhabdomyosarcoma. Genes Chromosomes Cancer 2000;28(2):220–6.

25. Barr FG, Nauta LE, Davis RJ, et al. In vivo amplification of the PAX3-FKHR and PAX7-FKHR fusion genes in alveolar rhabdomyosarcoma. Hum Mol Genet 1996;5(1):15–21.

26. Raney RB, Anderson JR, Barr FG, et al. Rhabdomyosarcoma and undifferentiated sarcoma in the first two decades of life: a selective review of intergroup rhabdomyosarcoma study group experience and rationale for Intergroup Rhabdomyosarcoma Study V. J Pediatr Hematol Oncol 2001;23(4):215–20.

27. Kelly KM, Womer RB, Sorensen PH, et al. Common and variant gene fusions predict distinct clinical phenotypes in rhabdomyosarcoma. J Clin Oncol 1997;15(5):1831–6.

28. Furlong MA, Mentzel T, Fanburg-Smith JC. Pleomorphic rhabdomyosarcoma in adults: a clinicopathologic study of 38 cases with emphasis on morphologic variants and recent skeletal muscle-specific markers. Mod Pathol 2001;14(6):595–603.

29. Schurch W, Begin LR, Seemayer TA, et al. Pleomorphic soft tissue myogenic sarcomas of adulthood. A reappraisal in the mid-1990s. Am J Surg Pathol 1996;20(2):131–47.

30. Stock N, Chibon F, Binh MB, et al. Adult-type rhabdomyosarcoma: analysis of 57 cases with clinicopathologic description, identification of 3 morphologic patterns and prognosis. Am J Surg Pathol 2009;33(12):1850–9.

31. Li G, Ogose A, Kawashima H, et al. Cytogenetic and real-time quantitative reverse-transcriptase polymerase chain reaction analyses in pleomorphic rhabdomyosarcoma. Cancer Genet Cytogenet 2009;192(1):1–9.

32. Cavazzana AO, Schmidt D, Ninfo V, et al. Spindle cell rhabdomyosarcoma. A prognostically favorable variant of rhabdomyosarcoma. Am J Surg Pathol 1992;16(3):229–35.

33. Leuschner I, Newton WA Jr, Schmidt D, et al. Spindle cell variants of embryonal rhabdomyosarcoma in the paratesticular region. A report of the Intergroup Rhabdomyosarcoma Study. Am J Surg Pathol 1993;17(3):221–30.

34. Mentzel T, Kuhnen C. Spindle cell rhabdomyosarcoma in adults: clinicopathological and immunohistochemical analysis of seven new cases. Virchows Arch 2006;449(5):554–60.

35. Nascimento AF, Fletcher CD. Spindle cell rhabdomyosarcoma in adults. Am J Surg Pathol 2005;29(8):1106–13.

36. Agaram NP, Chen CL, Zhang L, et al. Recurrent MYOD1 mutations in pediatric and adult sclerosing and spindle cell rhabdomyosarcomas: evidence for a common pathogenesis. Genes Chromosomes Cancer 2014;53(9):779–87.

37. Alaggio R, Zhang L, Sung YS, et al. A molecular study of pediatric spindle and sclerosing rhabdomyosarcoma: identification of novel and recurrent VGLL2-related fusions in infantile cases. Am J Surg Pathol 2016;40(2):224–35.

38. Mosquera JM, Sboner A, Zhang L, et al. Recurrent NCOA2 gene rearrangements in congenital/infantile spindle cell rhabdomyosarcoma. Genes Chromosomes Cancer 2013;52(6):538–50.

39. Szuhai K, de Jong D, Leung WY, et al. Transactivating mutation of the MYOD1 gene is a frequent event in adult spindle cell rhabdomyosarcoma. J Pathol 2014;232(3):300–7.

40. Kohsaka S, Shukla N, Ameur N, et al. A recurrent point mutation in MYOD1 defines a clinically aggressive subset of embryonal rhabdomyosarcoma. Mod Pathol 2014;27(Supplement 2):20A–1A, [abstract: 68].

41. Agaram NP, LaQuaglia MP, Alaggio R, et al. MYOD1-mutant spindle cell and sclerosing rhabdomyosarcoma: an aggressive subtype irrespective of age. A reappraisal for molecular classification and risk stratification. Mod Pathol 2018. https://doi.org/10.1038/s41379-018-0120-9.

42. de Saint Aubain Somerhausen N, Fletcher CD. Leiomyosarcoma of soft tissue in children: clinicopathologic analysis of 20 cases. Am J Surg Pathol 1999;23(7):755–63.

43. Gladdy RA, Qin LX, Moraco N, et al. Predictors of survival and recurrence in primary leiomyosarcoma. Ann Surg Oncol 2013;20(6):1851–7.

44. Wile AG, Evans HL, Romsdahl MM. Leiomyosarcoma of soft tissue: a clinicopathologic study. Cancer 1981;48(4):1022–32.

45. Leu HJ, Makek M. Intramural venous leiomyosarcomas. Cancer 1986;57(7):1395–400.

46. Oda Y, Miyajima K, Kawaguchi K, et al. Pleomorphic leiomyosarcoma: clinicopathologic and immunohistochemical study with special emphasis on its distinction from ordinary leiomyosarcoma and malignant fibrous histiocytoma. Am J Surg Pathol 2001;25(8):1030–8.

47. Bell SW, Kempson RL, Hendrickson MR. Problematic uterine smooth muscle neoplasms. A clinicopathologic study of 213 cases. Am J Surg Pathol 1994;18(6):535–58.

48. Guillou L, Aurias A. Soft tissue sarcomas with complex genomic profiles. Virchows Arch 2010;456(2):201–17.

49. Yang J, Du X, Chen K, et al. Genetic aberrations in soft tissue leiomyosarcoma. Cancer Lett 2009;275(1):1–8.

50. Agaram NP, Zhang L, LeLoarer F, et al. Targeted exome sequencing profiles genetic alterations in leiomyosarcoma. Genes Chromosomes Cancer 2016;55(2):124–30.

51. Larramendy ML, Kaur S, Svarvar C, et al. Gene copy number profiling of soft-tissue leiomyosarcomas by array-comparative genomic hybridization. Cancer Genet Cytogenet 2006;169(2):94–101.

52. Perot G, Derre J, Coindre JM, et al. Strong smooth muscle differentiation is dependent on myocardin gene amplification in most human retroperitoneal leiomyosarcomas. Cancer Res 2009;69(6):2269–78.

53. Cancer Genome Atlas Research Network. Electronic address: elizabeth.demicco@sinaihealthsystem.ca, Cancer Genome Atlas Research Network. Comprehensive and integrated genomic characterization of adult soft tissue sarcomas. Cell 2017;171(4):950–65.e28.

54. George S, Serrano C, Hensley ML, et al. Soft tissue and uterine leiomyosarcoma. J Clin Oncol 2018;36(2):144–50.

Pleomorphic Sarcomas
The State of the Art

Sofia Daniela Carvalho, MD[a,b], Daniel Pissaloux, PhD[c], Amandine Crombé, MD[d], Jean-Michel Coindre, MD[b,e], François Le Loarer, MD, PhD[a,e,*]

KEYWORDS

- Sarcoma • Undifferentiated pleomorphic sarcoma • Genomic instability • Liposarcoma
- Myxofibrosarcoma • Leiomyosarcoma • Rhabdomyosarcoma • Dedifferentiation

Key points

- Pleomorphic sarcomas encompass a group of mesenchymal malignancies associated with complex genetic features devoid of defining driver alterations.
- They may display a broad array of histologic lineages including myogenic, lipogenic, neurogenic, or none.
- They affect predominantly adult patients older than 50 years.
- Morphologically, they display variable levels of pleomorphism, although pleomorphism is not always a feature of malignancy.
- Prognostic stratification can be assessed with the 3-tier French grading system FNCLCC, taking into account morphologic features, mitotic activity, and tumor necrosis.

ABSTRACT

This article focuses on pleomorphic sarcomas, which are malignant mesenchymal tumors with complex genetic background at the root of their morphologic pleomorphism. They are poorly differentiated tumors that may retain different lines of differentiation, sometimes correlating with clinicopathological or prognostic features. Accurate diagnosis in this group of tumors relies on adequate sampling due to their heterogeneity and assessment with both microscopy and large panels of immunohistochemistry. Molecular analyses have a limited role in their diagnosis as opposed to translocation-related sarcomas but may provide theranostic and important prognostic information in the future.

OVERVIEW

Pleomorphic sarcomas refer to a heterogeneous group of malignant mesenchymal tumors characterized by morphologic pleomorphism, defined as having marked variations in the size and shape of tumor nuclei and/or cell shape, which is underlined by genetic instability. Pleomorphic sarcomas mostly affect patients older than 50 years and may display a wide array of histologic lineages, therefore a systematic immunohistochemical panel is

Disclosure Statement: Dr. Loarer is supported by a grant from Le Fil d'Oriane.
[a] Department of Pathology, Hospital de Braga, Sete Fontes-Sao Victor, 4710-243 Braga, Portugal;
[b] Department of Pathology, Institut Bergonié, 276 cours de l'Argonne, 33000, Bordeaux, France;
[c] Department of Pathology, Centre Leon Berard, Promenade Lea Bullukian, 69376 Lyon, France;
[d] Department of Radiology, Institut Bergonié, 276 cours de l'Argonne, 33000, Bordeaux, France;
[e] University of Bordeaux, Talence, France
* Corresponding author.
E-mail address: f.le-loarer@bordeaux.unicancer.fr

Box 1
Main types of pleomorphic sarcomas

Lines of differentiation in pleomorphic sarcomas
Lipogenic differentiation

  Dedifferentiated liposarcoma

  Pleomorphic liposarcoma

Myogenic differentiation

  Leiomyosarcoma

  Pleomorphic rhabdomyosarcoma

Neurogenic differentiation

  Malignant peripheral nerve sheath tumor

Osteogenic differentiation

  Extraskeletal osteosarcoma

Vascular differentiation

  Angiosarcoma

Pleomorphic sarcomas as a result of dedifferentiation

  Dedifferentiated liposarcoma

  Dedifferentiated gastrointestinal stromal tumor ("sarcoma")

  Dedifferentiated solitary fibrous tumor

No lineage of differentiation as yet identified

  Undifferentiated pleomorphic sarcoma

Unknown lineage of differentiation

  Myxofibrosarcoma

---

used to support their classification (**Box 1**). The most frequent subtypes of pleomorphic sarcomas include dedifferentiated liposarcomas, myxofibrosarcomas, and undifferentiated pleomorphic sarcomas. From a molecular standpoint, their initiating oncogenic events are unknown, and the most recurrent alterations affect commonplace tumor suppressor genes *TP53, RB1, PTEN,* and *CDKN2A.* The molecular classification of pleomorphic sarcomas mostly mirrors the histologic subtyping, except for myxofibrosarcomas, which are molecularly similar to undifferentiated pleomorphic sarcomas. Pleomorphic sarcomas are stratified into 3 grades with histologic grading schemes, the most widely used being the French sarcoma grading system (FNCLCC), which takes into account the type of differentiation, necrosis, and mitotic activity.

MORPHOLOGIC PLEOMORPHISM AND DIAGNOSTIC APPROACH OF PLEOMORPHIC SARCOMAS

Pleomorphic sarcomas have been historically defined based on their morphologic features using descriptive terms reflecting their heterogeneous features, and histotypes have been delineated based on immunohistochemical and molecular studies.[1]

Nuclear pleomorphism refers to marked variation in both size and shape of tumor cell nuclei, with frequent nuclear membrane irregularities, and nuclear hyperchromasia, hints toward complex underlying genetic features and genetic instability in tumors as opposed to the bland nuclei, referred to as "monomorphism," harbored by most translocation-related sarcomas. Pleomorphism is hardly a specific morphologic feature, as it is most often associated with high-grade advanced tumors, whatever their initial epithelial or mesenchymal lineage. In viscera, pleomorphic sarcomas remain a diagnosis of exclusion after a sarcomatoid carcinoma is ruled out on microscopy and immunohistochemistry. Conversely, the presence of pleomorphism in a tumor, although worrisome, does not equal to malignancy with the notable example of pleomorphic lipomas (**Box 2**).

Additionally, pleomorphism may occur as a marker of dedifferentiation in a specific type of sarcoma (see **Box 1**), such as dedifferentiated liposarcomas, solitary fibrous tumors or

> **Box 2**
> **Benign and locally aggressive mesenchymal tumors associated with pleomorphism**
>
> *Benign*
> Fibrous histiocytoma (so-called atypical variant)
>
> Tenosynovial giant cell tumor
>
> Pleomorphic lipoma
>
> Schwannoma ("ancient" schwannoma)
>
> Atypical neurofibroma
>
> *Intermediate (locally aggressive and rarely metastasizing) malignancy*
> Pleomorphic dermal sarcoma
>
> Atypical fibroxanthoma
>
> Pleomorphic hyalinizing angiectatic tumor
>
> Myxoinflammatory fibroblastic sarcoma

gastrointestinal stromal tumors (GISTs).[2–4] In this situation, microscopic assessment may help identify the presence of a coexisting nonpleomorphic component within tumor bulk, pointing toward the proper diagnosis, although the "dedifferentiated" (anaplastic) pleomorphic component dictates the prognosis.

For all reasons stated previously, the microscopic assessment of a pleomorphic tumor is systematically completed with a thorough immunohistochemical panel seeking for an overlooked histologic lineage, all the more if the tumor is not located in soft tissue.

An immunohistochemical panel supporting the diagnosis when facing a pleomorphic proliferation should at least include epithelial markers (AE1/E3, EMA, for instance), CD34, S100 protein, h-caldesmon, and desmin. Additional markers may be added depending on the location or the clinicopathological features, such as HMGA2/MDM2 (retroperitoneal mass lipogenic component), CD117/DOG1 (in gastrointestinal tract or prior history of GIST).

MOLECULAR FEATURES OF PLEOMORPHIC SARCOMAS

From a molecular standpoint, pleomorphic sarcomas are genetically complex with no identified initiating genetic alteration. Although they are considered of mesenchymal origin, pleomorphic sarcomas share with epithelial tumors the frequent inactivation of tumor suppressor genes *TP53, RB1,* and *CDKN2A* (p16).[5] This molecular overlap suggests the critical nature of these pathways in tumorigenesis, and mirrors the challenges pathologists may have to distinguish

sarcomatoid carcinomas from pleomorphic sarcomas and the artificial boundaries of these entities in some settings. Aside from these tumor suppressors, and rare cases with DNA mismatch repair defects, pleomorphic sarcomas have relatively low mutation burden and display mainly age-related types of mutations.[6] Instead, pleomorphic sarcomas are characterized by copy number alterations (CNAs) that are thought to drive tumorigenesis genomic studies have delineated 3 distinct molecular subgroups based on the patterns of genomic events, including (1) sarcomas with arm and whole chromosome alterations, (2) sarcomas with amplicons, and (3) sarcomas with segmental alterations.[7] However, this genomic subclassification has no practical interest. In contrast, the degree of genomic complexity present in mesenchymal tumors may well have both diagnostic and prognostic significance.

The concept of genomic complexity refers to rearranged genomic profiles with CNAs interspersed across tumor genomes. The level of genetic complexity can be quantified with the "genomic index," calculated with the square number of CNAs divided by the number of chromosomes involved.[7] Overall, the higher the genomic index, the higher the probability of malignancy and aggressiveness of the tumor. The genomic index can therefore be used as a marker of malignancy when dealing with pleomorphic tumors of uncertain malignant potential based on the sole morphologic findings, such as uterine/prostatic leiomyosarcomas versus smooth muscle tumor of uncertain malignant potential (STUMP)/atypical leiomyoma.[8] Furthermore, genomic complexity in sarcomas correlates with prognosis: the CINSARC (Complexity INdex in SARComas) signature can stratify patients with sarcoma into 2 prognostic groups, as opposed to the 3-tier histologic grading.[7,9] This signature incorporates the levels of expression of a set of 67 genes that are mostly involved in the maintenance of chromosome integrity and mitotic control. Interestingly, the level of nuclear pleomorphism in sarcomas correlates with the underlying genomic complexity of the tumor.[6] Additionally, the Genomic Grade Index, a signature of 108 genes initially identified in early-stage breast cancers, has been shown to predict outcomes in patients with resected sarcomas, outperforming the CINSARC signature in this setting.[10]

It is notable that next-generation sequencing studies have also highlighted the presence of gene fusions in a subset of pleomorphic sarcomas such as *TRIO* rearrangements, which most probably represent passenger translocations as opposed to the translocations underlying monomorphic sarcomas, such as synovial sarcomas.[11]

PROGNOSIS AND GRADING OF PLEOMORPHIC SARCOMAS

Pleomorphic sarcomas can be stratified with the 3-tier histologic grading system of the French sarcoma group.[12–14] It takes into account 3 parameters, including differentiation, mitotic activity, and necrosis (**Table 1**). Some investigators have advocated reliance on Ki67 staining rather than mitotic count on core needle biopsy specimens due to tumor heterogeneity and poor interobserver agreement in the counting of mitotic figures.[15]

Notably, myogenic differentiation, in particular rhabdomyosarcomas, has been associated with worse prognosis.[16–19]

GROSS EXAMINATION OF PLEOMORPHIC SARCOMAS

Most pleomorphic sarcomas do not display specific gross features, save for dedifferentiated liposarcomas, which may include both well-differentiated (fatty) and dedifferentiated components (**Fig. 1**). Macroscopic features reflect the high-grade nature of these tumors with presence of necrosis and hemorrhage.

Gross examination should be performed following the general recommendations for sarcomas. In surgical specimens, a thorough sampling should be performed to ensure the identification of lines of differentiation, which

Table 1
French Grading System for Sarcomas with updated criteria

Three-Tier French Grading System for Sarcomas (FNCLCC Grading)[12–14]

1-Tumor differentiation	*Score 1* normal-like tissue, low-grade cytological features *Score 2* certain histologic diagnosis based on morphology, low-grade cytologic features *Score 3* synovial sarcoma, clear cell, epithelioid, alveolar, undifferentiated sarcomas; high-grade cytological features
2-Mitotic activity (10 high-power fields assessed with a field of 0.174 mm^2) and/or Ki-67 staining on core needle biopsy	*Score 1* 0–9 mitotic figures or Ki-67 positive in 0%–9% *Score 2* 10–19 mitotic figures or Ki-67 positive in 10%–29% *Score 3* >19 mitotic figures or Ki-67 positive in ≥30%
3-Tumor necrosis	*Score 1* absent, note that in core needle biopsies, the score is upgraded to 1 if necrosis is present on MRI *Score 2* <50% of tumor surface *Score 3* >50% of tumor surface

Final grade: grade 1 (2–3), grade 2 (score 4–5), grade 3 (score 6–8).
Data from Refs.[12–14]

may be only focally present. We recommend sampling of a complete section of the tumor mass along its greatest axis to assess all sarcoma surgical specimens, with or without prior neoadjuvant chemotherapy or radiation therapy.[20] Additional sampling will focus on the assessment of margins, including areas of interest based on gross examination and indications provided by the surgeons. The presence of a fascia/aponeurosis should be mentioned in the report and its histologic status reported to adjust adjuvant therapy.

Fig. 1. Gross specimen of a dedifferentiated liposarcoma. Yellow differentiated fatty areas adjacent to solid, fleshy areas with necrosis.

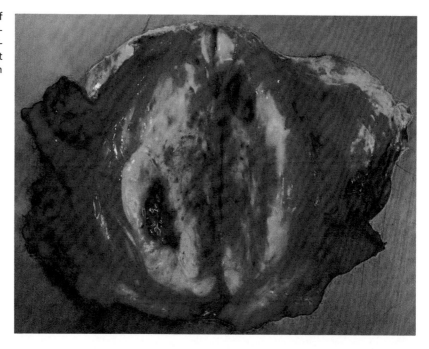

PLEOMORPHIC LIPOSARCOMA

Pleomorphic liposarcoma is the rarest subtype of liposarcoma, and is defined by the coexistence of undifferentiated sarcomatous areas admixed with a variable amount of pleomorphic lipoblasts.[21,22]

CLINICAL FEATURES

Pleomorphic liposarcomas affect most commonly the elderly, with a peak incidence in the sixth decade and a slight predominance in men. They show marked predilection for deep soft tissues of the extremities, particularly the thigh and limb girdles, but can be found in a wide variety of sites,[23,24] with the exception of the retroperitoneum in which the primary diagnosis to consider, if not the only one, is a dedifferentiated liposarcoma.

They do not have specific radiological features, but MRI may evidence necrosis or edema, in keeping with their high-grade features.

MICROSCOPIC FEATURES

By definition, pleomorphic liposarcomas are composed of areas of undifferentiated pleomorphic sarcoma admixed with pleomorphic lipoblasts. This lipogenic component may vary greatly in abundance. Pleomorphic lipoblasts correspond to multivacuolated or univacuolated tumor cells with pleomorphic scalloped nuclei (**Fig. 2**A). The nonlipogenic component may cover the wide morphologic spectrum of undifferentiated pleomorphic sarcoma (UPS), including fascicular, epithelioid, or myxoid histologic patterns.[22–25] Rare cases with extensive lipogenic differentiation have been reported[24] (**Fig. 2**B–D). The vascular network may even be prominently staghorn/pericytic.[24] Heterologous osteoid, chondroid, or striated muscle differentiation can be rarely observed,[24] and in practice, their presence should be mentioned in the report, as the presence of another line of mesenchymal differentiation may suggest the differential diagnosis of mesenchymoma.

IMMUNOHISTOCHEMICAL FEATURES

Immunohistochemistry helps in excluding any line of differentiation in the setting of a pleomorphic spindle proliferation. Lipoblasts can be highlighted with S100 protein staining or adipophilin, as proposed by a few groups.[26] Smooth muscle actin and CD34 are focally expressed in half of cases. Other markers that can be positive at least focally are HMGA2, desmin, pankeratin, and EMA, the last 2 in almost half of the epithelioid cases.[23–25,27] Staining for MDM2 and CDK4 is typically negative.[28]

MOLECULAR PATHOLOGY

Pleomorphic liposarcomas are not associated with *MDM2* amplification.[29] Molecular studies have highlighted they are close to UPS at the genomic level.[30]

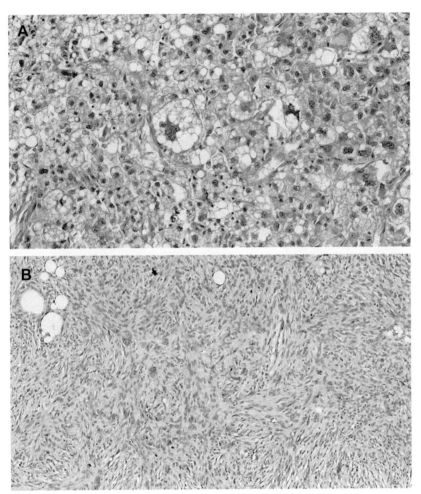

Fig. 2. Pleomorphic liposarcoma. (*A*) Pleomorphic lipoblasts. Different histologic patterns may be seen in these tumors with (*B*) spindle cell,

DIFFERENTIAL DIAGNOSIS

The differential diagnosis of pleomorphic liposarcomas is broad, including both other adipocytic and nonadipocytic neoplasms.

Dedifferentiated liposarcoma (DD-LPS) is the most important differential diagnosis to consider, especially in retroperitoneal location. The dedifferentiated component may indeed display pleomorphic lipoblasts, corresponding to persistence or reactivation of lipogenic differentiation, which is repressed during the dedifferentiation process.[31] The coexistence of a well-differentiated adipocytic component in the tumor hints toward the diagnosis of DD-LPS,[32] and the identification of *MDM2* amplification is confirmatory of this diagnosis.[32]

A subset of *spindle cell/pleomorphic lipoma* displays a striking level of pleomorphism, raising suspicion of malignancy. However, pleomorphic cells are never lipogenic. Pleomorphic cells are mostly multinucleated "floret cells" and may coexist with a spindled monomorphic component (**Fig.** 3A, B). Pleomorphic lipoma presents typically as a well-circumscribed subcutaneous mass, smaller than 6 cm. This lesion shows diffuse expression of CD34, and is associated with *RB1* inactivation at proteic level and heterozygous deletion of 13q spanning *RB1* locus at genomic level (**Fig.** 3C).

The epithelioid subtype of pleomorphic liposarcoma may be misinterpreted as *primary* or *metastatic carcinoma*, in particular renal cell carcinoma and adrenal cortical carcinoma, in which neoplastic cells can be similar to lipoblasts. Renal cell carcinoma has diffuse expression of

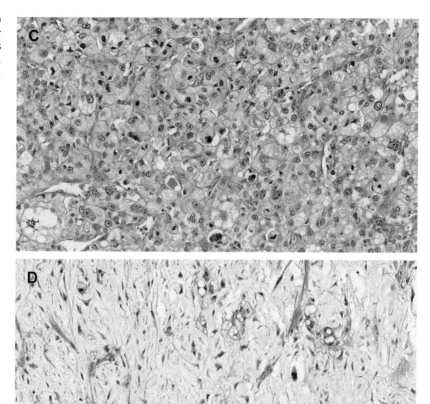

Fig. 2. (continued). (*C*) xanthomatous, (*D*) or myxoid morphologies (hematoxylin-eosin [H&E], original magnification, [*B, D*] ×10; [*A, C*] ×20).

keratins and EMA, in addition to being positive for PAX8, and the renal cell carcinoma antibody. In a series of epithelioid pleomorphic liposarcomas, EMA was absent in all cases.[25]

Pitfalls
PLEOMORPHIC LIPOSARCOMA

! Pleomorphic lipoblasts may be very scarce and not readily identified.

! Epithelioid pattern and rare expression of keratins may be misleading and raise suspicion of carcinoma.

! Myxoid stromal changes, for example, in myxofibrosarcoma may cause cytoplasmic vacuolation, which may resemble lipogenic differentiation but S100 protein is not expressed by tumor cells.

PROGNOSIS

Pleomorphic liposarcomas are aggressive neoplasms with both local recurrence and metastatic rates ranging from 30% to 50%. Five-year survival rate is estimated to 60%. Metastases occur primarily in the lungs and pleura. Clinical and histologic factors linked with worse prognosis are nonextremity location, size, and mitotic index.[23,24]

LEIOMYOSARCOMA AND PLEOMORPHIC SARCOMAS WITH PARTIAL MYOGENIC PHENOTYPE

Leiomyosarcomas (LMSs) are sarcomas displaying smooth muscle differentiation. They may be poorly differentiated with overt pleomorphism in fewer than 10% of cases, most commonly admixed with classic areas of LMS[33–35] (**Fig. 4**A–E). In this setting, the smooth muscle differentiation may be overlooked on microscopic

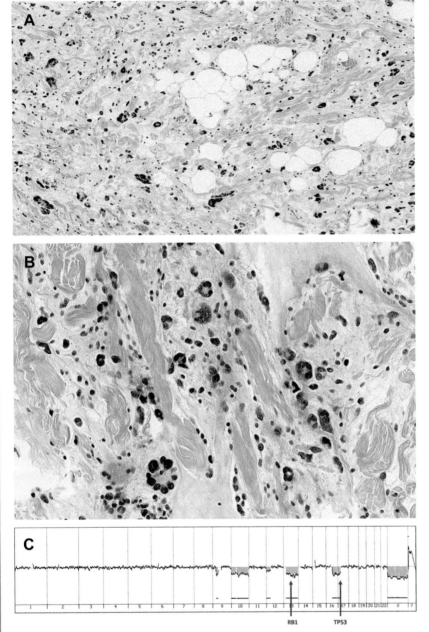

Fig. 3. Spindle/pleomorphic cell lipoma. (*A*) Floretlike multinucleate cells in a background of thick collagen fibers and adipocytes. (*B*) Cells present pleomorphic, hyperchromatic nuclei (H&E, original magnification, [*A*] ×10; [*B*] ×20). (*C*) aCGH profile showing heterozygous deletion of *RB1* and *TP53* compatible with a pleomorphic cell lipoma.

examination. Expression of smooth muscle markers (h-caldesmon AND smooth muscle actin or desmin or transgelin) should be positive in the well-differentiated component or partially retained in pleomorphic areas to render this diagnosis[33,34] (Fig. 4F–H).

Studies highlighted a subclass of pleomorphic sarcoma with incomplete myogenic phenotype, defined as tumors harboring morphologic features reminiscent of myogenic differentiation but with only focal expression of myogenic markers h-caldesmon, transgelin, calponin, and smooth muscle actin, or with diffuse expression of only 1 marker in the absence of all others. Tumors presenting partial myogenic phenotype may have a higher metastatic potential than UPS but lower than bona fide LMS.[36] From a molecular standpoint, pleomorphic sarcomas with partial myogenic phenotype are close to, if not indistinguishable from, UPS at the genomic level,[7,36–38] therefore this terminology is not widely used in clinical practice. Some investigators use the term dedifferentiated LMS to refer to LMS in which morphologically and phenotypically typical areas of LMS coexist along with pleomorphic areas negative for smooth muscle markers.[33,39]

MOLECULAR PATHOLOGY

LMSs represent a molecularly distinct subgroup of pleomorphic sarcomas enriched in myogenic factors.[6] Two subgroups of soft tissue LMS can be delineated, including a group with PTEN/AKT pathway deregulation and a second group expressing hypomethylated and inflammation signatures.[6] LMS genomes contain mainly losses and deletions (**Fig. 4I**) but rare amplifications with the exception of *MYOCD* amplicons.[40] Of note, soft tissue LMS can be distinguished from uterine LMS at the transcriptomic and methylation levels; these 2 tumor types belonging to distinct clusters.[6] Array-comparative genomic hybridization (aCGH) may be useful to distinguish benign smooth muscle proliferation from leiomyosarcoma, as homozygous deletions of *RB1* and/or *TP53* are not present in benign smooth muscle lesions and the overall genomic complexity is higher in malignant lesions.[36]

DIFFERENTIAL DIAGNOSIS

LMSs may focally express keratins and/or EMA[41] and are therefore misdiagnosed as *carcinomas*.

Myogenin or myoD1 staining should be performed when dealing with a pleomorphic tumor expressing desmin to rule out a *pleomorphic rhabdomyosarcoma*. Morphologically, they characteristically have large polygonal and pleomorphic cells. GISTs express h-caldesmon in 80% of cases and desmin in fewer than 1%[42] but not transgelin.[35] Expression of CD117 may be lost in dedifferentiated GIST.

Pitfalls
LEIOMYOSARCOMA

! h-caldesmon can be expressed in GIST and dedifferentiated GISTs may be negative for CD117.

! Sarcoma with partial myogenic phenotype are defined as spindled tumors reminiscent of LMS displaying focal or isolated expression of 1 myogenic marker.

! LMSs might display an epithelioid pattern and express keratins.

PROGNOSIS

LMS has a more aggressive clinical course than pleomorphic sarcomas without myogenic differentiation.[16,18,34] Reported metastasis and mortality rate are of 48% to 89% and 50% to 65%, respectively, with a median survival of 9 to 17 months. Lung is the most common site of metastasis.[33,34]

PLEOMORPHIC RHABDOMYOSARCOMA

Pleomorphic rhabdomyosarcomas are high-grade pleomorphic sarcomas showing an isolated rhabdomyosarcomatous phenotype without any other line of differentiation. They are the most common subtype of rhabdomyosarcoma in adults.[21]

CLINICAL FEATURES

Pleomorphic rhabdomyosarcomas arise predominantly in the lower extremities of elderly men, most commonly in the sixth to seventh decades of life.[43,44] Cases occurring in pediatric patients may be associated with Li-Fraumeni syndrome[45]

MICROSCOPIC FEATURES

These tumors are mainly composed of a pleomorphic high-grade "UPS-like" proliferation. Some cases may contain scattered large atypical cells with abundant polygonal and eosinophilic cytoplasm, reminiscent of rhabdomyoblasts. These cells are frequently multinucleated, harboring vesicular nuclei with prominent nucleoli (**Fig. 5A, B**). High mitotic count and extensive necrosis are frequent, in keeping with their high-grade features.[43]

IMMUNOHISTOCHEMICAL FEATURES

Desmin expression is multifocal in most cases, restricted to the scattered polygonal cells, but may be diffuse (**Fig. 5C**). By definition, they express at least 1 skeletal muscle–specific marker; for example, MyoD1 and/or myf4/myogenin at the nuclear level (**Fig. 5D**). The expression of 1 of these 2 markers is required for unequivocal diagnosis.[43,46] Variable smooth muscle actin and focal keratin AE1/AE3 and EMA positivity also can be observed.[43,44] MDM2 nuclear labeling without *MDM2* amplification has been reported.[44]

MOLECULAR PATHOLOGY

No large series are available regarding this histotype. They are not associated with *MDM2*

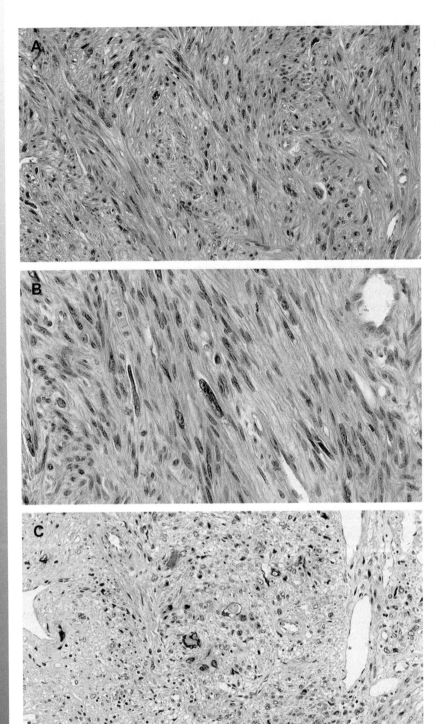

Fig. 4. Leiomyosarcoma. (*A*) Intersecting fascicles of spindle cells with eosinophilic cytoplasm and (*B*) tapered end nuclei (*C*) admix with pleomorphic spindle, multinucleated bizarre cells, and rarely

Fig. 4. (continued). (*D*) epithelioid cells. (*E*) Multinucleated cells can be prominent in this group of tumors. (*F*) Diffuse and

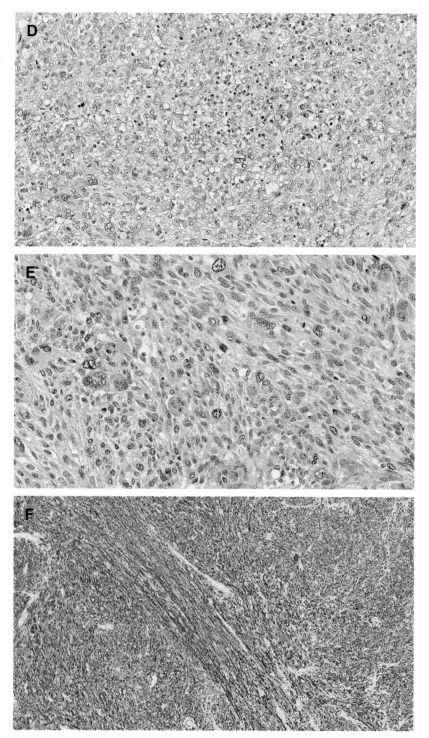

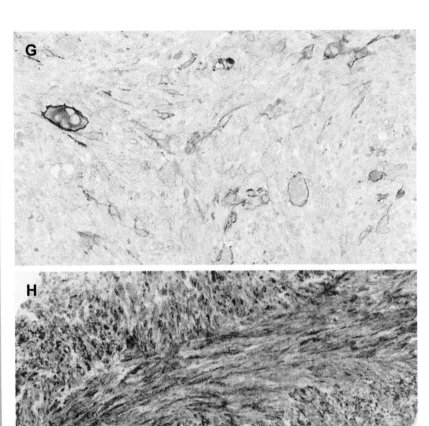

Fig. 4. (*continued*). (*G*) focal expression of h-caldesmon. (*H*) A subset of leiomyosarcomas are positive for EMA (H&E, original magnification, [*F*] ×10; [*A, C–E, G, H*] ×20; [*B*] ×40). (*I*) aCGH analyses of a smooth muscle neoplasm showing a complex genomic profile containing numerous deletions in chromosomes 10, 16, 1p, and 6q, consistent with the diagnosis of leiomyosarcoma. Deletions in chromosomes 13 and 17 are also a frequent finding in LMS but were absent in this case. Homozygous deletion in *DMD* was also present. This profile is highly suggestive of leiomyosarcoma.

amplification[44] and their genomic profiles are indistinguishable from those of UPS (unpublished data).

DIFFERENTIAL DIAGNOSIS

On small biopsy specimens, the rhabdomyosarcomatous component may represent a heterologous component part of a complex tumor, such as a sarcomatoid carcinoma, a malignant peripheral nerve sheath tumor (also known as Triton tumor), dedifferentiated liposarcoma, or a malignant mesenchymoma.

Pitfalls
PLEOMORPHIC RHABDOMYOSARCOMA

! Desmin expression is mostly focal, restricted to polygonal/epithelioid tumor cells.

! Rhabdomyosarcoma may represent the heterologous component of a complex high-grade tumor that may be overlooked on a core needle biopsy.

! Rhabdomyosarcoma might express MDM2 without underlying amplification.

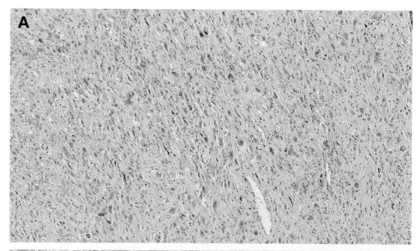
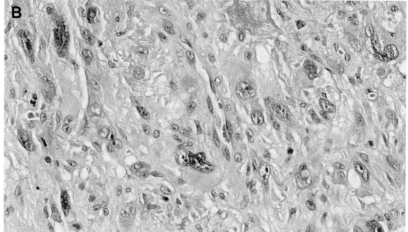

Fig. 5. Pleomorphic rhabdomyosarcoma. (*A*) Scattered large eosinophilic cells (*B*) with vesicular nuclei and prominent nucleoli, in a background with UPS-like morphology.

PROGNOSIS

Pleomorphic rhabdomyosarcoma portends a worse prognosis than other pleomorphic sarcomas. Tumors have a relapse rate of 53.8% and more than 80% metastasize within 5 years. Median survival at local and metastatic stage are 12.8 months and 7.1 months, respectively. Older patients have higher risk of adverse outcome.[44,47]

PLEOMORPHIC SARCOMAS AS A RESULT OF DEDIFFERENTIATION

Dedifferentiation, or anaplastic change, refers to tumor progression involving the transformation of a low-grade sarcoma to a higher-grade sarcoma.[2–4,39,48] The dedifferentiated component mainly displays a pleomorphic morphology, distinct from the low-grade component,[49]

and the identification of this higher-grade "differentiated" component is required to render the diagnosis. This dedifferentiation process has been best described in liposarcomas, solitary fibrous tumors, and GISTs.

DEDIFFERENTIATED LIPOSARCOMA

Dedifferentiated liposarcomas (DD-LPSs) are malignant adipocytic tumors underlined by *MDM2* amplification with coexistent lipogenic and nonlipogenic differentiated components. They develop from a known well-differentiated liposarcoma or de novo. Dedifferentiation occurs in up to 10% of well-differentiated liposarcomas.[2]

CLINICAL FEATURES

DD-LPS affects predominantly adults older than 50 years but not exclusively. Retroperitoneum is

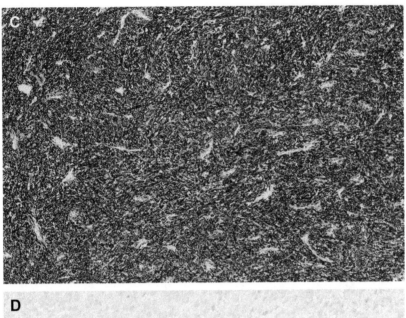

the most frequent location. Other common sites include extremities, trunk, and scrotum/spermatic cord.[2,50]

Their radiological features are diagnostic with coexistent fatty and nonfatty solid components within the tumor bulk (**Fig. 6**).

MICROSCOPIC FEATURES

The lipogenic "well-differentiated" and nonlipogenic components often display abrupt transition (**Fig. 7**A, B). The dedifferentiated component is highly plastic, and spans a wide morphologic spectrum from low-grade to high-grade pleomorphic sarcomas[2,22,51–53] (**Fig. 7**C–G). Rarely, the lipogenic differentiation may persist in the

dedifferentiated component with the presence of pleomorphic lipoblasts resembling a pleomorphic liposarcoma.[32,54]

IMMUNOHISTOCHEMICAL FEATURES

DD-LPSs display diffuse nuclear expression of HMGA2 and MDM2 in 67% and 85% of cases, respectively[27,28,32] (**Fig. 7**H, I). *MDM2* amplification should be demonstrated by fluorescence in situ hybridization (FISH) (**Fig. 7**J), especially if MDM2 is only focally expressed or the location of the tumor is other than retroperitoneum.[55] Eleven percent of DD-LPSs show nuclear STAT6 staining, as the *STAT6* locus is

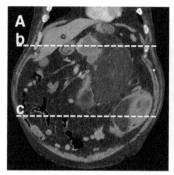
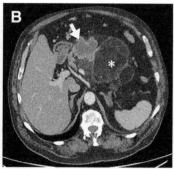
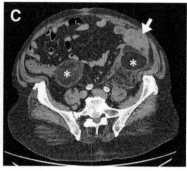

Fig. 6. Imaging features in a retroperitoneal dedifferentiated liposarcoma. Imaging distinguished 2 distinct components in this tumor. Computed tomography with iodine contrast-agent intravenous injection, acquisition at portal phase, axial (*B,C*) and coronal view (*A*). The levels of the axial slices are reported in white dashed lines on the coronal view. Well-differentiated areas typically show very low attenuation consistent with fat (*white asterisks*) whereas dedifferentiated areas (*white arrows*) display higher, tissular attenuation and enhancement after contrast-agent injection.

located close to *MDM2* and may be coamplified.[56,57]

MOLECULAR PATHOLOGY

DD-LPSs are defined by the amplification of the *MDM2* oncogene.[50] Most DD-LPSs harbor additional genetic alterations that turn off pathways involved in lipogenesis, such as *peroxisome proliferator-activated receptor* gamma signaling through *JUN* and *ASK* amplifications[31] or *VGLL3, DDIT3,* and *CEBPA*[6,58] (**Fig.** 7K).

DIFFERENTIAL DIAGNOSIS

Any mesenchymal pleomorphic tumor developing in the retroperitoneum should be considered as DD-LPS until proven otherwise.[59] An immunohistochemical screening with HMGA2 or CDK4 and MDM2 should at least be performed to test this hypothesis and, as MDM2 immunohistochemistry has a sensitivity of 85% for the diagnosis of DD-LPS, although not being entirely specific,[28,60,61] positive cases should be confirmed with FISH testing for MDM2 amplification.

MPNST can occasionally show extensive pleomorphism and, in 60% of cases, display MDM2 staining. However, amplification of *MDM2* is absent.[62]

As a great mimicker, DD-LPS can have solitary fibrous tumor (SFT)-like features, show diffuse expression of CD34, and may even overexpress STAT6.[63] In these cases, search for *MDM2* amplification is mandatory, as it is not observed in SFTs[56,57] (**Fig.** 8).

Pitfalls
DEDIFFERENTIATED LIPOSARCOMA

! DD-LPSs span a wide morphologic spectrum and may mimic many sarcoma histotypes.

! DD-LPS may express STAT6, leading to potentially misinterpretation as fat-forming SFT.

! MDM2 staining is not entirely specific for DD-LPS and should be correlated with genetic status (presence of amplification).

PROGNOSIS

DD-LPSs have lower metastatic potential than other pleomorphic sarcomas, but are associated with important morbidity, especially retroperitoneal tumors.[64] Local recurrence occurs in 40% to 80% of cases. Distant metastases account for 19% of cases and disease-related mortality is of 42%.[65]

The histologic grade of the dedifferentiated component correlates with survival.[64,66]

Both smooth muscle and rhabdomyoblastic differentiation (**Fig.** 9) correlate with aggressive clinical behavior in DD-LPS.[53,66]

DEDIFFERENTIATED GASTROINTESTINAL STROMAL TUMOR

GIST is the most common primary mesenchymal tumor in the gastrointestinal tract, deriving from the interstitial cell of Cajal. They may behave in a benign or malignant manner.[21] Dedifferentiation in GIST is extremely uncommon, being mainly secondary to

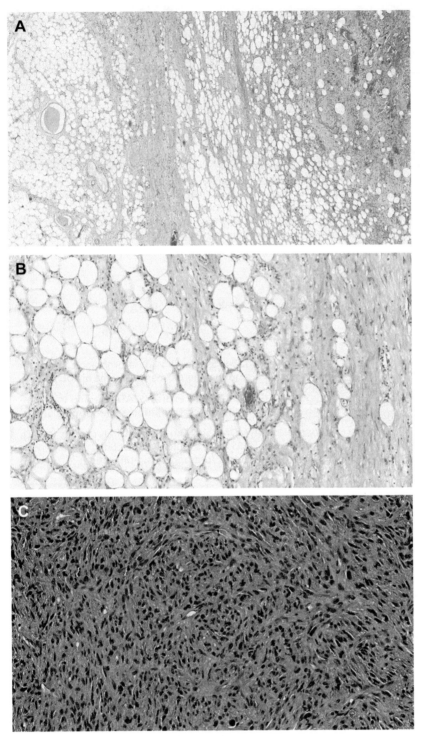

Fig. 7. Dedifferentiated liposarcoma. (*A*) Sharp transition between (*B*) well-differentiated component and (*C*) dedifferentiated component is highly variable with examples of spindled,

Fig. 7. (*continued*). (*D*) epithelioid, (*E*) myxoid, (*F*) UPS-like,

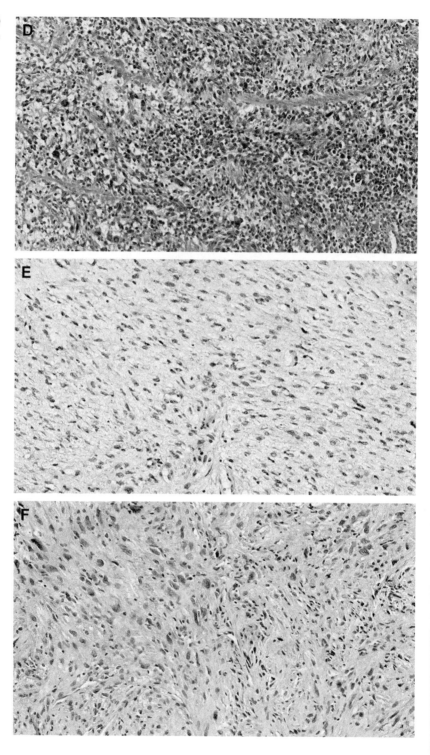

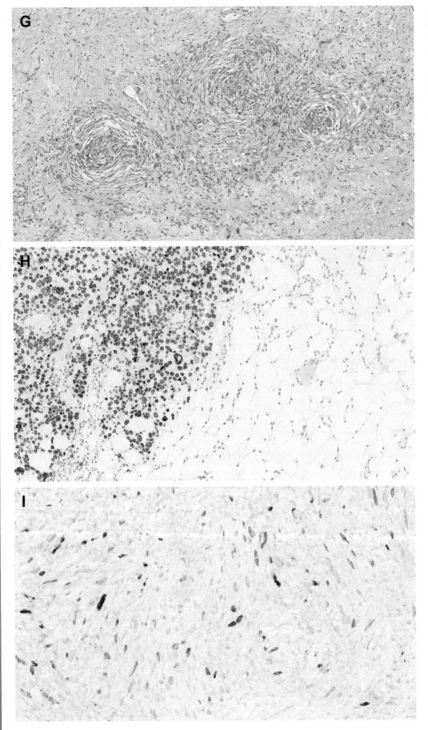

Fig. 7. (continued). (*G*) and meningothelial-like appearances. (*H*) HMGA2 staining in both components (*I*) and MDM2 expression in the dedifferentiated component (H&E, original magnification, [*A*] ×2,5; [*B, G, H*] ×10; [*C–F, I*] ×20).

Fig. 7. (continued). (*J*) FISH screening showing strong amplification of *MDM2* forming clusters (probes targeting *MDM2* locus and chromosome 12 centromere are labeled in *green* and *red*, respectively). (*K*) aCGH analyses of a dedifferentiated liposarcoma with characteristic amplification of *MDM2, CDK4* and *JUN*. DD-LPS typically display amplicons in their genome.

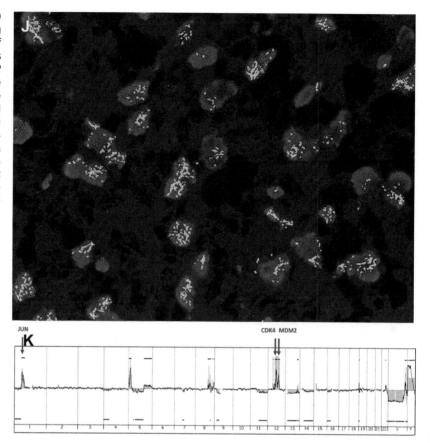

chronic imatinib therapy and secondary resistance to therapy, but may develop de novo.[3]

MICROSCOPIC FEATURES

Dedifferentiated GIST (DD-GIST) displays 2 components in abrupt transition, including a morphologically classic area of GIST and a high-grade anaplastic/pleomorphic proliferation (**Fig. 10**A, B). The dedifferentiated component is highly variable with reports of angiosarcomatous,[3] epithelioid/rhabdoid, rhabdomyosarcomatous, and chondrosarcomatous differentiation.[67]

Fig. 8. Fat-forming SFT. Hemangiopericytomalike vessels and adipocytic component (H&E, original magnification, ×10).

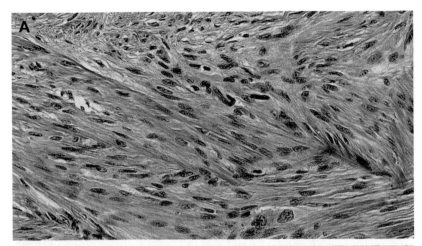

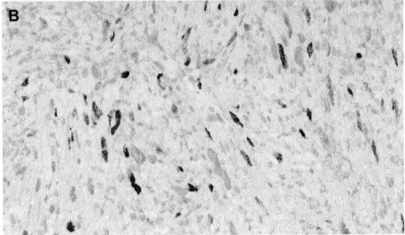

Fig. 9. Dedifferentiated liposarcoma with myogenic differentiation. (*A*) Spindle cell proliferation with eosinophilic cytoplasm somewhat reminiscent of myogenic differentiation. Expression of MDM2 (*B*), desmin

IMMUNOHISTOCHEMICAL FEATURES

The dedifferentiated components lose expression of CD117 and CD34[3] and may express variable markers depending on the line of differentiation[67] (**Fig. 10**C–E).

MOLECULAR PATHOLOGY

Despite differences in the immunophenotype, both conventional and dedifferentiated components have the same *KIT, BRAF,* and *TP53* mutational profile.[3,67] DD-GIST may be wild-type, but the corresponding conventional area is wild-type as well in these cases.[3]

DEDIFFERENTIATED SOLITARY FIBROUS TUMOR

SFT is a fibroblastic mesenchymal tumor of intermediate malignancy defined by intrachromosomic *NAB2-STAT6* fusions. SFT may remain local or metastasize ("malignant SFT").[21] They may rarely undergo dedifferentiation. Dedifferentiated SFTs (DD-SFTs) are mostly diagnosed de novo,[4,68] but dedifferentiation can occur at the time of recurrence.[68]

MICROSCOPIC FEATURES

DD-SFT shows a conventional SFT component admixed to a dedifferentiated component with high-grade and pleomorphic features (**Fig. 11**).[4,68,69] The dedifferentiated component may even exhibit pseudorosettes[4] or heterologous rhabdomyosarcomatous, osteosarcomatous, or chondrosarcomatous differentiation.[68,70]

IMMUNOHISTOCHEMICAL FEATURES

The dedifferentiated component loses expression of CD34 in half of the cases[4,68] and has decreased or absent expression of STAT6.[71]

Fig. 9. (continued). (*C*) and myogenin (*D*) Myogenic differentiation correlates with adverse outcome in DD-LPS (H&E, original magnification, [*A, B*] ×25, [*C*] ×10, [*D*] ×10).

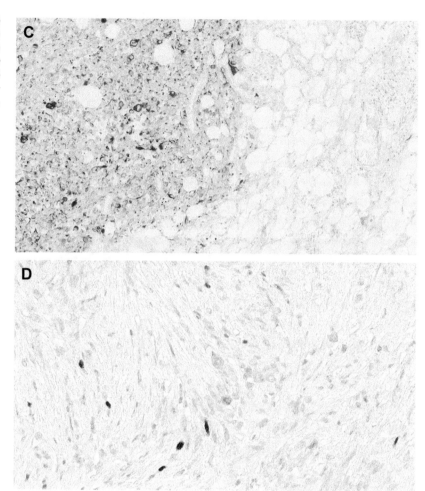

MOLECULAR PATHOLOGY

SFTs are underlined by recurrent *NAB2-STAT6* fusions.[72] Interestingly, DD-SFTs retain the fusion in the dedifferentiated component, although the expression of STAT6 is dramatically decreased at the proteic level.[71]

DD-SFTs display unstable genomic profile with CNAs, contrasting with the simple diploid profiles of conventional SFT. CNAs include constant loss of chromosome 13 and in 16q.[4,71] Malignant SFTs harbor genomic profiles of intermediate complexity between benign SFT and DD-SFT with gains of whole chromosomes and loss of chromosome 13.

PROGNOSIS

Dedifferentiation in SFT portends a worse prognosis with a high risk of metastasis in up to 50%

of cases, affecting primarily lung but also brain, liver, and bone.[68] In the risk stratification model study by Demicco and colleagues,[73] all 3 included cases of dedifferentiated SFT, which were accounted as high-risk tumors, metastasized.

MYXOFIBROSARCOMA

Myxofibrosarcoma is a clinicopathological entity arising in limbs and trunk of the elderly associated with a longitudinal spreading of malignant cells along fascial planes. They span a wide morphologic spectrum with variable levels of myxoid stromal changes, cellularity, and pleomorphism.[21]

CLINICAL FEATURES

Myxofibrosarcoma (MFS) is one of the most common sarcomas in the elderly individuals,

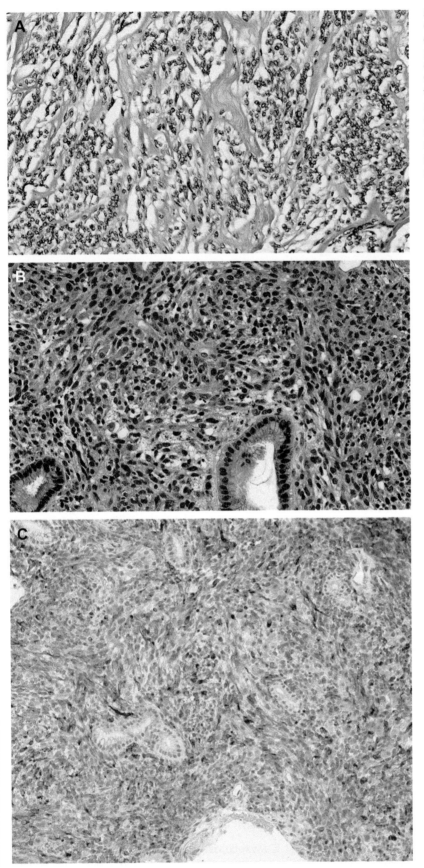

Fig. 10. Dedifferentiated GIST. (*A*) Primary lesion displayed an epithelioid pattern. (*B*) After 2 years of adjuvant therapy with KIT inhibitor, patient developed a recurrence. Tumor mass contained a high-grade dedifferentiated component. (*C*) Diffuse expression of CD117 was retained but not DOG1

Fig. 10. (continued). (D).
(E) The dedifferentiated
component expressed
desmin and myogenin
(not shown), in keeping
with a rhabdomyosar-
comatous differentiation
(H&E, original magnifica-
tion, [C] ×10; [A–E] ×20).

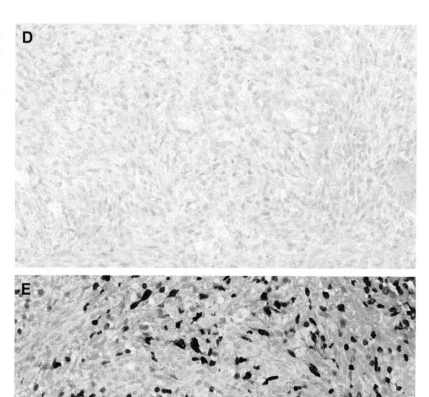

MICROSCOPIC FEATURES

MFSs are composed of nodules (Fig. 13A) of pleomorphic cells embedded in a myxoid stroma
(conventionally representing at least 20% of tumor
surface), richly vascularized with typical curvilinear
capillaries[74] (Fig. 13B).

Like UPS, MFS is a tumor with no specific line of
differentiation, and it can be a challenge to
discriminate between the 2 entities, particularly
as myxoid changes may occur in UPS. Attempts
at setting a quantitative threshold of myxoid
changes necessary to reach a diagnosis of MFS
have proposed values from 10% to 50% of the tumor surface.[74] Retrospective clinical studies have
evidenced improved outcomes with as low as 5%
of myxoid changes, although clinical outcomes are
even better with myxoid changes beyond 70%.[75]
Pragmatically, we render the diagnosis of MFS

with a peak at the sixth to eighth decades. There
is a slight predominance in men. Tumors
commonly present as a slow-growing subcutaneous mass in limbs and limb girdles.[74] They
develop within muscles and in close vicinity
with fascia.

RADIOLOGICAL AND GROSS FEATURES

MRIs reveal ill-defined tumors with peritumoral
infiltration, beyond apparent tumor borders. This
infiltration is referred to as "tail sign" when located
along fascia and is correlated with the presence of
satellite tumor cells. Radiologists must inform the
surgeon of these findings to include the tissue
with peritumoral enhancement within the surgical
margins (Fig. 12).

At gross examination, MFS presents as a myxoid multinodulated mass.

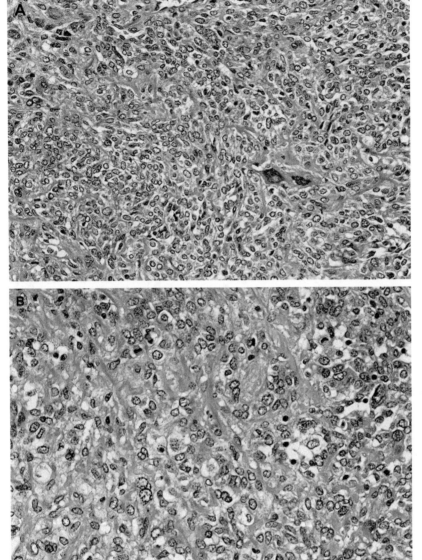

Fig. 11. Dedifferentiated SFT. (*A*) Well-differentiated component with monotonous proliferation of cells with round uniform nuclei and few scattered pleomorphic cells. (*B*) Pleomorphic areas with high mitotic activity (H&E, original magnification, [*A*, *B*] ×20) STAT6 expression was focally and weakly expressed in the dedifferentiated component (not shown).

without quantifying precisely the amount of myxoid changes, but by taking into account the clinical setting (mass of limb or trunk) and presence of the typical vascular network within the myxoid stroma.

MFSs may display variable levels of cellularity, atypia, and proliferation (Fig. 13C–E). Lower grade lesions may progress to higher grade at time of recurrence. Tumor cells are stellate to ovoid with hyperchromatic nuclei[74] (Fig. 13F). Cytoplasmic vacuolation may occur due to the myxoid stroma, giving to tumor cells a pseudolipoblastic appearance (Fig. 17B). MFSs also may display a focal or diffuse epithelioid appearance.[76]

IMMUNOHISTOCHEMICAL FEATURES

S100 protein is negative, whereas CD34 highlights the vascular network. MDM2 can be focally expressed by immunohistochemistry.[28]

MOLECULAR PATHOLOGY

Clustering analysis has highlighted the vicinity of MFS and UPS. These entities may be part of a phenotypic spectrum of tumors sharing a common histogenesis, although further studies are required to confirm this concept.[6] They do not harbor

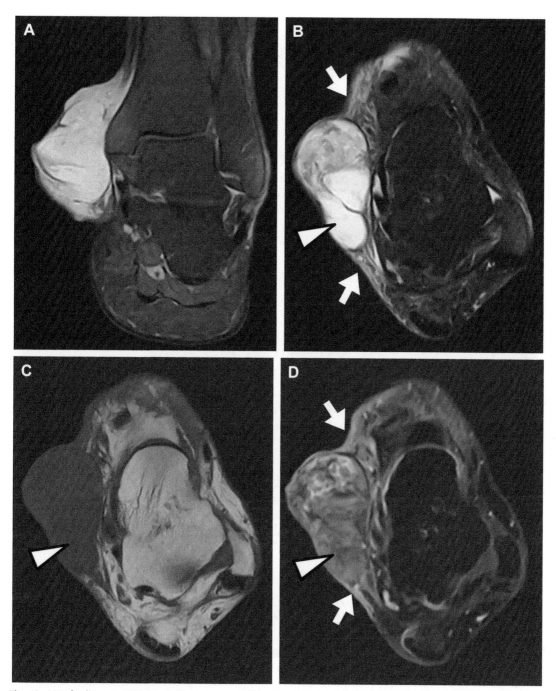

Fig. 12. MRI findings in MFS. Myxofibrosarcoma of the internal face of the left ankle. T2-weighted imaging with coronal (*A*) and axial (*B*) views, axial T1-weighted imaging (*C*) and axial T1-weighted imaging with suppression of fat signal and after a gadolinium chelates intravenous injection (*D*). The tumor is ill-defined with presence of peritumoral infiltration (*white arrows*, bright signal and contrast enhancement), spreading beyond apparent tumor borders. Myxoid component (*white arrowhead*) displays bright fluidlike signal on T2-weighted imaging, low signal on T1-weighted and enhancement after contrast-agent injection.

specific genetic hits that would be defining or represent therapeutic targets.[77,78] On methylation profiling, 3 molecular subgroups of MFS can be delineated, each defined by different sets of deregulated pathways. One subgroup, defined by *MDM2* amplification and alteration of chromatin modifiers, is associated with excellent outcome (no disease-related death).[79] These data further

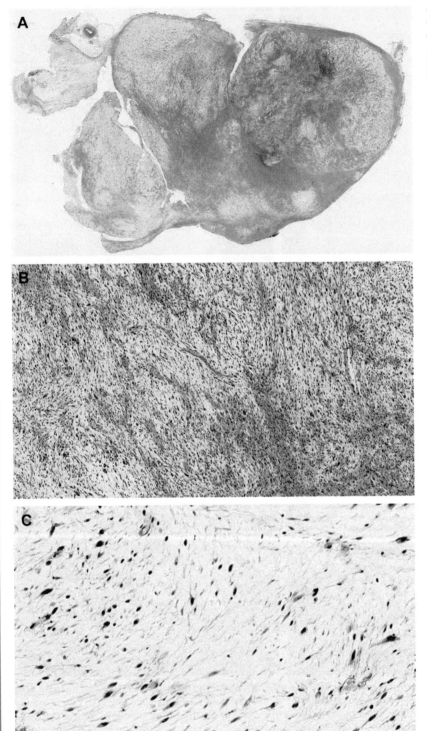

Fig. 13. Myxofibrosarcoma. (*A*) Multinodular architecture, (*B*) abundant myxoid stroma with abundant curvilinear blood vessels characteristic of MFS.

Fig. 13. (*continued*). (*C–E*) MFS may display variable cellularity from low to solid UPS-like areas (*F*) Pleomorphic elongated cells with hyperchromatic atypical nuclei. Mitotic figures may be scant in low-grade MFS. aCGH may be helpful in this setting, evidencing complex genetic profiles similar to those of UPS (H&E, original magnification, [*A*] ×0.5; [*B*] ×5; [*C–E*] ×20; [*F*] ×40).

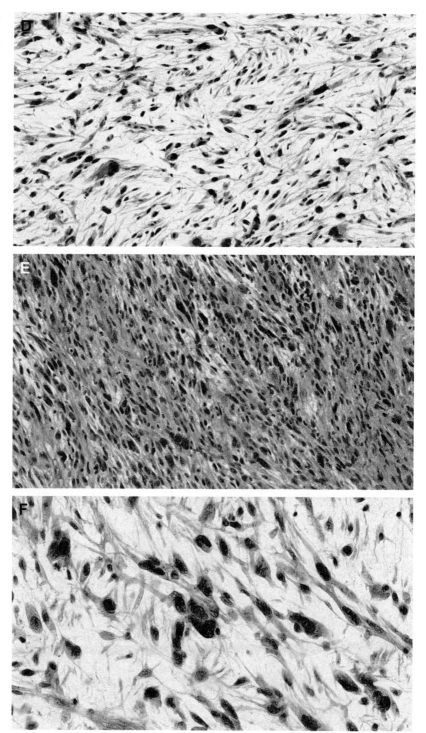

fuel the hypothesis that *MDM2*-amplified pleomorphic sarcomas in limbs or trunk represent dedifferentiated liposarcomas rather than MFS or UPS.[79] The 2 other subgroups are defined by high-frequency of *TP53* alterations and homozygous deletions of *CDKN2A*, respectively. The latter group harbors the worse overall survival.[78] In this study, no correlation was performed between the histologic grading and the molecular classifications. Notably, the deregulated pathways include commonplace tumor suppressor genes, namely *RB1* axis, *TP53,* and RAS-PI3K axis.[78]

DIFFERENTIAL DIAGNOSIS

For most of the differential diagnosis of MFS, immunostaining will be of limited interest with

antibodies of poor specificity, thereby the differential relies on the clinical vignette, morphologic clues, and the use of molecular tools.

Myxoinflammatory fibroblastic sarcomas are mesenchymal tumors of intermediate malignancy (locally aggressive) arising in the extremities (typically acral location in hands and feet) of middle-aged adults. This tumor has a multinodular architecture composed of larger atypical cells with viral-like vesicular nuclei (**Fig. 14**) embedded in a myxoid stroma, admixed with a prominent inflammatory infiltrate of histiocytes and lymphocytes. Emperipolesis of inflammatory elements may be present. The diagnosis can be confirmed by the identification of TGFBR3-MGEA5 translocations by FISH, reverse-transcriptase polymerase chain reaction, or aCGH.[80] Alternatively, translocations

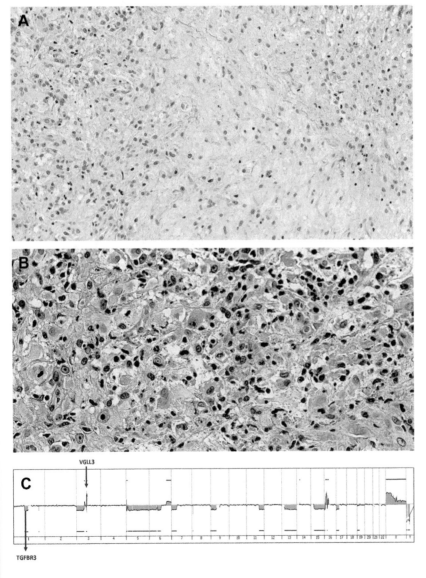

Fig. 14. Myxoinflammatory fibroblastic sarcoma. (*A*) Large atypical cells with large nucleoli within a myxoid and inflammatory background. (*B*) "Virocyte"-like cells and emperipolesis of inflammatory cells seeming engulfed in the cytoplasm of tumor cells (H&E, original magnification, [*A*] ×20; [*B*] ×40). (*C*) aCGH profile of a myxoinflammatory fibroblastic sarcoma showing breakpoint within *TGFBR3* locus and amplification of *VGLL3*. This sarcoma is commonly associated with unbalanced translocation, which can be evidenced by aCGH.

may involve *BRAF* in *TGFBR3* non-rearranged cases[81] or remain unidentified in a subset of cases.

Pleomorphic liposarcoma may display focal to extensive myxoid changes. Careful sampling and identification of pleomorphic lipoblasts will secure the diagnosis

Additional tumors with prominent myxoid stroma may enter the differential, including myxoma (**Fig. 15**), extraskeletal myxoid chondrosarcoma (**Fig. 16**), and myxoid liposarcoma (**Fig. 17**A). However, although they can be hypercellular or show degenerative atypia, pleomorphism is absent. The differential diagnosis of cellular myxoma versus myxofibrosarcoma may sometimes be difficult with the sole morphology. This differential can be supported by aCGH, as higher genetic complexity and oncogene amplification or homozygous deletions of tumor suppressor genes *RB1* and *TP53* are absent in myxomas.

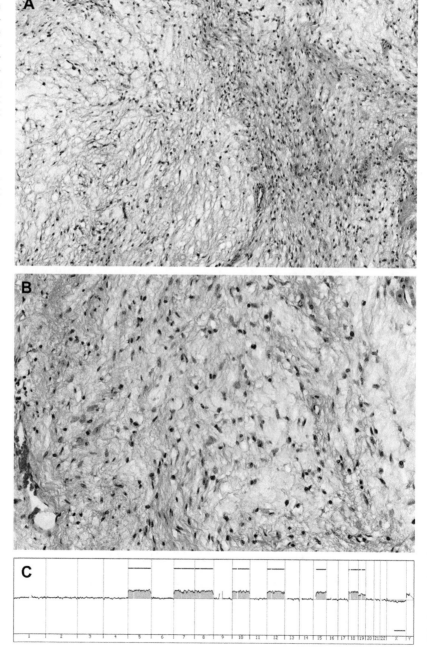

Fig. 15. Myxoma. (*A*) Extensive myxoid stroma with rare capillaries. Variable cellularity may be seen, especially in recurrent myxomas. (*B*) Tumor cell nuclei may display irregular contours and be hyperchromatic but do not display overt pleomorphism (H&E, original magnification, [*A*] ×10; [*B*] ×20). (*C*) aCGH profile showing CNAs (gains of whole chromosomes) consistent but not specific of myxoma. aCGH may be helpful in recurrent myxoma on core needle biopsy to rule out myxofibrosarcoma.

Pitfalls
MYXOFIBROSARCOMA

! Low-grade lesions with intermediate cellularity and limited pleomorphism may raise the differential diagnosis of myxoma.

! Artifacts of vacuolation may be interpreted as lipoblasts, raising suspicion for pleomorphic liposarcoma.

! MDM2 may be overexpressed by MFS but *MDM2* amplification is absent.

PROGNOSIS

MFS displays a longitudinal mode of spreading, and can infiltrate microscopically far beyond what is grossly apparent, warranting careful surgical resection. MFSs are characterized by high local recurrence rates of 50% to 60%. Metastatic potential is reliably predicted by histologic grade: low-grade MFS almost never metastasizes, whereas intermediate-grade and high-grade neoplasms may develop metastases in approximately 20% to 35% of cases.[16,74] The overall 5-year survival rate is 70%.[82]

Apart from classic clinical predictors (tumor size, histologic grade, and margin status), the percentage of myxoid component correlates with disease-specific survival and recurrence-free survival: more than 5% of the myxoid component correlates with better outcome.[75]

UNDIFFERENTIATED PLEOMORPHIC SARCOMA

UPSs are pleomorphic tumors devoid of line of differentiation,[21] accounting for 15% to 20% of soft tissue sarcomas.[16]

CLINICAL FEATURES

UPSs mostly arise in deep soft tissue of limbs and trunk, and predominantly affect male adults older

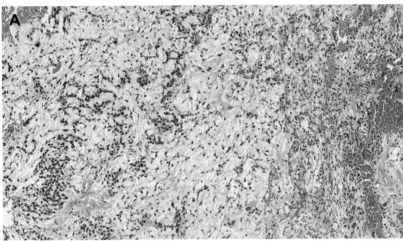

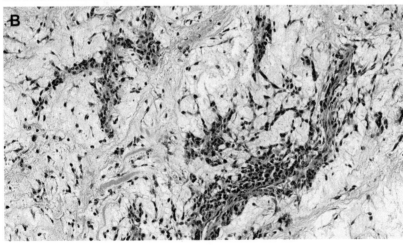

Fig. 16. Extraskeletal myxoid chondrosarcoma. (*A*) Prominent myxoid stroma and neoplastic cells arranged in a cord-like pattern. (*B*) Small, ovoid and hyperchromatic neoplastic cells, without pleomorphism (H&E, original magnification, [*A*] ×10; [*B*] ×20).

Fig. 17. Myxoid liposarcoma versus myxofibrosarcoma. (*A*) Lipoblasts in a myxoid liposarcoma compared with (*B*) pseudolipoblasts in myxofibrosarcoma (H&E, original magnification, [*A, B*] ×40).

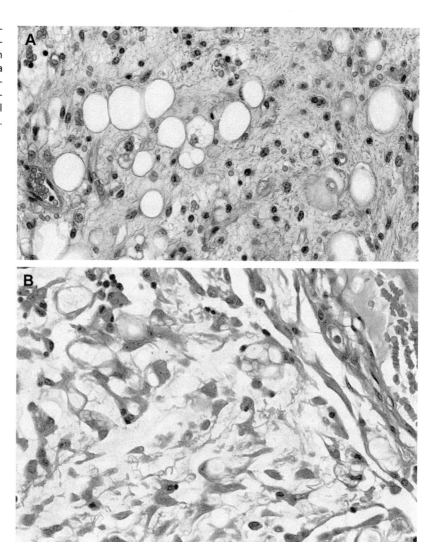

than 40 years, although they may occur at any age. They may occasionally occur in the setting of prior radiation therapy (being the most frequent histotype of radiation-associated sarcomas[83–85]), or of tumor predisposition syndrome, such as Li-Fraumeni syndrome.

Radiological features are poorly specific, reflecting their high-grade nature (**Fig. 18**).

MICROSCOPIC FEATURES

Histologically, UPSs are morphologically heterogeneous and by definition devoid of line of differentiation. They are pleomorphic tumors with high-grade features, commonly combining several architectural patterns, the most frequent presentation being a mixture of storiform and fascicular. Their stroma may vary from myxoid to hyaline, verging on the formation of osteoid matrix. Tumor cells are pleomorphic and may display a wide array of cytologic appearance: spindled, epithelioid, or be multinucleated. The level of pleomorphism is variable, sometimes striking with presence of giant pleomorphic cells (**Fig. 19A–D**).

Malignant mesenchymomas refer to pleomorphic sarcomas harboring at least 2 different types of mesenchymal differentiation in the setting of a "UPS-like" proliferation.[86] They are not singled out as a specific entity in the World Health Organization (WHO) classification.

IMMUNOHISTOCHEMICAL FEATURES

The poorly specific morphologic features of UPS warrant the systematic use of immunostaining to rule out melanoma, sarcomatoid carcinoma, or

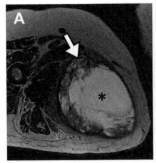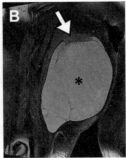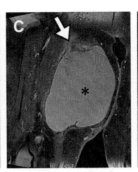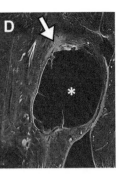

Fig. 18. MRI findings in a UPS. Deep-seated UPS of the right thigh. Axial T2-weighted imaging (*A*); coronal T1-weighted imaging with suppression of fat signal before (*B*) and after (*C*) a gadolinium chelates contrast-agent injection; subtracted images (*D* = *C–B*). Necrotic area (*asterisk*) typically demonstrates high signal intensity on T2-weighted imaging and no enhancement after contrast-agent injection. Persistence of viable tumor component within tumor mass after neoadjuvant chemotherapy within tumor mass (high signal intensity on T1-weighted imaging, *white arrow*).

identify a line of differentiation overlooked by the microscopic examination (including AE1/E3, EMA, CD34, S100 or SOX10, h-caldesmon, desmin/myoD1, MDM2). Their immunophenotype is plastic and they may even focally express keratins, EMA, or p63.[87] Therefore, it is mandatory to integrate the clinical context before rendering this diagnosis of exclusion. It is worth noting that UPSs are commonly infiltrated by histiocytes/macrophages, which may result in difficulty in the interpretation of certain immunostains, including CD31.

MOLECULAR PATHOLOGY

Genomically, UPSs display complex genomic profiles. Two molecular subtypes can be delineated: a less rearranged group with CNAs of chromosome arms, and a second, more genetically complex group, displaying whole chromosome gains and losses.[7] This molecular subclassification is of limited practical interest. Commonplace tumor suppressor genes *TP53, RB1,* and *PTEN* are frequently inactivated in UPS, emphasizing pathways that are shared with many tumor types, including epithelial ones (**Fig. 19E**).

DIFFERENTIAL DIAGNOSIS

Overall, it should be kept in mind that UPSs are a diagnosis of exclusion, which should be made cautiously outside of soft tissue, especially in viscera, considering the phenotypic plasticity of high-grade undifferentiated tumors, whatever their epithelial or mesenchymal origin.

Facing tumors developed in viscera, the diagnosis of *sarcomatoid carcinoma* should always be the first to be considered. Recognition of an intraepithelial dysplastic component and the use of several epithelial markers and p63 are required. The differential is all the more challenging, as UPSs may focally express cytokeratins.

Pleomorphic tumors located near large joints (knees) of the elderly should always raise suspicion for a *tenosynovial giant cell tumor,* which may display degenerative atypia, although these lesions are classically not mitotic (**Fig. 20**).

In the retroperitoneum, UPS-like tumors are *dedifferentiated liposarcomas* until proven otherwise.

Extraskeletal osteosarcoma can pose a particularly difficult differential diagnosis, as it resembles UPS except for the presence of osteoid matrix (**Fig. 21**). The osteoid nature of a matrix may be difficult to assess in tumors with fibrohyaline stroma and SATB2 staining may help ascertain this suspicion, if strongly and diffusely expressed.[88]

The presence of a myxoid component may entertain the differential with *MFS,* which may be difficult to ascertain on core needle biopsy. Presence of a myxoid component as low as 5% may be associated with better outcome[75] but the current WHO classification recommendation is to use a 20% threshold for the diagnosis of MFS.[21]

PROGNOSIS

Local recurrence and metastatic rates in UPS range between 20% and 30% and 30% and 35%, respectively.[89] Both local recurrence and distant metastasis often develop within 12 to 24 months after initial diagnosis. Metastatic sites include lung, bone, and liver. The reported 5-year overall survival is 65% to 70%. Prognostic factors include tumor size, grade, and distant metastases at initial presentation. UPS arising in limbs or trunk have improved 5-year metastases-free survival

Fig. 19. UPS. Morphologic spectrum of UPS, including (*A*) spindle, (*B*) epithelioid/rhabdoid, (*C*) osteoclastlike giant cells, and

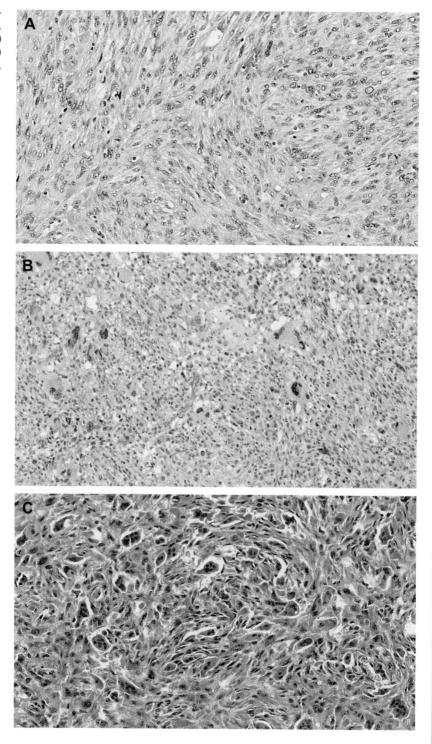

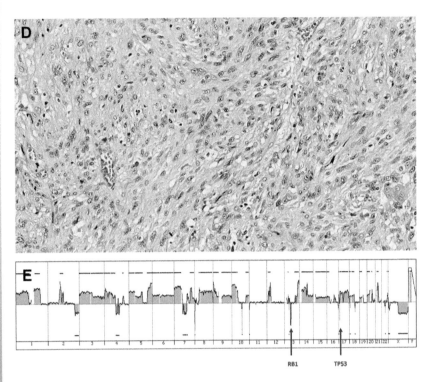

Fig. 19. (*continued*). (*D*) slightly myxoid stroma with no criteria for myxo-fibrosarcoma (H&E, original magnification, [*A–D*] ×20). (*E*) aCGH profile of a high-grade UPS showing homozygous deletion of both *RB1* and *TP53* genes.

rate of 83%.[90,91] Reported survival in children is 70% to 75%,[92,93] suggesting that UPS in this age group may have a different tumorigenesis.

SUPERFICIAL PLEOMORPHIC SARCOMAS

ATYPICAL FIBROXANTHOMA AND PLEOMORPHIC DERMAL SARCOMA

Atypical fibroxanthomas (AFXs) are cutaneous tumors of intermediate malignancy devoid of line of differentiation.[21] Pleomorphic dermal sarcoma (PDS) refers to dermal-based pleomorphic tumors indistinguishable from AFX but associated with invasion of deep subcutaneous tissue, tumor necrosis, lymphovascular invasion, or perineurial infiltration.[94,95] These tumors are part of a disease spectrum with partial overlap, but PDSs are associated with a low metastatic potential as opposed to AFX.[96,97]

Clinical Features

Both tumors occur in the same clinical setting, affecting elderly men in sun-damaged skin, particularly head (scalp) and neck regions. Presentation at younger age can be seen in patients with xeroderma pigmentosum.[94] By definition, AFX

measures less than 2 to 3 cm, whereas PDS lesions can be larger.[95]

Microscopic Features

AFXs present as cutaneous nodules often associated with epidermal ulceration. Epidermal collarette and marked solar elastosis in the adjacent dermis are common (**Fig. 22**A, B). The most frequent morphologic pattern is an admixture of pleomorphic epithelioid, spindled, and multinucleated tumor cells in varying proportions (**Fig. 22**C, D), often admixed with a chronic inflammatory infiltrate. Nuclear pleomorphism is marked and there is brisk and atypical mitotic activity.[94,96,98] However, AFXs are morphologically heterogeneous, with reports of pseudoangiomatous, osteoclastlike giant cells, clear cell, and granular cell patterns.[94,98]

By definition, all 3 criteria should be present to render the diagnosis of AFX: (1) <2 to 3 cm, (2) no significant involvement of hypodermis/fascia, and (3) no vascular/neural invasion. In case only 1 of these criteria is present, the diagnosis of PDS should be favored.[95] The final diagnosis can be reached only on total excision specimens to assess the level of extension of the lesion.

Key Features OF PLEOMORPHIC SARCOMAS					
Histotype	Frequency[80]	Clinical Context	Morphologic Features	Immunostains	Molecular Features
Pleomorphic liposarcoma	1.6%	Limb, trunk	Multivacuolated pleomorphic lipoblasts	S100 protein in lipoblasts	Complex karyotypes with TP53 and RB1 inactivation
Leiomyosarcoma	14.9%	—	Cytoplasmic eosinophilia and tapered end nuclei	h-caldesmon	Complex karyotypes, MYOCD amplification, PTEN deletion
Pleomorphic rhabdomyosarcoma	1.3%	Li-Fraumeni or old patients	Large cells with eosinophilic cytoplasm	Desmin, Myogenin, and MyoD1	Complex karyotypes
MPNST	3.2%	Neurofibromatosis 1 patient	Highly variable from monomorphic to pleomorphic features	Foci of S100 and SOX10 expression, loss of H3K27me3	NF1 inactivation, CDKN2A deletion; mutations of PRC2 subunits SUZ12 or EED
Extraskeletal osteosarcoma	1%	Elderly	Osteoid matrix	SATB2	Complex karyotypes
Dedifferentiated liposarcoma	8.7%	Retroperitoneum	Abrupt transition between well-differentiated and high-grade components	HMGA2 and MDM2	Amplification of MDM2
Dedifferentiated GIST	Extremely rare	Chronic imatinib therapy and secondary resistance	Abrupt transition between well-differentiated and high-grade components	—	KIT/PDGFRA mutation
Dedifferentiated SFT	Rare	—	Presence of conventional SFT areas	STAT6 expression retained in conventional SFT areas	NAB2-STAT6 fusion
Myxofibrosarcoma	5.6%	Elderly, limb, and limb girdles	Myxoid stroma composes 20% of the tumor, curvilinear vasculature	—	Complex karyotypes

Immunohistochemical Features

By definition, AFXs are devoid of line of differentiation. The immunohistochemical panel should exclude epidermal (AE1/E3 and p63/p40), melanocytic (SOX10), smooth muscle (h-caldesmon), and vascular (ERG or CD31) origins. Tumor cells may express less-specific markers focally, including smooth muscle actin, CD68, and EMA. Melan A and HMB-45 expression

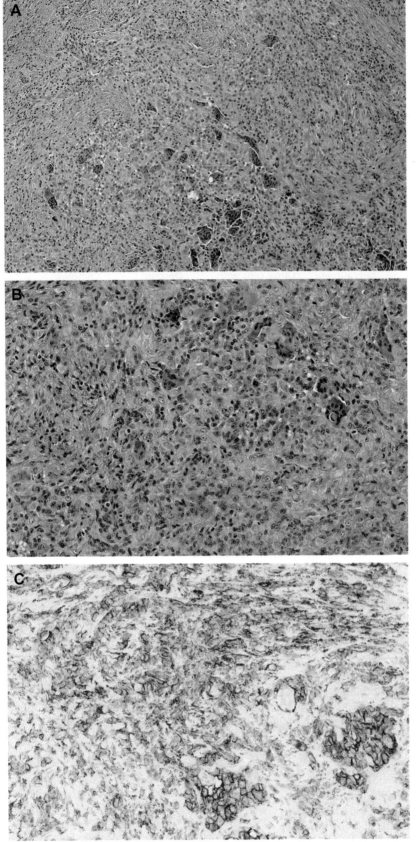

Fig. 20. Tenosynovial giant cell tumor. (*A*) Numerous osteoclastlike giant cells admixed with atypical cells in a background with hemorrhage and hemosiderin deposition. (*B*) There is variation in size and shape of cell nuclei but not overt pleomorphism. (*C*) Strong and diffuse expression of CD163 confirming the histiocytic phenotype of the proliferation (H&E, original magnification, [*A*] ×20; [*B, C*] ×20).

Fig. 21. Extraskeletal osteosarcoma. (*A*) Tumor composed of sheets of polyedric atypical cells intimately associated with neoplastic bone. (*B*) Nuclear expression of SATB2 confirming the osteogenic phenotype of tumor cells (H&E, original magnification, [*A, B*] ×20).

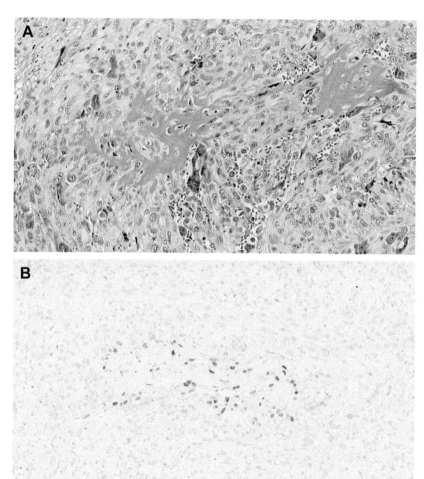

has also been documented in a minority of AFXs, largely restricted to tumor giant cells.[96,98,99]

Molecular Pathology

From a genomic standpoint, AFX and DPS are indistinguishable, sharing similar mutational profiles and CNA patterns. Furthermore, they display UV-related types of mutation, acknowledging their common UV-related pathogenesis.[100–102]

Differential Diagnosis

Both AFX and PDS are diagnosis of exclusion rendered in the absence of line of differentiation on morphology and immunohistochemistry, including immunostains against melanoma, carcinoma, angiosarcoma, and leiomyosarcoma.

p63 is a helpful marker for distinguishing poorly differentiated squamous cell carcinomas from AFX.[96] AFX may display hemorrhagic areas surrounding pseudoangiomatous spaces lined by the pleomorphic cells; however, neither CD31 nor ERG are diffusely expressed by tumor cells. CD31 may be difficult to assess due to abundant histiocytic infiltrate, so the combination with ERG staining is helpful. Smooth muscle actin is frequently expressed in AFX; however, the diagnosis of *leiomyosarcoma* should be rendered only if more specific markers, such as desmin and h-caldesmon, are expressed.[95,96,98]

Prognosis

AFX, as defined by strict criteria, is entirely benign. Local recurrence is a consequence of

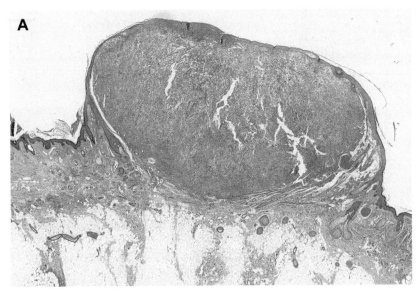

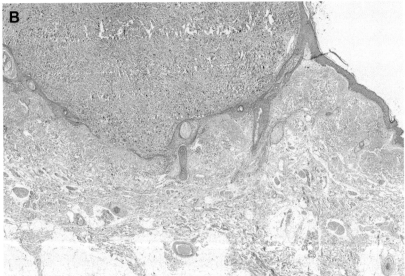

Fig. 22. Atypical fibrox-anthoma. (*A*) Well-circumscribed symmetrical tumor nodule (*B*) with solar elastosis surrounding the lesion in upper dermis.

incomplete excision. Metastases are exceptional, with only 1 believable case reported in the literature.[103]

PDS is best regarded as a tumor of low-grade malignant behavior, as shown by a local recurrence risk of 28% and a metastatic risk of 10%. Metastatic disease mainly affects skin and lymph nodes. Disease-related mortality is extremely rare. Local recurrence is a risk factor for the development of subsequent metastasis.[95]

THERAPEUTIC MANAGEMENT OF PLEOMORPHIC SARCOMAS

At nonmetastatic stage, management consists of surgical resection in a tertiary care center combined with radiotherapy.[104] Neoadjuvant chemotherapy has proven beneficial in terms of survival in high-grade pleomorphic sarcomas.[105] At advanced metastatic stage, patients have poor outcome and chemotherapy regimens, including doxorubicin alone or in combination, is the standard of care.[89]

Fig. 22. (*continued*). (*C*) Morphology is highly variable, the most frequent patterns being epithelioid, associated here with multinucleation (*D*) and spindled patterns (H&E, original magnification, [*A*] ×2.5; [*B*] ×5; [*C, D*] ×20).

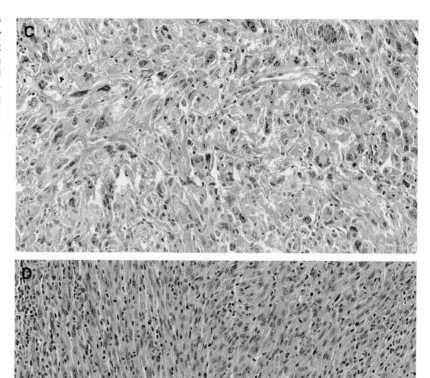

REFERENCES

1. Guillou L, Aurias A. Soft tissue sarcomas with complex genomic profiles. Virchows Arch 2010;456(2): 201–17.

2. Henricks WH, Chu YC, Goldblum JR, et al. Dedifferentiated liposarcoma: a clinicopathological analysis of 155 cases with a proposal for an expanded definition of dedifferentiation. Am J Surg Pathol 1997;21(3):271–81.

3. Antonescu CR, Romeo S, Zhang L, et al. Dedifferentiation in gastrointestinal stromal tumor to an anaplastic KIT-negative phenotype: a diagnostic pitfall: morphologic and molecular characterization of 8 cases occurring either de novo or after imatinib therapy. Am J Surg Pathol 2013;37(3):385–92.

4. Mosquera J-M, Fletcher CDM. Expanding the spectrum of malignant progression in solitary fibrous tumors: a study of 8 cases with a discrete anaplastic component–is this dedifferentiated SFT? Am J Surg Pathol 2009;33(9):1314–21.

5. Derré J, Lagacé R, Nicolas A, et al. Leiomyosarcomas and most malignant fibrous histiocytomas share very similar comparative genomic hybridization imbalances: an analysis of a series of 27 leiomyosarcomas. Lab Invest 2001;81(2):211–5.

6. Cancer Genome Atlas Research Network. Comprehensive and integrated genomic characterization of adult soft tissue sarcomas. Cell 2017;171(4): 950–65.e28.

7. Chibon F, Lagarde P, Salas S, et al. Validated prediction of clinical outcome in sarcomas and multiple types of cancer on the basis of a gene expression signature related to genome complexity. Nat Med 2010;16(7):781–7.

8. Croce S, Ribeiro A, Brulard C, et al. Uterine smooth muscle tumor analysis by comparative genomic hybridization: a useful diagnostic tool in challenging lesions. Mod Pathol 2015;28(7):1001–10.

9. Le Guellec S, Lesluyes T, Sarot E, et al. Validation of the Complexity INdex in SARComas prognostic signature on formalin-fixed, paraffin-embedded,

soft-tissue sarcomas. Ann Oncol 2018;29(8): 1828–35.

10. Bertucci F, De Nonneville A, Finetti P, et al. The Genomic Grade Index predicts postoperative clinical outcome in patients with soft-tissue sarcoma. Ann Oncol 2018;29(2):459–65.

11. Delespaul L, Lesluyes T, Pérot G, et al. Recurrent TRIO fusion in nontranslocation-related sarcomas. Clin Cancer Res 2017;23(3):857–67.

12. Guillou L, Coindre JM, Bonichon F, et al. Comparative study of the National Cancer Institute and French Federation of Cancer Centers Sarcoma Group grading systems in a population of 410 adult patients with soft tissue sarcoma. J Clin Oncol 1997;15(1):350–62.

13. Trojani M, Contesso G, Coindre JM, et al. Soft-tissue sarcomas of adults; study of pathological prognostic variables and definition of a histopathological grading system. Int J Cancer 1984;33(1):37–42.

14. Coindre JM, Terrier P, Guillou L, et al. Predictive value of grade for metastasis development in the main histologic types of adult soft tissue sarcomas: a study of 1240 patients from the French Federation of Cancer Centers Sarcoma Group. Cancer 2001; 91(10):1914–26.

15. Tanaka K, Hasegawa T, Nojima T, et al. Prospective evaluation of Ki-67 system in histological grading of soft tissue sarcomas in the Japan Clinical Oncology Group Study JCOG0304. World J Surg Oncol 2016;14:110.

16. Fletcher CD, Gustafson P, Rydholm A, et al. Clinicopathologic re-evaluation of 100 malignant fibrous histiocytomas: prognostic relevance of subclassification. J Clin Oncol 2001;19(12):3045–50.

17. Deyrup AT, Haydon RC, Huo D, et al. Myoid differentiation and prognosis in adult pleomorphic sarcomas of the extremity: an analysis of 92 cases. Cancer 2003;98(4):805–13.

18. Oshiro Y, Shiratsuchi H, Oda Y, et al. Rhabdoid features in leiomyosarcoma of soft tissue: with special reference to aggressive behavior. Mod Pathol 2000;13(11):1211–8.

19. Massi D, Beltrami G, Capanna R, et al. Histopathological re-classification of extremity pleomorphic soft tissue sarcoma has clinical relevance. Eur J Surg Oncol 2004;30(10):1131–6.

20. Wardelmann E, Haas RL, Bovée JVMG, et al. Evaluation of response after neoadjuvant treatment in soft tissue sarcomas; the European Organization for Research and Treatment of Cancer-Soft Tissue and Bone Sarcoma Group (EORTC-STBSG) recommendations for pathological examination and reporting. Eur J Cancer 2016;53:84–95.

21. Fletcher CDM. WHO classification of tumours of soft tissue and bone. Lyon (France): IARC press World Health Organization; 2013.

22. Dei Tos AP. Liposarcomas: diagnostic pitfalls and new insights. Histopathology 2014;64(1):38–52.

23. Hornick JL, Bosenberg MW, Mentzel T, et al. Pleomorphic liposarcoma: clinicopathologic analysis of 57 cases. Am J Surg Pathol 2004;28(10): 1257–67.

24. Gebhard S, Coindre J-M, Michels J-J, et al. Pleomorphic liposarcoma: clinicopathologic, immunohistochemical, and follow-up analysis of 63 cases. Am J Surg Pathol 2002;26(5):601–16.

25. Miettinen M, Enzinger FM. Epithelioid variant of pleomorphic liposarcoma: a study of 12 cases of a distinctive variant of high-grade liposarcoma. Mod Pathol 1999;12(7):722–8.

26. Ramírez-Bellver JL, López J, Macías E, et al. Primary dermal pleomorphic liposarcoma: utility of adipophilin and MDM2/CDK4 immunostainings. J Cutan Pathol 2017;44(3):283–8.

27. Dreux N, Marty M, Chibon F, et al. Value and limitation of immunohistochemical expression of HMGA2 in mesenchymal tumors: about a series of 1052 cases. Mod Pathol 2010;23(12):1657–66.

28. Binh MBN, Sastre-Garau X, Guillou L, et al. MDM2 and CDK4 immunostainings are useful adjuncts in diagnosing well-differentiated and dedifferentiated liposarcoma subtypes: a comparative analysis of 559 soft tissue neoplasms with genetic data. Am J Surg Pathol 2005;29(10):1340–7.

29. Wang L, Ren W, Zhou X, et al. Pleomorphic liposarcoma: a clinicopathological, immunohistochemical and molecular cytogenetic study of 32 additional cases. Pathol Int 2013;63(11):523–31.

30. Idbaih A, Coindre J-M, Derré J, et al. Myxoid malignant fibrous histiocytoma and pleomorphic liposarcoma share very similar genomic imbalances. Lab Invest 2005;85(2):176–81.

31. Mariani O, Brennetot C, Coindre J-M, et al. JUN oncogene amplification and overexpression block adipocytic differentiation in highly aggressive sarcomas. Cancer Cell 2007;11(4):361–74.

32. Mariño-Enríquez A, Fletcher CDM, Dal Cin P, et al. Dedifferentiated liposarcoma with "homologous" lipoblastic (pleomorphic liposarcoma-like) differentiation: clinicopathologic and molecular analysis of a series suggesting revised diagnostic criteria. Am J Surg Pathol 2010;34(8): 1122–31.

33. Nicolas MM, Tamboli P, Gomez JA, et al. Pleomorphic and dedifferentiated leiomyosarcoma: clinicopathologic and immunohistochemical study of 41 cases. Hum Pathol 2010;41(5):663–71.

34. Oda Y, Miyajima K, Kawaguchi K, et al. Pleomorphic leiomyosarcoma: clinicopathologic and immunohistochemical study with special emphasis on its distinction from ordinary leiomyosarcoma and malignant fibrous histiocytoma. Am J Surg Pathol 2001;25(8):1030–8.

35. Robin Y-M, Penel N, Pérot G, et al. Transgelin is a novel marker of smooth muscle differentiation that improves diagnostic accuracy of leiomyosarcomas: a comparative immunohistochemical reappraisal of myogenic markers in 900 soft tissue tumors. Mod Pathol 2013;26(4):502–10.

36. Pérot G, Mendiboure J, Brouste V, et al. Smooth muscle differentiation identifies two classes of poorly differentiated pleomorphic sarcomas with distinct outcome. Mod Pathol 2014;27(6):840–50.

37. Colombo C, Miceli R, Collini P, et al. Leiomyosarcoma and sarcoma with myogenic differentiation: two different entities or 2 faces of the same disease? Cancer 2012;118(21):5349–57.

38. Demicco EG, Boland GM, Brewer Savannah KJ, et al. Progressive loss of myogenic differentiation in leiomyosarcoma has prognostic value. Histopathology 2015;66(5):627–38.

39. Chen E, O'Connell F, Fletcher CDM. Dedifferentiated leiomyosarcoma: clinicopathological analysis of 18 cases. Histopathology 2011;59(6):1135–43.

40. Pérot G, Derré J, Coindre J-M, et al. Strong smooth muscle differentiation is dependent on myocardin gene amplification in most human retroperitoneal leiomyosarcomas. Cancer Res 2009;69(6): 2269–78.

41. Iwata J, Fletcher CDM. Immunohistochemical detection of cytokeratin and epithelial membrane antigen in leiomyosarcoma: a systematic study of 100 cases. Pathol Int 2000;50(1):7–14.

42. Miettinen M, Lasota J. Gastrointestinal stromal tumors: review on morphology, molecular pathology, prognosis, and differential diagnosis. Arch Pathol Lab Med 2006;130(10):1466–78.

43. Furlong MA, Mentzel T, Fanburg-Smith JC. Pleomorphic rhabdomyosarcoma in adults: a clinicopathologic study of 38 cases with emphasis on morphologic variants and recent skeletal muscle-specific markers. Mod Pathol 2001;14(6):595–603.

44. Stock N, Chibon F, Binh MBN, et al. Adult-type rhabdomyosarcoma: analysis of 57 cases with clinicopathologic description, identification of 3 morphologic patterns and prognosis. Am J Surg Pathol 2009;33(12):1850–9.

45. Hettmer S, Archer NM, Somers GR, et al. Anaplastic rhabdomyosarcoma in TP53 germline mutation carriers. Cancer 2014;120(7):1068–75.

46. Kumar S, Perlman E, Harris CA, et al. Myogenin is a specific marker for rhabdomyosarcoma: an immunohistochemical study in paraffin-embedded tissues. Mod Pathol 2000;13(9):988–93.

47. Noujaim J, Thway K, Jones RL, et al. Adult pleomorphic rhabdomyosarcoma: a multicentre retrospective study. Anticancer Res 2015;35(11):6213–7.

48. Dahlin DC, Beabout JW. Dedifferentiation of low-grade chondrosarcomas. Cancer 1971;28(2): 461–6.

49. Montgomery E, Fisher C. Myofibroblastic differentiation in malignant fibrous histiocytoma (pleomorphic myofibrosarcoma): a clinicopathological study. Histopathology 2001;38(6):499–509.

50. Coindre J-M, Hostein I, Maire G, et al. Inflammatory malignant fibrous histiocytomas and dedifferentiated liposarcomas: histological review, genomic profile, andMDM2 andCDK4 status favour a single entity. J Pathol 2004;203(3):822–30.

51. Fanburg-Smith JC, Miettinen M. Liposarcoma with meningothelial-like whorls: a study of 17 cases of a distinctive histological pattern associated with dedifferentiated liposarcoma. Histopathology 1998;33(5):414–24.

52. Nascimento AG, Kurtin PJ, Guillou L, et al. Dedifferentiated liposarcoma: a report of nine cases with a peculiar neurallike whorling pattern associated with metaplastic bone formation. Am J Surg Pathol 1998;22(8):945–55.

53. Binh MBN, Guillou L, Hostein I, et al. Dedifferentiated liposarcomas with divergent myosarcomatous differentiation developed in the internal trunk. Am J Surg Pathol 2007;31(10):1557–66.

54. Boland JM, Weiss SW, Oliveira AM, et al. Liposarcomas with mixed well-differentiated and pleomorphic features: a clinicopathologic study of 12 cases. Am J Surg Pathol 2010;34(6):837–43.

55. Sirvent N, Coindre J-M, Maire G, et al. Detection of MDM2-CDK4 amplification by fluorescence in situ hybridization in 200 paraffin-embedded tumor samples: utility in diagnosing adipocytic lesions and comparison with immunohistochemistry and real-time PCR. Am J Surg Pathol 2007;31(10): 1476–89.

56. Doyle LA, Tao D, Mariño-Enríquez A. STAT6 is amplified in a subset of dedifferentiated liposarcoma. Mod Pathol 2014;27(9):1231–7.

57. Demicco EG, Harms PW, Patel RM, et al. Extensive survey of STAT6 expression in a large series of mesenchymal tumors. Am J Clin Pathol 2015; 143(5):672–82.

58. Pissaloux D, Le Loarer F, Decouvelaere A-V, et al. MDM4 amplification in a case of de-differentiated liposarcoma and in-silico data supporting an oncogenic event alternative to MDM2 amplification in a subset of cases. Histopathology 2017;71(6): 1019–23.

59. Coindre J-M, Mariani O, Chibon F, et al. Most malignant fibrous histiocytomas developed in the retroperitoneum are dedifferentiated liposarcomas: a review of 25 cases initially diagnosed as malignant fibrous histiocytoma. Mod Pathol 2003;16(3):256–62.

60. Thway K, Flora R, Shah C, et al. Diagnostic utility of p16, CDK4, and MDM2 as an immunohistochemical panel in distinguishing well-differentiated and dedifferentiated liposarcomas from other adipocytic tumors. Am J Surg Pathol 2012;36(3):462–9.

61. Kammerer-Jacquet S-F, Thierry S, Cabillic F, et al. Differential diagnosis of atypical lipomatous tumor/well-differentiated liposarcoma and dedifferentiated liposarcoma: utility of p16 in combination with MDM2 and CDK4 immunohistochemistry. Hum Pathol 2017;59:34–40.

62. Makise N, Sekimizu M, Kubo T, et al. Clarifying the distinction between malignant peripheral nerve sheath tumor and dedifferentiated liposarcoma: a critical reappraisal of the diagnostic utility of MDM2 and H3K27me3 status. Am J Surg Pathol 2018;42(5):656–64.

63. Creytens D, Libbrecht L, Ferdinande L. Nuclear expression of STAT6 in dedifferentiated liposarcomas with a solitary fibrous tumor-like morphology. Appl Immunohistochem Mol Morphol 2015;23(6):462–3.

64. Mussi C, Collini P, Miceli R, et al. The prognostic impact of dedifferentiation in retroperitoneal liposarcoma. Cancer 2008;113(7):1657–65.

65. Keung EZ, Hornick JL, Bertagnolli MM, et al. Predictors of outcomes in patients with primary retroperitoneal dedifferentiated liposarcoma undergoing surgery. J Am Coll Surg 2014;218(2):206–17.

66. Gronchi A, Collini P, Miceli R, et al. Myogenic differentiation and histologic grading are major prognostic determinants in retroperitoneal liposarcoma. Am J Surg Pathol 2015;39(3):383–93.

67. Zhu P, Fei Y, Wang Y, et al. Recurrent retroperitoneal extra-GIST with rhabdomyosarcomatous and chondrosarcomatous differentiations: a rare case and literature review. Int J Clin Exp Pathol 2015; 8(8):9655–61.

68. Collini P, Negri T, Barisella M, et al. High-grade sarcomatous overgrowth in solitary fibrous tumors: a clinicopathologic study of 10 cases. Am J Surg Pathol 2012;36(8):1202–15.

69. Olson NJ, Linos K. Dedifferentiated solitary fibrous tumor: a concise review. Arch Pathol Lab Med 2018;142(6):761–6.

70. Thway K, Hayes A, Ieremia E, et al. Heterologous osteosarcomatous and rhabdomyosarcomatous elements in dedifferentiated solitary fibrous tumor: further support for the concept of dedifferentiation in solitary fibrous tumor. Ann Diagn Pathol 2013; 17(5):457–63.

71. Dagrada GP, Spagnuolo RD, Mauro V, et al. Solitary fibrous tumors: loss of chimeric protein expression and genomic instability mark dedifferentiation. Mod Pathol 2015;28(8):1074–83.

72. Mohajeri A, Tayebwa J, Collin A, et al. Comprehensive genetic analysis identifies a pathognomonic NAB2/STAT6 fusion gene, nonrandom secondary genomic imbalances, and a characteristic gene expression profile in solitary fibrous tumor. Genes Chromosomes Cancer 2013;52(10):873–86.

73. Demicco EG, Park MS, Araujo DM, et al. Solitary fibrous tumor: a clinicopathological study of 110 cases and proposed risk assessment model. Mod Pathol 2012;25(9):1298–306.

74. Mentzel T, Calonje E, Wadden C, et al. Myxofibrosarcoma. Clinicopathologic analysis of 75 cases with emphasis on the low-grade variant. Am J Surg Pathol 1996;20(4):391–405.

75. Lee AY, Agaram NP, Qin L-X, et al. Optimal percent myxoid component to predict outcome in high-grade myxofibrosarcoma and undifferentiated pleomorphic sarcoma. Ann Surg Oncol 2016; 23(3):818–25.

76. Nascimento AF, Bertoni F, Fletcher CDM. Epithelioid variant of myxofibrosarcoma: expanding the clinicomorphologic spectrum of myxofibrosarcoma in a series of 17 cases. Am J Surg Pathol 2007; 31(1):99–105.

77. Barretina J, Taylor BS, Banerji S, et al. Subtype-specific genomic alterations define new targets for soft-tissue sarcoma therapy. Nat Genet 2010; 42(8):715–21.

78. Ogura K, Hosoda F, Arai Y, et al. Integrated genetic and epigenetic analysis of myxofibrosarcoma. Nat Commun 2018;9(1):2765.

79. Le Guellec S, Chibon F, Ouali M, et al. Are peripheral purely undifferentiated pleomorphic sarcomas with MDM2 amplification dedifferentiated liposarcomas? Am J Surg Pathol 2014;38(3):293–304.

80. Hallor KH, Sciot R, Staaf J, et al. Two genetic pathways, t(1;10) and amplification of 3p11-12, in myxoinflammatory fibroblastic sarcoma, haemosiderotic fibrolipomatous tumour, and morphologically similar lesions. J Pathol 2009;217(5):716–27.

81. Kao Y-C, Ranucci V, Zhang L, et al. Recurrent BRAF gene rearrangements in myxoinflammatory fibroblastic sarcomas, but not hemosiderotic fibrolipomatous tumors. Am J Surg Pathol 2017;41(11):1456–65.

82. Penel N, Coindre J-M, Giraud A, et al. Presentation and outcome of frequent and rare sarcoma histologic subtypes: a study of 10,262 patients with localized visceral/soft tissue sarcoma managed in reference centers. Cancer 2018;124(6):1179–87.

83. Pitcher ME, Davidson TI, Fisher C, et al. Post irradiation sarcoma of soft tissue and bone. Eur J Surg Oncol 1994;20(1):53–6.

84. Berrington de Gonzalez A, Kutsenko A, Rajaraman P. Sarcoma risk after radiation exposure. Clin Sarcoma Res 2012;2(1):18.

85. Mark RJ, Poen J, Tran LM, et al. Postirradiation sarcomas. A single-institution study and review of the literature. Cancer 1994;73(10):2653–62.

86. Newman PL, Fletcher CD. Malignant mesenchymoma. Clinicopathologic analysis of a series with evidence of low-grade behaviour. Am J Surg Pathol 1991;15(7):607–14.

87. Jo VY, Fletcher CDM. p63 immunohistochemical staining is limited in soft tissue tumors. Am J Clin Pathol 2011;136(5):762–6.

88. Conner JR, Hornick JL. SATB2 is a novel marker of osteoblastic differentiation in bone and soft tissue tumours. Histopathology 2013;63(1):36–49.

89. Widemann BC, Italiano A. Biology and management of undifferentiated pleomorphic sarcoma, myxofibrosarcoma, and malignant peripheral nerve sheath tumors: state of the art and perspectives. J Clin Oncol 2018;36(2):160–7.

90. Engellau J, Anderson H, Rydholm A, et al. Time dependence of prognostic factors for patients with soft tissue sarcoma: a Scandinavian Sarcoma Group Study of 338 malignant fibrous histiocytomas. Cancer 2004;100(10):2233–9.

91. Belal A, Kandil A, Allam A, et al. Malignant fibrous histiocytoma: a retrospective study of 109 cases. Am J Clin Oncol 2002;25(1):16–22.

92. Somers GR, Gupta AA, Doria AS, et al. Pediatric undifferentiated sarcoma of the soft tissues: a clinicopathologic study. Pediatr Dev Pathol 2006;9(2): 132–42.

93. Alaggio R, Collini P, Randall RL, et al. Undifferentiated high-grade pleomorphic sarcomas in children: a clinicopathologic study of 10 cases and review of literature. Pediatr Dev Pathol 2010;13(3):209–17.

94. Brenn T. Pleomorphic dermal neoplasms: a review. Adv Anat Pathol 2014;21(2):108–30.

95. Miller K, Goodlad JR, Brenn T. Pleomorphic dermal sarcoma: adverse histologic features predict aggressive behavior and allow distinction from atypical fibroxanthoma. Am J Surg Pathol 2012; 36(9):1317–26.

96. Beer TW, Drury P, Heenan PJ. Atypical fibroxanthoma: a histological and immunohistochemical review of 171 cases. Am J Dermatopathol 2010; 32(6):533–40.

97. McCalmont TH. Correction and clarification regarding AFX and pleomorphic dermal sarcoma. J Cutan Pathol 2012;39(1):8.

98. Luzar B, Calonje E. Morphological and immunohistochemical characteristics of atypical fibroxanthoma with a special emphasis on potential diagnostic pitfalls: a review. J Cutan Pathol 2010; 37(3):301–9.

99. Folpe AL, Cooper K. Best practices in diagnostic immunohistochemistry: pleomorphic cutaneous spindle cell tumors. Arch Pathol Lab Med 2007; 131(10):1517–24.

100. Sakamoto A, Oda Y, Itakura E, et al. Immunoexpression of ultraviolet photoproducts and p53 mutation analysis in atypical fibroxanthoma and superficial malignant fibrous histiocytoma. Mod Pathol 2001;14(6):581–8.

101. Griewank KG, Schilling B, Murali R, et al. TERT promoter mutations are frequent in atypical fibroxanthomas and pleomorphic dermal sarcomas. Mod Pathol 2014;27(4):502–8.

102. Griewank KG, Wiesner T, Murali R, et al. Atypical fibroxanthoma and pleomorphic dermal sarcoma harbor frequent NOTCH1/2 and FAT1 mutations and similar DNA copy number alteration profiles. Mod Pathol 2018;31(3):418–28.

103. Wang W-L, Torres-Cabala C, Curry JL, et al. Metastatic atypical fibroxanthoma: a series of 11 cases including with minimal and no subcutaneous involvement. Am J Dermatopathol 2015;37(6): 455–61.

104. Blay J-Y, Soibinet P, Penel N, et al. Improved survival using specialized multidisciplinary board in sarcoma patients. Ann Oncol 2017;28(11): 2852–9.

105. Gronchi A, Ferrari S, Quagliuolo V, et al. Histotype-tailored neoadjuvant chemotherapy versus standard chemotherapy in patients with high-risk soft-tissue sarcomas (ISG-STS 1001): an international, open-label, randomised, controlled, phase 3, multicentre trial. Lancet Oncol 2017;18(6):812–22.

Beyond Smooth Muscle— Other Mesenchymal Neoplasms of the Uterus

Brendan C. Dickson, BA, BSc, MD, MSc, FRCPC[a,b,*]

KEYWORDS

- Endometrial stromal sarcoma • Uterine tumor resembling ovarian sex cord tumor
- Undifferentiated uterine sarcoma • PEComa • Inflammatory myofibroblastic tumor

---

Key points

- Numerous mesenchymal neoplasms may contain morphologic and immunohistochemical overlap with uterine smooth muscle neoplasms. Differences in outcome and clinical management warrant accurate classification.

- Endometrial stromal sarcomas are subclassified into low-grade and high-grade tumors based on their underlying gene fusion product. Morphology and immunohistochemistry alone do not always reliably permit accurate subclassification.

- Sex cord–like differentiation occurs in several primary uterine tumors. It may occur as a minor line of differentiation (eg, endometrial stromal sarcoma) or an intrinsic feature (eg, uterine tumor resembling ovarian sex cord tumor).

- Undifferentiated uterine sarcoma may originate from either the endometrium or myometrium. These tumors lack morphologic, immunohistochemical, and molecular support for a specific line of differentiation and represent a diagnosis of exclusion.

- In many cases of perivascular epithelioid cell tumor, less than 5% of tumor cells are positive for melanocytic markers by immunohistochemistry.

- The pattern of anaplastic lymphoma kinase (ALK) expression varies in inflammatory myofibroblastic tumor. Staining may involve specific areas of the cytoplasm or nucleus. A significant subset of cases is negative for ALK because they possess an altogether different molecular driver.

ABSTRACT

Mesenchymal tumors of the uterus comprise a heterogeneous group of neoplasms of varied biologic potential. In addition to being host to several anatomically unique entities, the uterus may contain mesenchymal neoplasms typically found elsewhere in the body. Although smooth muscle neoplasms are common, other mesenchymal neoplasms in this location are relatively rare. Many of these neoplasms exhibit morphologic overlap. In addition to a careful histomorphologic review, definitive classification frequently depends on the judicious application of ancillary immunohistochemical and molecular testing. The intent of this review is to offer a basic approach to the classification of primary uterine mesenchymal neoplasms.

Disclosures: Not applicable.
[a] Department of Pathology and Laboratory Medicine, Mount Sinai Hospital, 600 University Avenue, Toronto, Ontario M5G 1X5, Canada; [b] Department of Laboratory Medicine and Pathobiology, University of Toronto, Toronto, Ontario, Canada
* Department of Pathology and Laboratory Medicine, Mount Sinai Hospital, 600 University Avenue, Toronto, Ontario M5G 1X5, Canada.
E-mail address: Brendan.Dickson@sinaihealthsystem.ca

OVERVIEW

Mesenchymal tumors are ubiquitous throughout the body. The uterus is host to a subset of tumors unique to this anatomic location; however, it may also contain tumors more frequently identified at other sites of the body. Complicated by the fact that many of these tumors are rare and contain overlapping morphologic and immunohistochemical attributes, definitive classification is often challenging for pathologists. Clinical history and diagnostic imaging are occasionally helpful in guiding the differential diagnosis. Nevertheless, with trends toward more limited sampling techniques and treatments that are increasingly based on targeting underlying genetic drivers, ancillary immunohistochemical and molecular testing is often warranted. In and of themselves, uterine smooth muscle neoplasms—leiomyoma, leiomyosarcoma, and borderline cases—have the potential for an impressive spectrum of histomorphologic findings; there are several excellent reviews dedicated to this topic.[1–3] Several other primary uterine mesenchymal neoplasms are gaining increasing recognition for their importance in terms of differing clinical behavior and treatment implications. The purpose of this review is to discuss a diagnostic approach to several recently recognized and/or clinically relevant mesenchymal neoplasms arising within the uterus.

ENDOMETRIAL STROMAL SARCOMA

OVERVIEW

In recent years there has been significant revision to the classification of endometrial stromal neoplasms, largely the result of a recent seminal publication elucidating the molecular pathogenesis of high-grade endometrial stromal tumors.[4] As a result, the World Health Organization currently divides tumors of endometrial stromal derivation into several types: endometrial stromal nodule, low-grade endometrial stromal sarcoma, and high-grade endometrial stromal sarcoma.[5] An awareness of the molecular pathogenesis of these tumors is crucial to providing a robust diagnostic foundation. Many of these cases contain extremely rare genetic drivers, whereas in other cases the molecular pathogenesis has yet to be characterized; consequently, it is conceivable that classification schemes may undergo subtle refinement in the future. Admittedly, the rarity of these cases, combined with their varied molecular underpinnings, poses a challenge in attempting to accrue clinical cohorts of sufficient sizes to draw meaningful inferences.

LOW-GRADE ENDOMETRIAL STROMAL SARCOMA

OVERVIEW

Low-grade endometrial stromal sarcoma is a malignant mesenchymal tumor resembling endometrial stroma.[6] Most tumors occur in the uterus, with occasional extrauterine cases arising in the setting of endometriosis.[7,8] This is the second most common uterine sarcoma but rare relative to other uterine malignancies.[9] There is a broad range of age involvement, with most women premenopausal or perimenopausal.[6,10] Patients most often present with symptoms of abnormal bleeding and/or pain.[6,10]

GROSS FEATURES

Tumors range from approximately 1 cm to well over 15 cm.[6,11] They may be intramural or project into the uterine cavity.[6,11,12] The margins are, by definition, infiltrative,[6] and extension into myometrial veins is occasionally seen.[5,12] The cut surface is soft and fleshy. It ranges from yellow-orange to white-tan[6]; areas of hemorrhage, cystic degeneration, and necrosis are common.[6]

MICROSCOPIC FEATURES

The histomorphologic appearance of low-grade endometrial stromal sarcoma varies. The prototypic morphology is that of a tumor resembling normal endometrial stroma (**Fig. 1**),[6,12] that is, uniform ovoid-spindle cells with variable pale cytoplasm,[11] with a vague nested to fascicular pattern. The cytoplasm is eosinophilic and frequently scant.[11] The nuclei are small, round-ovoid, and monomorphic; mitotic activity is generally less than 10 per 10 high-power fields (HPFs) (increased mitotic activity does not seem to preclude classification of a tumor as low grade).[6,10] The vasculature is often arteriole-like and is enveloped by a concentric layering of tumor cells.[12] Tumors often invade myometrium with a so-called tongue-like growth pattern (**Fig. 2**). Necrosis may be identified, and lymphovascular space invasion is frequently present.[10] Although many reports describe tumors as reminiscent of proliferative-type endometrial stroma, low-grade endometrial stromal sarcoma is morphologically heterogeneous. For example, some cases have smooth muscle differentiation (often associated with nodules containing central hyalinization and centrifugally radiating collagen bundles [**Fig. 3**]),[13,14] fibromyxoid differentiation,[14,15] and epithelioid[16] and rhabdoid[17] morphologies, glandular differentiation,[18] and sex cord–like differentiation (**Fig. 4**).[12,19–21] Collagen plaques and bundles

Fig. 1. (*A, B*) Low-grade endometrial stromal sarcoma, resembling proliferative-type endometrium (RNA sequencing: *JAZF1-SUZ12* fusion product). (*A*) There is a prominent vasculature resembling arterioles (H&E, original magnification ×200). (*B*) Sheets of ovoid cells with monomorphic nuclei; mitotic activity is not conspicuous (H&E, original magnification ×400).

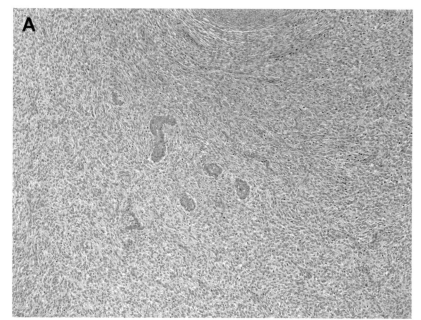

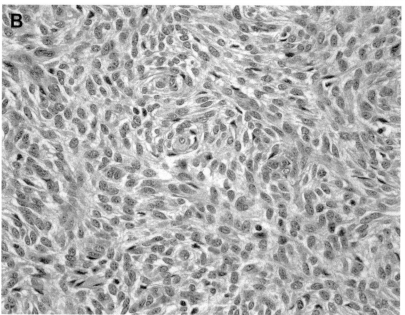

are often prominently interspersed (**Fig. 5**), and in some cases hyalinization may be extensive (**Fig. 6**). Tumors are usually diffusely positive for CD10[22–25] and estrogen receptor and progesterone receptor (**Fig. 7**).[26–30] Areas of smooth muscle differentiation may additionally contain smooth muscle actin and desmin expression, although reports of h-caldesmon expression are more variable.[14,23,31,32] Tumors, notably those with epithelioid cells and/or sex cord differentiation, can express keratin.[33,34]

MOLECULAR FEATURES

Approximately half of cases are characterized by fusion genes involving *JAZF1-SUZ12* (formerly *JJAZ1*).[35,36] A subset of tumors contains fusion genes involving *PHF1*, including *BRD8-PHF1*,[37] *EPC1-PHF1*,[38] *EPC2-PHF1*,[39] *JAZF1-PHF1*,[38] and *MEAF6-PHF1*.[40] The author's group recently identified an endometrial stromal sarcoma with foci that seemed morphologically low grade, containing an *EPC1-SUZ12* fusion.[41] Finally, there are

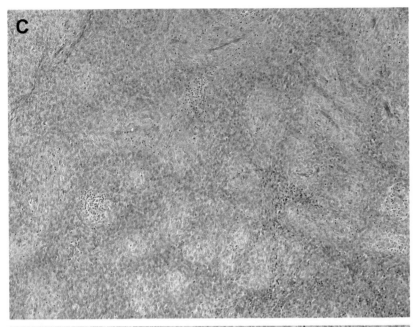

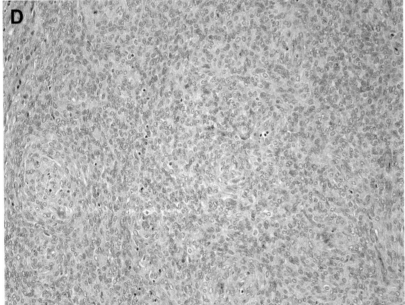

Fig. 1. (*continued*). (*C, D*) Low-grade endometrial stromal sarcoma, resembling proliferative-type endometrium (RNA sequencing: *MEAF6-PHF1* fusion product). (*C*) Prominent whorling of tumor cells around small vessels (H&E, original magnification ×100). (*D*) Despite possessing a completely different fusion gene from that in (*A*) and (*B*), the cells have a similar morphology (H&E, original magnification ×200).

also reported fusions involving seemingly unrelated genes, such as *MBTD1-CXorf67*.[42]

DIFFERENTIAL DIAGNOSIS AND DIAGNOSIS

When confined to the uterus, the differential diagnosis is usually straightforward. The primary differential diagnosis includes other endometrial stromal neoplasms—endometrial stromal nodule and high-grade endometrial stromal sarcoma. Other considerations include smooth muscle tumors (eg, leiomyoma and leiomyosarcoma) and low-grade fibromyxoid sarcoma.

The World Health Organization classifies endometrial stromal nodule as a benign neoplasm resembling proliferative-phase endometrial stroma, with a well-circumscribed margin.[5] It is characterized by a morphology, immunophenotype, and

Fig. 2. Same patient as in Fig. 1A, B. (*A*) and (*B*) images highlighting so-called tongue-like pattern of myometrial infiltration (H&E, original magnification [*A*] ×50; [*B*] ×100).

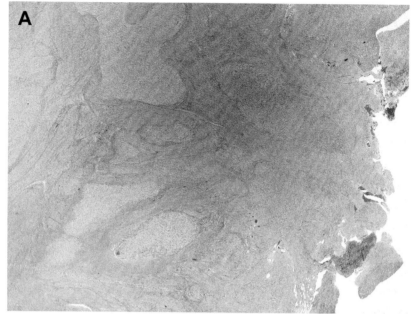

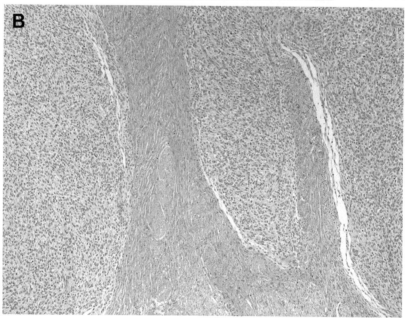

molecular signature analogous to low-grade endometrial stromal sarcoma; however, it is distinguished solely based on the—outwardly arbitrary—presence of less than 3 foci of myometrial invasion (<3 mm in greatest extent) and/or lymphovascular invasion. By definition, a diagnosis of endometrial stromal nodule cannot be made on curetted samples. Moreover, there are no clear guidelines on the extent of margin sampling necessary to evaluate invasive growth in endometrial stromal nodule and/or endometrial stromal sarcoma.

Low-grade endometrial stromal sarcoma and high-grade endometrial stromal sarcoma are ultimately differentiated based on their underlying molecular pathogenesis (discussed later).[5,43,44] Nevertheless, tumors frequently can be recognized based on their differing morphologies and

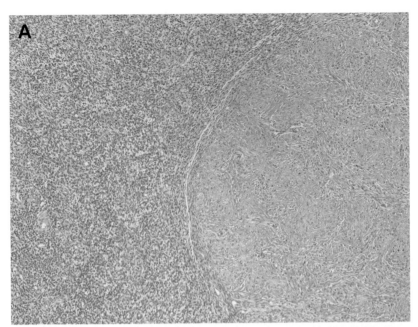

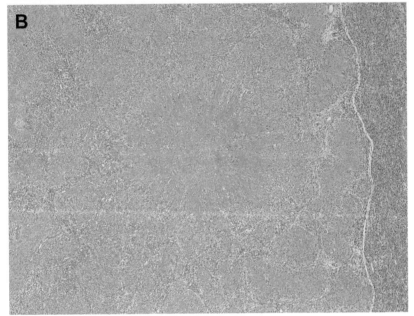

Fig. 3. Low-grade endometrial stromal sarcoma with myoid nodules (RNA sequencing: *JAZF1-SUZ12* fusion product). (*A*) Myoid nodules are often morphologically well demarcated, with an immunophenotype similar to smooth muscle. (*B*) Nodules may contain central hyalinization and centrifugally radiating collagen bundles (H&E, original magnification [*A–B*] ×100).

immunophenotype. For example, in contrast to low-grade endometrial stromal sarcoma, high-grade tumors frequently contain round cells with brisk mitotic activity,[4] and immunoreactivity for cyclin D1,[45] CD117,[46] and BCOR.[47] That said, there are reports of cases resembling low-grade tumors yet possessing molecular attributes of high-grade tumors[48,49] and vice versa.[50,51] As a result, in addition to morphology and immunohistochemistry, molecular testing is increasingly important in stratifying patients.[49]

Smooth muscle tumors, such as leiomyoma and leiomyosarcoma, can generally be readily differentiated from low-grade endometrial stromal sarcoma based on the expression of h-caldesmon[32]; however, careful attention to morphology is also required so as not to confuse a smooth muscle tumor with endometrial stromal sarcoma with

Fig. 4. Low-grade endometrial stromal sarcoma with sex cord–like differentiation (RNA sequencing: *EPC1-PHF1* fusion product). (*A*, *B*) Cords and nests of epithelioid cells resembling ovarian sex cord tumors (H&E, original magnification [*A*] ×100; [*B*] ×200).

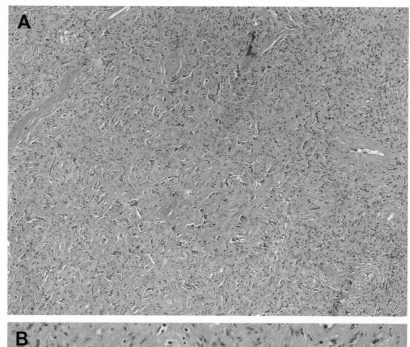

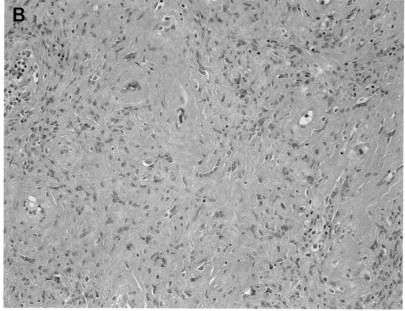

smooth muscle differentiation.[1] Low-grade fibromyxoid sarcoma, in particular the morphologic variant "hyalinizing spindle cell tumor with giant rosettes", bears a striking resemblance to low-grade endometrial stromal sarcoma with myoid differentiation (see **Figs.** 3B and 6).[52] The latter has not, to date, been reported as a uterine primary, although visceral involvement is well recognized, and tumors have been reported to originate in the pelvis[53] and vulva.[54] The possibility of low-grade fibromyxoid sarcoma can be confirmed based on

immunoreactivity for MUC4[55] or demonstration of the presence of a fusion gene involving *FUS-CREB3L1*,[56] *FUS-CREB3L2*,[57] or *EWSR1-CREB3L1*.[58]

PROGNOSIS

Low-grade endometrial stromal sarcoma is considered indolent.[1,10,44] Surgical stage is the most important prognostic factor.[9,10] Approximately half of patients with stage I disease recur[10];

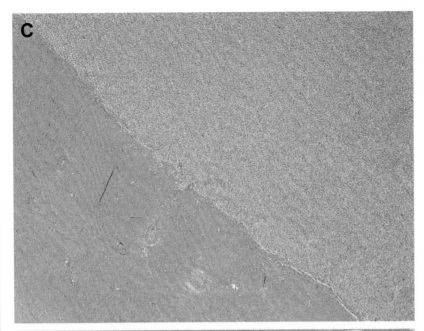

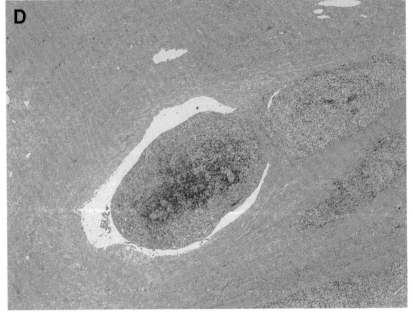

Fig. 4. (continued). (*C*) This tumor was originally sharply circumscribed; (*D*) however, lymphovascular invasion was present, and this tumor ultimately metastasized 6 years later (H&E, original magnification [*A*] ×50; [*B*] ×100).

the 5-year and 10-year overall survival rates are 69% to 84% and 65% to 76%, respectively.[1]

HIGH-GRADE ENDOMETRIAL STROMAL SARCOMA

OVERVIEW

The World Health Organization defines high-grade endometrial stromal sarcoma as a malignant tumor of endometrial stromal derivation morphologically composed of round cells. Tumors also may be associated with a low-grade spindle cell component[5] that resembles endometrial stroma. There is a broad range of involvement, but most patients tend to be perimenopausal.[50,59,60] Patients usually present with of abnormal bleeding[59] and/or a mass.

GROSS FEATURES

Tumors range from approximately 1 cm to more than 10 cm.[59,60] They may be intramural or

Fig. 5. (*A, B*) Low-grade endometrial stromal sarcoma showing prominent collagen plaques and bands (RNA sequencing: *JAZF1-SUZ12* fusion product) (H&E, original magnification [*A*] ×200; [*B*] ×400).

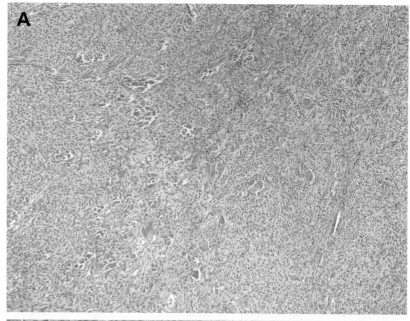

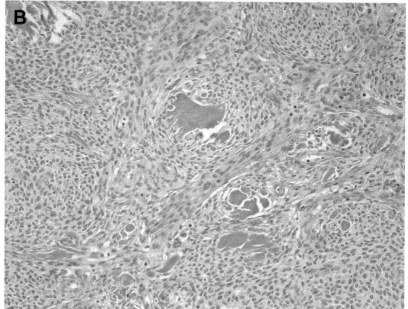

polypoid with infiltrative margins.[60] The cut surface is soft and fleshy and/or rubbery. It ranges from white to tan to pink to yellow.[60] Lymph node metastases are common.[60]

MICROSCOPIC FEATURES

Morphologically, tumors are undifferentiated and variably composed of a spectrum of round-spindle cells, of varying proportions.[50,59]

Round cell areas tend to be cellular and arranged in nests (**Fig. 8**).[59] The cytoplasm is scant-moderate and eosinophilic.[59] The nuclei are round-ovoid, angulated, and relatively monomorphic; mitotic activity is typically conspicuous (>10 per 10 HPFs).[59] Necrosis and lymphovascular space invasion are usually present.[59] Spindle cell areas tend to be composed of fascicles of variable cellularity[61] and fibrous-myxoid background.[60] It has been suggested

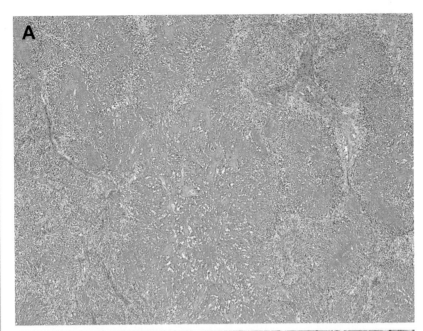

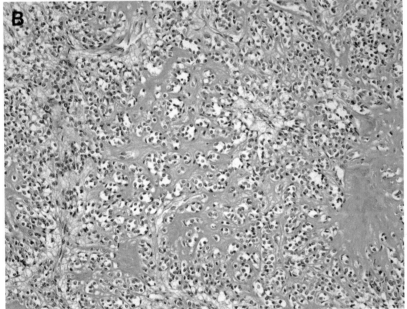

Fig. 6. (*A, B*) Low-grade endometrial stromal sarcoma with extensive hyalinization (RNA sequencing: *JAZF1-SUZ12* fusion product) (H&E, original magnification [*A*] ×100; [*B*] ×400).

that fusion gene status may correspond to differences in tumor morphology; for example, the spindle cell component of *YWHAE-NUTM2* fusion-associated tumors tends to be bland, with low-grade nuclei containing minimal mitotic activity, whereas those harboring *BCOR* abnormalities (*ZC3H7B–BCOR* or *BCOR* internal tandem duplication) tend to be composed of cellular fascicles of ovoid-spindle cells with mild-to-moderate pleomorphism and conspicuous mitoses (**Fig. 9**). Sex cord–like,[59] pseudopapillary,[59] pseudoglandular,[59] and heterologous differentiation[50] are reported in a minority of cases. Immunohistochemistry is usually positive for cyclin D1 (see **Fig. 8**),[45] CD117,[46] and BCOR,[47] with variable immunoreactivity for CD10 (often negative in tumors with *YWHAE-NUTM2* fusion products but positive in *BCOR*-associated cases)[59,60] and estrogen receptor and progesterone receptor.[59,60]

Fig. 7. Low-grade endometrial stromal sarcoma (RNA sequencing: *HCFC1-PHF1* fusion product [heretofore unreported fusion]). (*A*) Morphology resembling proliferative-type endometrium. (*B*) Immunohistochemistry for CD10. (*C*) Immunohistochemistry for estrogen receptor (H&E, original magnification [*A*] ×100; [*B*] ×200; [*C*] ×200).

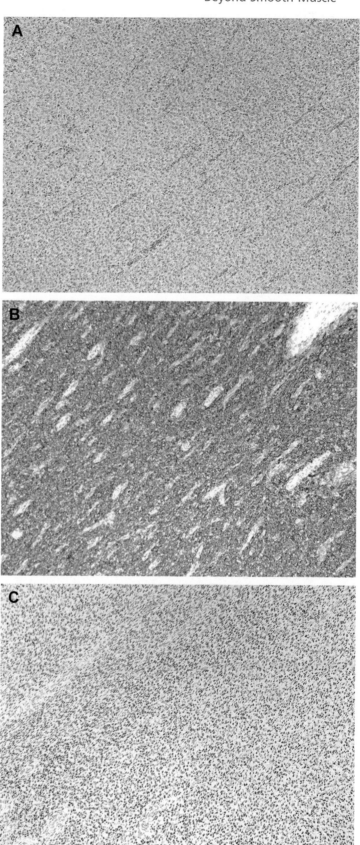

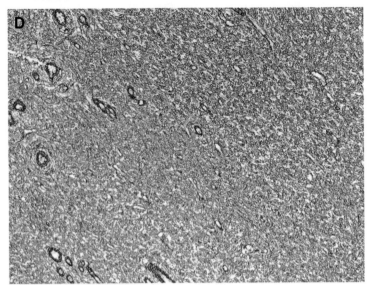

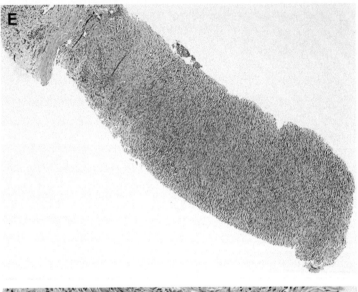

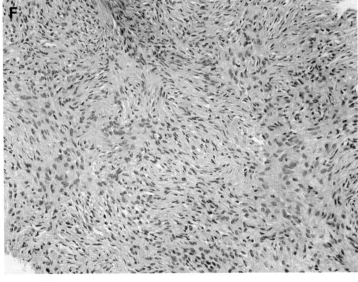

Fig. 7. (*continued*). (*D*) Immunohistochemistry for smooth muscle actin. Metastatic low-grade endometrial stromal sarcoma to the abdominal wall (RNA sequencing: *BRD8-PHF1* fusion product). (*E, F*) Similar to the primary tumor, the metastasis is composed of spindle cells with a fascicular-storiform pattern and monomorphic nuclei (H&E, original magnification [*D*] ×200; [*E*] ×100; [*F*] ×400).

Fig. 7. (*continued*). (*G*) Immuno-histochemistry for estrogen receptor. (*H*) Although the primary tumor was positive for CD10, this was lost in the metastasis (H&E, original magnification [*G*] ×100; [*H*] ×200).

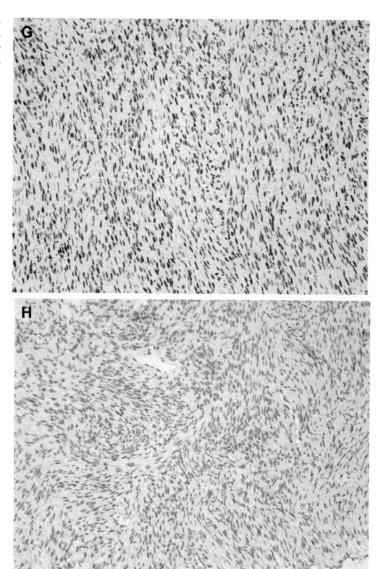

MOLECULAR FEATURES

Multiple disease-defining translocations have been reported; the most common fusions, to date, involve *YWHAE-NUTM2*.[4,62] A subset of cases harbors *ZC3H7B–BCOR* fusions[47,60] and *BCOR* internal tandem duplication.[63] The author and colleagues recently identified an endometrial stromal sarcoma with microcystic-reticulated morphology and abundant myxoid stroma containing an *EPC1-BCOR* fusion.[41] There is also a recent report of *JAZF1-BCORL1* in endometrial stromal sarcoma,[64] which likely corresponds to high-grade endometrial stromal sarcoma.[44]

DIFFERENTIAL DIAGNOSIS AND DIAGNOSIS

The differential diagnosis includes low-grade endometrial stromal sarcoma and undifferentiated uterine sarcoma. An approach to the distinction from low-grade endometrial stromal sarcoma is discussed previously. A more significant challenge may be separating high-grade endometrial stroma sarcoma from undifferentiated uterine sarcoma. The former tends to be morphologically primitive, although, in most cases, the nuclei are paradoxically uniform (monomorphic)—an attribute that is often a clue to the presence of a simple underlying genetic event (eg, translocation or mutation). In contrast, the nuclei in undifferentiated endometrial

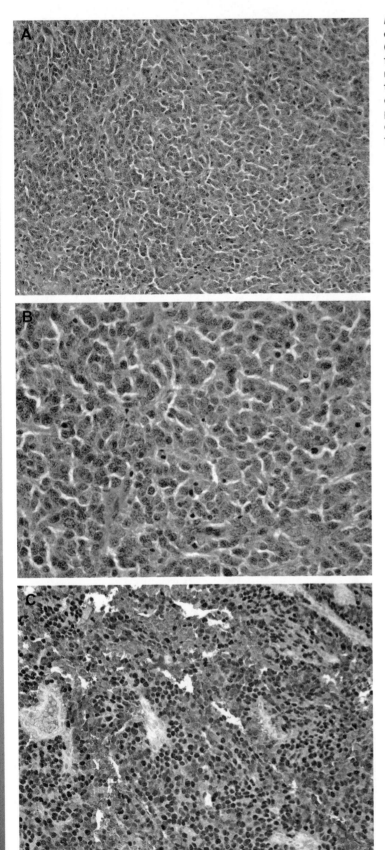

Fig. 8. Prototypical high-grade endometrial stromal sarcoma (RNA sequencing: *YWHAE-NUTM2* fusion product). (*A*) Sheets and nests of round cells. (*B*) Despite the morphologic absence of differentiation, the nuclei are monomorphic. (*C*) Immunohistochemistry for cyclin D1 (H&E, original magnification [*A*] ×200; [*B*] x400; [*C*] ×200).

Fig. 9. High-grade endometrial stromal sarcoma (RNA sequencing: *ZC3H7B-BCOR* fusion product). (*A*) Spindle cell fascicles, with area of myxoid stroma. (*B*) Relatively monomorphic ovoid nuclei with brisk mitotic activity. (*C*) Immuno-histochemistry for estrogen receptor (H&E, original magnification [*A*] ×100; [*B*] ×400; [*C*] ×200).

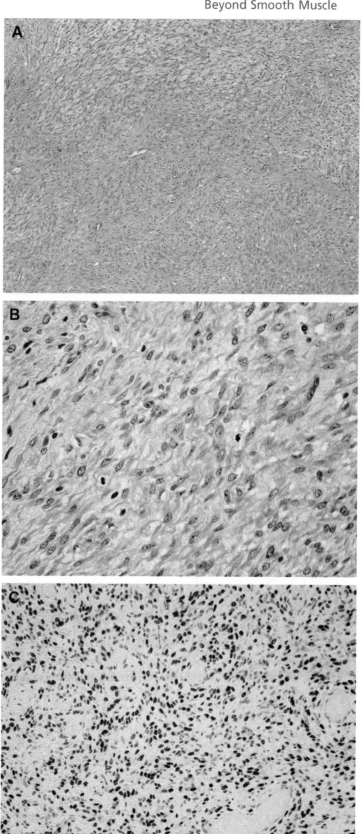

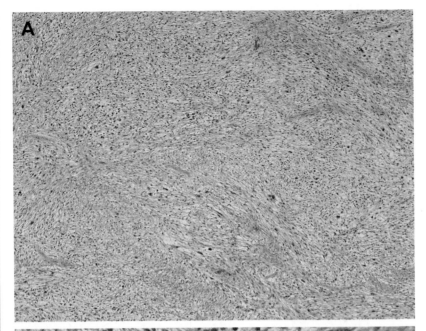

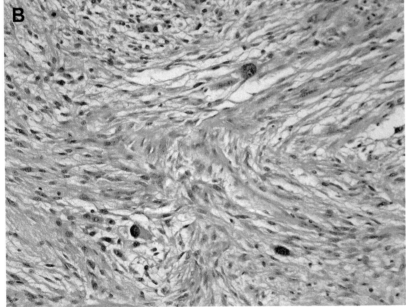

Fig. 10. Undifferentiated uterine sarcoma. (*A*, *B*) Spindle cell neoplasm with a vague fascicular-storiform pattern. The nuclei are ovoid and contain areas of marked pleomorphism and conspicuous mitotic activity. After extensive sampling, immunohistochemistry of this primary uterine tumor showed only focal immunoreactivity for CD34; it was negative for smooth muscle actin, desmin, h-caldesmon, estrogen receptor, ALK1, S100, MDM2, and keratin (AE1/AE3). RNA sequencing failed to identify any known fusion associated with endometrial stromal sarcoma (H&E, original magnification [*A*] ×100; [*B*] ×400).

stromal sarcoma tend to be pleomorphic. That said, genetically confirmed cases with nuclear pleomorphism have been reported.[47,65] The role of immunohistochemistry in differentiating high-grade endometrial stromal sarcoma from undifferentiated uterine sarcoma remains poorly characterized; both may contain staining for CD10,[60,65,66] but there are insufficient studies evaluating markers of high-grade endometrial stromal sarcoma (eg, cyclin D1, CD117, and BCOR) in undifferentiated uterine sarcoma. The

detection of a known fusion event remains the gold standard in the diagnosis of high-grade endometrial stromal sarcoma.

PROGNOSIS

High-grade endometrial stromal sarcoma with *YWHAE-NUTM2* fusion is suggested to have a malignant potential intermediate between low-grade endometrial stromal sarcoma and undifferentiated uterine sarcoma.[59] Tumors with *ZC3H7B-BCOR* fusions likewise seem to have a worse prognosis than low-grade endometrial stromal sarcoma.[60] That said, in view of the rarity of molecular-confirmed cases, multi-institutional studies are required to better delineate these issues in the future.[60]

UNDIFFERENTIATED UTERINE SARCOMA

OVERVIEW

Under the rubric of endometrial stromal and related tumors, the World Health Organization recognizes a forth category of tumors—undifferentiated uterine sarcoma. These tumors may originate from either the endometrium or myometrium, and they lack resemblance to endometrial stroma or any specific line of differentiation.[5] This category is presumed to represent a heterogeneous group of tumors.[67] In the past, endometrial tumors have been divided into undifferentiated tumors with either uniform or pleomorphic nuclei.[51] Tumors with uniform features are increasingly being evaluated molecularly and, unsurprisingly, reclassified into other categories, such as low-grade endometrial stromal sarcoma,[68] high-grade endometrial stromal sarcoma,[50] SMARCA4-deficient undifferentiated uterine sarcoma,[69] and NTRK-fusion positive uterine spindle cell sarcoma[67]; this occurs, albeit to a much lesser extent, in those tumors with pleomorphic nuclei. Analogous to pleomorphic undifferentiated sarcoma in the soft tissue, undifferentiated uterine sarcoma represents a diagnosis of exclusion.[67] These are rare and aggressive tumors. Patients tend to be postmenopausal.[70,71] Patients usually present with abnormal bleeding.[71]

GROSS FEATURES

Few details have been published on the gross attributes of bona fide cases of undifferentiated uterine sarcomas. Tumors tend to be greater than 8 cm[71] and intramural or polypoi,[51] with infiltrative margins.

MICROSCOPIC FEATURES

Morphologically, tumors consist of sheets of spindle-epithelioid-rhabdoid cells[1] with fascicular-herringbone-storiform-nested patterns (Fig. 10).[1] The cytoplasm ranges from scant to voluminous. The nuclei are pleomorphic and frequently hyperchromatic; mitotic activity is brisk. Necrosis and lymphovascular space invasion are frequent.[1] Immunohistochemistry is usually noncontributory, with variable immunoreactivity for CD10, cyclin D1, muscle markers, estrogen receptor, and progesterone receptor.

MOLECULAR FEATURES

Limited in-depth molecular studies exist for this neoplasm. Fluorescence in situ hybridization may show a pattern compatible with polysomy.[70]

DIFFERENTIAL DIAGNOSIS AND DIAGNOSIS

Undifferentiated uterine sarcoma is not a pure entity; instead, it is presumed to represent a heterogeneous collection of undifferentiated malignancies. This remains a diagnosis of exclusion, and the presence of a specific fusion, or mutation, by molecular testing precludes this diagnosis. Similarly, extensive tumor sampling may reveal evidence of a lower-grade counterpart, thereby suggesting a more specific diagnosis. In time, with refined molecular classification techniques, this category will presumably narrow. It assumed that a subset of cases represent dedifferentiated uterine neoplasms, such as leiomyosarcoma[72] and endometrial carcinoma.[73] It is likewise anticipated that, in the future, a subset of these cases will be found to harbor novel genetic identifiers.

PROGNOSIS

The prognosis is typically poor, with a mean survival of less than 2 years.[71,74]

Diagnostic Algorithm

Primary uterine tumor that is morphologically undifferentiated.

1. Sample the lesion and surrounding uterus extensively. Can a better differentiated component be identified? Proceed to step 2 for diagnostic confirmation or further investigation.

2. Perform a broad immunohistochemical screening panel, encompassing (A) smooth muscle and myofibroblastic differentiation (eg, desmin, smooth muscle actin, h-caldesmon, ALK, +/−estrogen receptor); (B) skeletal muscle differentiation (myogenin); (C) endometrial stroma (eg, CD10, CD117, cyclin D1, BCOR, +/−estrogen receptor); (D) epithelial and sex cord–stromal differentiation (keratin, GATA3, calretinin); (E) perivascular epithelioid cell tumor (PEComa) (HMB45, melanA, cathepsin K); and (F) consider the possibility the tumor may be invading from an adjacent tissue, such as (i)

gastrointestinal stromal tumor (CD34, CD117, DOG1) or (ii) dedifferentiated liposarcoma (MDM2, CDK4).

3. The presence of significant staining in each of these categories ostensibly excludes undifferentiated uterine sarcoma and, assuming there is no morphologic, immunohistochemical, or molecular evidence to support a particular line of differentiation, classification as an undifferentiated uterine sarcoma is warranted.

UTERINE TUMOR RESEMBLING OVARIAN SEX CORD TUMOR

OVERVIEW

The World Health Organization classifies uterine tumors with a predominant morphology reminiscent of sex cord tumors and lacking recognizable areas of endometrial stroma as so-called uterine tumor resembling ovarian sex cord tumor.[5] These tumors occur in middle-aged women. Patients generally present with abnormal bleeding, pain, and/or an enlarged uterus.[75–77]

GROSS FEATURES

Grossly, tumors may be intramural, submucosal and polypoid, or subserosal.[78–80] They tend to be circumscribed with minimal infiltration of surrounding stroma,[78–80] although invasive growth is occasionally reported.[81] They range from less than 1 cm to more than 20 cm.[79,80] The cut surface has been reported to be solid and fleshy and yellow to off-white.[78,79]

MICROSCOPIC FEATURES

Morphologically heterogeneous, tumors are composed of epithelioid cells with an admixture of patterns, including anastomosing trabeculae, cords and tubules, retiform gland-like, nests, and diffuse sheets (Fig. 11).[77–81] The cytoplasm ranges from scant to ample and clear-eosinophilic-amphophilic.[77,78] The nuclei are round with vesicular chromatin and small nucleoli; mitotic activity is not conspicuous (<5 per 10 HPFs),[80] and clefts are notably absent.[77,79] Foamy cells are occasionally present.[77,82] Necrosis and lymphovascular invasion are rarely observed.[83] The immunohistochemical profile is polyphenotypic. Tumors are generally positive for keratins (AE1/AE3, Cam5.3), calretinin, WT-1 (nuclear), estrogen and progesterone receptors, and vimentin, with variable immunoreactivity for epithelial membrane antigen, inhibin, FOXL2, steroidogenic factor-1, desmin, smooth muscle actin, calponin, h-caldesmon, CD10, CD56, and melan-A; tumors are usually negative for CD34 and CD117.[77–79,81,84,85]

MOLECULAR FEATURES

There is cytogenetic evidence showing a case of t(X;6) (p22.3;q23.1) and t(4;18) (q21.1;q21.3).[86] Genome-wide copy number analysis was found to show recurrent gain in chromosome 1q.[87] More directed molecular interrogation shows these tumors lack JAZF1-SUZ12 fusions[80,88] and PHF1 rearrangement,[89] characteristic of endometrial stromal sarcoma. Furthermore, they lack mutations involving FOXL2 and DICER1,[85,90] typifying ovarian adult granulosa cell tumor and Sertoli-Leydig cell tumor, respectively. The author's group has recently shown that most tumors contain fusions involving NCOA2 and NCOA3.[91]

DIFFERENTIAL DIAGNOSIS AND DIAGNOSIS

Sex cord–like differentiation may occur as a secondary phenomenon in several uterine mesenchymal neoplasms, including smooth muscle neoplasms,[92] endometrial stromal sarcoma,[19,93] and mullerian adenosarcoma.[94,95] Differentiation from adenosarcoma and smooth muscle neoplasms is generally not problematic. Sex cord–like differentiation is typically focal in smooth muscle neoplasms, and the background morphology and immunophenotype remain consistent with smooth muscle. Similarly, sex cord–like differentiation tends to be only focal in adenosarcoma; in addition, the glandular epithelium is often endocervical-type and surrounded by a characteristic cellular periglandular cuff.[5] Uterine tumor resembling ovarian sex cord tumor and endometrial stromal sarcoma may show tremendous morphologic overlap[75]; however, similar to other mimics, the latter tends to be focal (<50% of the tumor). In limited samples, molecular testing to confirm the presence or absence of a translocation typical of endometrial stromal sarcoma may be necessary to confirm the diagnosis.

PROGNOSIS

Most cases are reported to have an indolent clinical course; however, a recent large series demonstrated that 23.5% of patients developed metastases and 8.8% of patients died of their tumor. For this reason, it has been proposed that uterine tumor resembling ovarian sex cord tumor be considered of uncertain malignant potential.[83]

Fig. 11. Uterine tumor resembling ovarian sex cord tumor. (*A*) Anastomosing trabeculae of epithelioid cells. (*B*) Retiform-tubular pattern of epithelioid cells. (*C*) Nests of plump epithelioid cells (H&E, original magnification ×200).

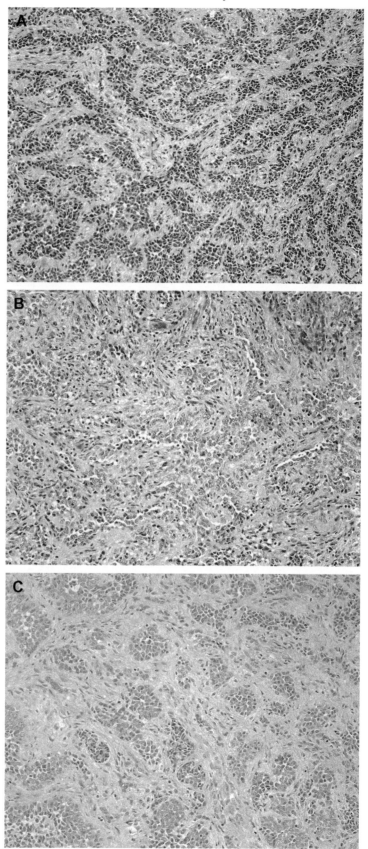

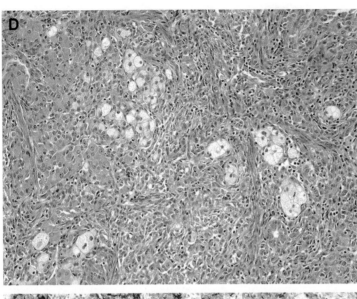

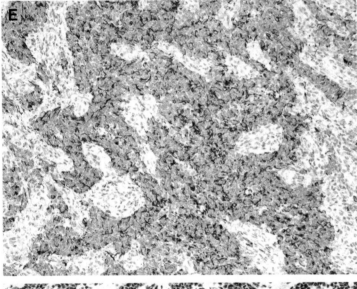

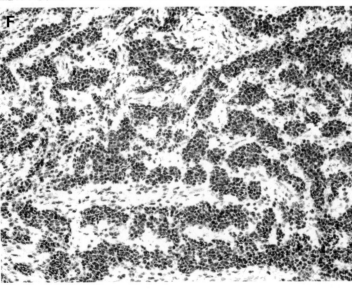

Fig. 11. (continued). (*D*) Aggregates of foamy cells are frequently present. (*E*) Immunohistochemistry for keratin (AE1/AE3). (*F*) Immunohistochemistry for estrogen receptor (H&E, original magnification [*D–F*] ×200).

Pathologic Key Features

- Tumors are generally circumscribed and may be centered in myometrium or involve endometrium.
- Tumors predominantly/entirely are composed of sex cord–like differentiation.
- Epithelioid cells are arranged in trabeculae, cords and tubules, nests, and/or sheets.
- Immunohistochemistry usually is diffusely positive for keratin, calretinin, and estrogen/progesterone. Patchy staining for muscle and melanocytic markers is often present.
- Tumors are frequently characterized by fusions involving NCOA, as well as other genes.

Fig. 12. Benign PEComa. (*A*) Small circumscribed nodule centered within the myometrium. (*B*) Sheets of epithelioid-polygonal cells with abundant cytoplasm. The nuclei are round and monomorphic (H&E, original magnification [*A*] ×100; [*B*] ×200).

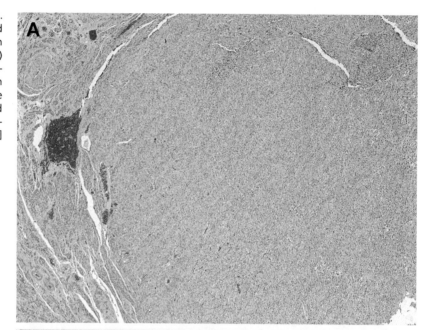

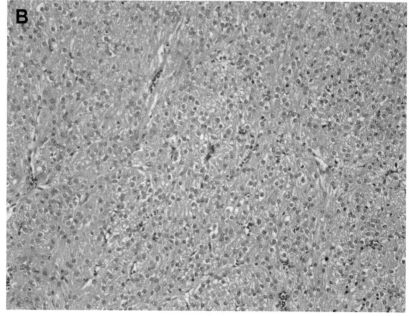

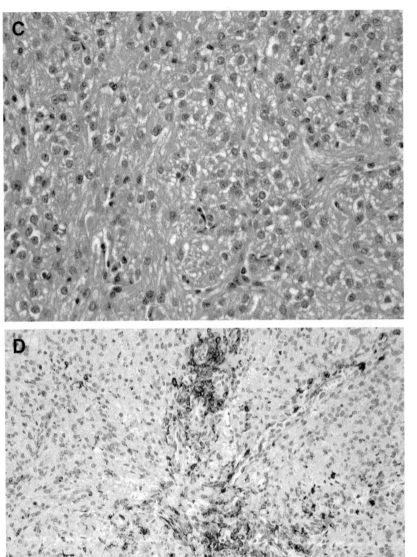

Fig. 12. (continued). (*C*) Occasional cells have cytoplasmic retraction yielding so-called spider cells. (*D*) Immunohisto-chemistry for HMB45; note, in this case, staining is largely found within cells centered around the vessel (H&E, original magnification [*C*] ×400; [*D*] ×200).

PERIVASCULAR EPITHELIOID CELL TUMOR

OVERVIEW

PEComa is a mesenchymal neoplasm exhibiting both smooth muscle and melanocytic differentia-tion.[5] Tumors can occur throughout the body; how-ever, they are considered rare in the gynecologic tract, where the most common site of involvement is the uterus.[96,97] Patients tend to present in mid-adulthood to late adulthood.[96,98] Presentation may be prompted by symptoms of abnormal bleeding and/or pelvic pain.[96,98] Although most tu-mors are sporadic, a minority of cases occur in the context of tuberous sclerosis.[96,99–101]

GROSS FEATURES

Tumors sizes range from subcentimeter to more than 15 cm.[96–98] The cut surface is soft, fleshy, and white-tan-yellow.[98]

MICROSCOPIC FEATURES

Tumors may be circumscribed or infiltrative.[96–98] Morphologically they are composed of sheets, nests, and/or fascicles of epithelioid-spindle cells,[96–98] often with a perivascular distribution (**Fig. 12**).[98] The cytoplasm is clear to eosinophilic and frequently granular; occasionally, enlarged cells with wispy cytoplasmic retractions from the cell membrane (so-called spider cells) can be identified.[96–98] Melanin pigmentation may be present in a subset of cases.[96] The nuclei are round-ovoid and often atypical, with occasional macronucleoli and pseudonuclear inclusions; mitotic activity is variable.[96] Necrosis, lymphovascular invasion, and lymph node metastases may be encountered (**Fig. 13**).[96–98] Multinucleated giant cells are occasionally present.[96,97] Stromal hyalinization and/or sclerosis is a common finding.[96,98] Immunohistochemistry is generally positive for

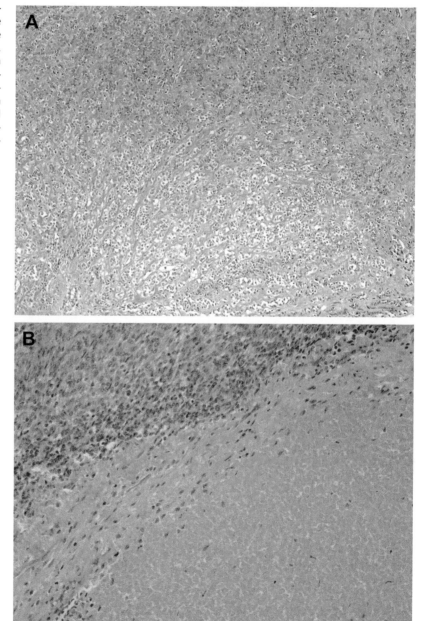

Fig. 13. Malignant PEComa. (*A*) This is a large tumor with infiltrative margins (not shown). The cells are arranged in cords and nests with sclerotic stroma. The cytoplasm ranges from eosinophilic to clear, and the nuclei have mild atypia (H&E, original magnification ×100).

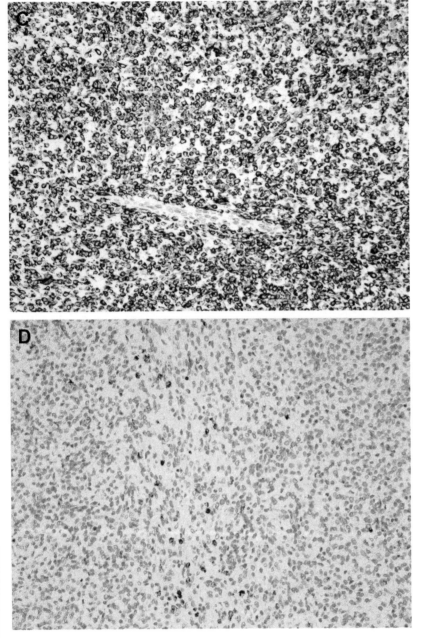

Fig. 13. (*continued*). (*B*) Necrosis is present. (*C*) Immunohistochemistry for desmin. (*D*) Immuno-histochemistry for HMB45; it is important to recognize that many cases contain less than 5% staining for melano-cytic markers (H&E, original magnification [*B–D*] ×200).

cathepsin K, HMB45, melan-A, MiTF, TFE3, desmin, smooth muscle actin, and h-caldesmon.[96–98] It should be emphasized that staining may occasionally be patchy or focal.[96–98]

MOLECULAR FEATURES

PEComas are genetically heterogeneous. Approximately half of cases are associated with underlying *TSC2* mutations, and approximately 23% of cases contain fusion genes associated with *TFE3* rearrangement.[102]

DIFFERENTIAL DIAGNOSIS AND DIAGNOSIS

Morphologically, the differential diagnosis largely includes epithelioid leiomyoma. It was previously suggested that uterine PEComa represents an epithelioid smooth muscle tumors with melanocytic differentiation, and this was the subject of some debate.[98,100,103] Currently, most investigators accept that tumors with morphologic features of PEComa, with at least focal immunoreactivity for 2 melanocytic markers and at least 1 smooth muscle marker, warrant classification as PEComa rather than an epithelioid smooth muscle tumor.[96] Where there is a history of melanoma, the possibility of metastasis should be excluded. Similarly, the presence of extrauterine involvement warrants exclusion of clear cell sarcoma.

PROGNOSIS

PEComa of the uterus is rare, and criteria for malignancy have only recently been proposed.

The presence of 2 or more of the following attributes merits classification as malignant: large size (≥5 cm), infiltrative growth, significant pleomorphism, mitotic activity (≥1 per 50 HPFs), necrosis, and/or lymphovascular invasion.[96,97]

Differential Diagnosis

- Epithelioid smooth muscle tumor
- Clear cell sarcoma
- Metastatic melanoma

INFLAMMATORY MYOFIBROBLASTIC TUMOR

OVERVIEW

Inflammatory myofibroblastic tumor is a mesenchymal neoplasm of (myo)-fibroblastic differentiation that is typically associated with an admixed inflammatory cell component.[5] Tumors may occur in the soft tissues and viscera; the uterus is a rare site of involvement.[104] Although patients span a broad range of age involvement, tumors predominate in early adulthood to mid-adulthood.[104–107] Clinical presentation may be prompted by abnormal bleeding, pain, mass, fatigue, and/or fever.[104,106,107]

GROSS FEATURES

Tumors range in size from 1 cm to 20 cm[104–107] Although most uterine cases are confined to the corpus, a minority show extrauterine involvement.[104] A majority of tumors are submucosal, although mural or subserosal involvement is possible.[104] The cut surface is soft, and tumors range from white-tan to yellow and pink.[104,106] Some tumors contain areas that are gelatinous, myxoid, and/or edematous.[106] Hemorrhage and necrosis may be identified.[104,106] Most cases have an infiltrative border, which is similar to endometrial stromal sarcoma.[104]

MICROSCOPIC FEATURES

Microscopically tumors may exhibit 1 or more of the characteristic morphologies originally described by Coffin and colleagues,[108] including myxoid, dense collagenous, and compact spindle cell patterns.[104,106,107] The cells range from spindle to epithelioid[104] and are occasionally arranged in fascicles (**Fig. 14**).[104] The cytoplasm is pale and eosinophilic; rarely, a decidual-like appearance may be present.[104] The nuclei are round-ovoid with variable atypia[104,106]; mitotic activity ranges from absent to brisk. The intervening stroma ranges from myxoid to collagenous. A lymphoplasmacytic inflammatory infiltrate is almost invariably present and may be supplemented with histiocytes, eosinophils, neutrophils, and/or multinucleated giant cells.[104] Necrosis and lymphovascular space invasion may be encountered. In contrast to other anatomic sites, a somewhat greater proportion of uterine cases—77% to 100%—expresses ALK[106] (the staining pattern is most often granular and cytoplasmic, but uniform cytoplasmic, membranous cytoplasmic, and perinuclear accentuation patterns may be observed), with variable immunoreactivity for desmin, smooth muscle actin, h-caldesmon, and CD10.[104–107]

MOLECULAR FEATURES

In cases of *ALK* rearrangement, there is a diverse array of potential partners that differs somewhat from tumors at other anatomic locations (eg, *DES, FN1, IGFBP5, SEC31, THBS1,* and *TIPM3*).[104,105] Alternate drivers (eg, *ROS1*) are presumed to account for a subset of the *ALK*-negative cases; there is a recent report of a case containing a *ETV6-NTRK3* fusion gene.[109]

DIFFERENTIAL DIAGNOSIS AND DIAGNOSIS

The differential diagnosis includes myxoid smooth muscle tumors[110] Accurate classification is essential because inflammatory myofibroblastic tumors may benefit from targeted therapy (eg, crizotinib). Distinction can, at times, be challenging, because hydropic degeneration, degenerative change, and smooth muscle neoplasms with myxoid stroma may show morphologic

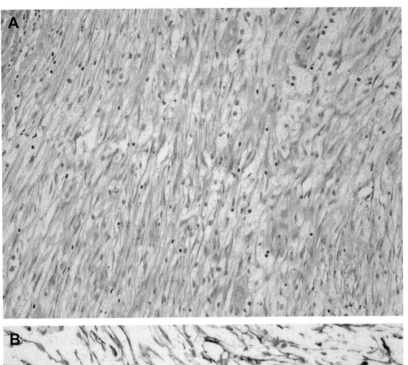

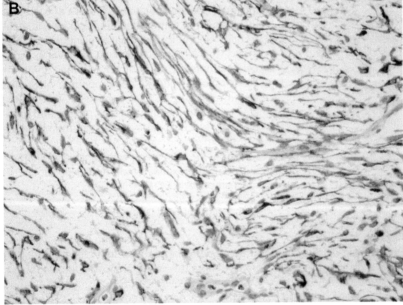

Fig. 14. Inflammatory myofibroblastic tumor (RNA sequencing: THBS1-ALK fusion product). (A) Spindle-stellate cells with vague fascicular pattern. The intervening stroma is myxoid-collagenous, with scattered interspersed lymphocytes. The nuclei are ovoid with prominent small nucleoli (H&E, original magnification ×200) (B) Immunohistochemistry for ALK1 shows a cytoplasmic pattern of staining (original magnification ×200).

overlap. Morphologic clues to the correct diagnosis include the presence of an inflammatory component and more slender spindle cell morphology. Immunohistochemistry for ALK and/or molecular testing, however, facilitate the correct diagnosis in a majority of cases where the possibility of inflammatory myofibroblastic tumor is suspected.

PROGNOSIS

Most cases are cured by surgery. As elsewhere in the body, however, a subset of tumors may pursue an aggressive clinical course. This seems, in part, to be associated with older patient age, larger tumors, and increased mitoses.[104,106]

Pitfalls

! Myxoid change may occur in smooth muscle neoplasms (leiomyoma and leiomyosarcoma). Although inflammatory myofibroblastic tumor often shows myoid differentiation, smooth muscle markers do not contain ALK or related fusion events.

! The location of ALK expression varies. Some cases and/or fusions are associated with cytoplasmic patterns, whereas others may involve the nucleus. Be aware of membranous patterns, which can be subtle.

! Given a large and growing number of potential gene fusions, reverse transcription–polymerase chain reaction–based assays are impractical and likely to miss actionable mutations.

REFERENCES

1. Chew I, Oliva E. Endometrial stromal sarcomas: a review of potential prognostic factors. Adv Anat Pathol 2010;17(2):113–21.

2. Oliva E. Practical issues in uterine pathology from banal to bewildering: the remarkable spectrum of smooth muscle neoplasia. Mod Pathol 2016; 29(Suppl 1):S104–20.

3. Mills AM, Longacre TA. Smooth muscle tumors of the female genital tract. Surg Pathol Clin 2009; 2(4):625–77.

4. Lee CH, Ou WB, Marino-Enriquez A, et al. 14-3-3 fusion oncogenes in high-grade endometrial stromal sarcoma. Proc Natl Acad Sci U S A 2012; 109(3):929–34.

5. Oliva E, Carcangiu ML, Carinelli SG, et al. Mesenchymal tumours. In: Kurman RJ, Carcangiu ML, Herrington CS, et al, editors. WHO classification of tumours of female reproductive organs. Lyon (France): International Agency for Research on Cancer; 2014. p. 142–4.

6. Norris HJ, Taylor HB. Mesenchymal tumors of the uterus. I. A clinical and pathological study of 53 endometrial stromal tumors. Cancer 1966;19(6):755–66.

7. Mostoufizadeh M, Scully RE. Malignant tumors arising in endometriosis. Clin Obstet Gynecol 1980;23(3):951–63.

8. Masand RP, Euscher ED, Deavers MT, et al. Endometrioid stromal sarcoma: a clinicopathologic study of 63 cases. Am J Surg Pathol 2013;37(11): 1635–47.

9. Chan JK, Kawar NM, Shin JY, et al. Endometrial stromal sarcoma: a population-based analysis. Br J Cancer 2008;99(8):1210–5.

10. Chang KL, Crabtree GS, Lim-Tan SK, et al. Primary uterine endometrial stromal neoplasms. A clinicopathologic study of 117 cases. Am J Surg Pathol 1990;14(5):415–38.

11. Yoonessi M, Hart WR. Endometrial stromal sarcomas. Cancer 1977;40(2):898–906.

12. Evans HL. Endometrial stromal sarcoma and poorly differentiated endometrial sarcoma. Cancer 1982; 50(10):2170–82.

13. Oliva E, Clement PB, Young RH, et al. Mixed endometrial stromal and smooth muscle tumors of the uterus: a clinicopathologic study of 15 cases. Am J Surg Pathol 1998;22(8):997–1005.

14. Yilmaz A, Rush DS, Soslow RA. Endometrial stromal sarcomas with unusual histologic features: a report of 24 primary and metastatic tumors emphasizing fibroblastic and smooth muscle differentiation. Am J Surg Pathol 2002;26(9): 1142–50.

15. Oliva E, Young RH, Clement PB, et al. Myxoid and fibrous endometrial stromal tumors of the uterus: a report of 10 cases. Int J Gynecol Pathol 1999;18(4): 310–9.

16. Oliva E, Clement PB, Young RH. Epithelioid endometrial and endometrioid stromal tumors: a report of four cases emphasizing their distinction from epithelioid smooth muscle tumors and other oxyphilic uterine and extrauterine tumors. Int J Gynecol Pathol 2002;21(1):48–55.

17. Kim YH, Cho H, Kyeom-Kim H, et al. Uterine endometrial stromal sarcoma with rhabdoid and smooth muscle differentiation. J Korean Med Sci 1996; 11(1):88–93.

18. Clement PB, Scully RE. Endometrial stromal sarcomas of the uterus with extensive endometrioid glandular differentiation: a report of three cases that caused problems in differential diagnosis. Int J Gynecol Pathol 1992;11(3):163–73.

19. McCluggage WG, Date A, Bharucha H, et al. Endometrial stromal sarcoma with sex cord-like areas and focal rhabdoid differentiation. Histopathology 1996;29(4):369–74.

20. Fukunaga M, Miyazawa Y, Ushigome S. Endometrial low-grade stromal sarcoma with ovarian sex cord-like differentiation: report of two cases with an immunohistochemical and flow cytometric study. Pathol Int 1997;47(6):412–5.

21. D'Angelo E, Ali RH, Espinosa I, et al. Endometrial stromal sarcomas with sex cord differentiation are associated with PHF1 rearrangement. Am J Surg Pathol 2013;37(4):514–21.

22. Chu P, Arber DA. Paraffin-section detection of CD10 in 505 nonhematopoietic neoplasms. Frequent expression in renal cell carcinoma and endometrial stromal sarcoma. Am J Clin Pathol 2000;113(3):374–82.

23. Chu PG, Arber DA, Weiss LM, et al. Utility of CD10 in distinguishing between endometrial stromal sarcoma and uterine smooth muscle tumors: an immunohistochemical comparison of 34 cases. Mod Pathol 2001;14(5):465–71.

24. Agoff SN, Grieco VS, Garcia R, et al. Immunohistochemical distinction of endometrial stromal sarcoma and cellular leiomyoma. Appl Immunohistochem Mol Morphol 2001;9(2):164–9.

25. McCluggage WG, Sumathi VP, Maxwell P. CD10 is a sensitive and diagnostically useful immunohistochemical marker of normal endometrial stroma and of endometrial stromal neoplasms. Histopathology 2001;39(3):273–8.

26. Lantta M, Kahanpaa K, Karkkainen J, et al. Estradiol and progesterone receptors in two cases of endometrial stromal sarcoma. Gynecol Oncol 1984;18(2):233–9.

27. Sutton GP, Stehman FB, Michael H, et al. Estrogen and progesterone receptors in uterine sarcomas. Obstet Gynecol 1986;68(5):709–14.

28. Sabini G, Chumas JC, Mann WJ. Steroid hormone receptors in endometrial stromal sarcomas. A biochemical and immunohistochemical study. Am J Clin Pathol 1992;97(3):381–6.

29. Reich O, Regauer S, Urdl W, et al. Expression of oestrogen and progesterone receptors in low-grade endometrial stromal sarcomas. Br J Cancer 2000;82(5):1030–4.

30. Park JY, Baek MH, Park Y, et al. Investigation of hormone receptor expression and its prognostic value in endometrial stromal sarcoma. Virchows Arch 2018;473(1):61–9.

31. Rush DS, Tan J, Baergen RN, et al. a novel smooth muscle-specific antibody, distinguishes between cellular leiomyoma and endometrial stromal sarcoma. Am J Surg Pathol 2001;25(2):253–8.

32. Nucci MR, O'Connell JT, Huettner PC, et al. h-Caldesmon expression effectively distinguishes endometrial stromal tumors from uterine smooth muscle tumors. Am J Surg Pathol 2001;25(4):455–63.

33. Bhargava R, Shia J, Hummer AJ, et al. Distinction of endometrial stromal sarcomas from 'hemangiopericytomatous' tumors using a panel of immunohistochemical stains. Mod Pathol 2005;18(1):40–7.

34. Adegboyega PA, Qiu S. Immunohistochemical profiling of cytokeratin expression by endometrial stroma sarcoma. Hum Pathol 2008;39(10):1459–64.

35. Koontz JI, Soreng AL, Nucci M, et al. Frequent fusion of the JAZF1 and JJAZ1 genes in endometrial stromal tumors. Proc Natl Acad Sci U S A 2001;98(11):6348–53.

36. Nucci MR, Harburger D, Koontz J, et al. Molecular analysis of the JAZF1-JJAZ1 gene fusion by RT-PCR and fluorescence in situ hybridization in endometrial stromal neoplasms. Am J Surg Pathol 2007; 31(1):65–70.

37. Micci F, Brunetti M, Dal Cin P, et al. Fusion of the genes BRD8 and PHF1 in endometrial stromal sarcoma. Genes Chromosomes Cancer 2017;56(12): 841–5.

38. Micci F, Panagopoulos I, Bjerkehagen B, et al. Consistent rearrangement of chromosomal band 6p21 with generation of fusion genes JAZF1/PHF1 and EPC1/PHF1 in endometrial stromal sarcoma. Cancer Res 2006;66(1):107–12.

39. Brunetti M, Gorunova L, Davidson B, et al. Identification of an EPC2-PHF1 fusion transcript in low-grade endometrial stromal sarcoma. Oncotarget 2018;9(27):19203–8.

40. Panagopoulos I, Micci F, Thorsen J, et al. Novel fusion of MYST/Esa1-associated factor 6 and PHF1 in endometrial stromal sarcoma. PLoS one 2012;7(6):e39354.

41. Dickson BC, Lum A, Swanson D, et al. Novel EPC1 gene fusions in endometrial stromal sarcoma. Genes Chromosomes Cancer 2018;57(11): 598–603.

42. Dewaele B, Przybyl J, Quattrone A, et al. Identification of a novel, recurrent MBTD1-CXorf67 fusion in low-grade endometrial stromal sarcoma. Int J Cancer 2014;134(5):1112–22.

43. Lee CH, Nucci MR. Endometrial stromal sarcoma–the new genetic paradigm. Histopathology 2015; 67(1):1–19.

44. Hoang L, Chiang S, Lee CH. Endometrial stromal sarcomas and related neoplasms: new developments and diagnostic considerations. Pathology 2017;50(2):162–77.

45. Lee CH, Ali RH, Rouzbahman M, et al. Cyclin D1 as a diagnostic immunomarker for endometrial stromal sarcoma with YWHAE-FAM22 rearrangement. Am J Surg Pathol 2012;36(10):1562–70.

46. Lee CH, Hoang LN, Yip S, et al. Frequent expression of KIT in endometrial stromal sarcoma with YWHAE genetic rearrangement. Mod Pathol 2014; 27(5):751–7.

47. Chiang S, Lee CH, Stewart CJR, et al. BCOR is a robust diagnostic immunohistochemical marker of genetically diverse high-grade endometrial stromal sarcoma, including tumors exhibiting variant morphology. Mod Pathol 2017;30(9):1251–61.

48. Attygalle AD, Vroobel K, Wren D, et al. An unusual case of YWHAE-NUTM2A/B endometrial stromal sarcoma with confinement to the endometrium

and lack of high-grade morphology. Int J Gynecol Pathol 2017;36(2):165–71.

49. Aisagbonhi O, Harrison B, Zhao L, et al. YWHAE rearrangement in a purely conventional low-grade endometrial stromal sarcoma that transformed over time to high-grade sarcoma: importance of molecular testing. Int J Gynecol Pathol 2018; 37(5):441–7.

50. Sciallis AP, Bedroske PP, Schoolmeester JK, et al. High-grade endometrial stromal sarcomas: a clinicopathologic study of a group of tumors with heterogenous morphologic and genetic features. Am J Surg Pathol 2014;38(9):1161–72.

51. Kurihara S, Oda Y, Ohishi Y, et al. Endometrial stromal sarcomas and related high-grade sarcomas: immunohistochemical and molecular genetic study of 31 cases. Am J Surg Pathol 2008;32(8):1228–38.

52. Kolson Kokohaare E, Strauss DC, Jones RL, et al. Endometrial stromal sarcoma with hyalinizing giant rosettes, mimicking low-grade fibromyxoid sarcoma. Int J Surg Pathol 2018;26(6):525–7.

53. Ud Din N, Ahmad Z, Zreik R, et al. Abdominopelvic and retroperitoneal low-grade fibromyxoid sarcoma: a clinicopathologic study of 13 cases. Am J Clin Pathol 2018;149(2):128–34.

54. VanSandt AM, Bronson J, Leclair C, et al. Low-grade fibromyxoid sarcoma of the vulva: a case report. J Low Genit Tract Dis 2013;17(1):79–81.

55. Doyle LA, Moller E, Dal Cin P, et al. MUC4 is a highly sensitive and specific marker for low-grade fibromyxoid sarcoma. Am J Surg Pathol 2011;35(5): 733–41.

56. Mertens F, Fletcher CD, Antonescu CR, et al. Clinicopathologic and molecular genetic characterization of low-grade fibromyxoid sarcoma, and cloning of a novel FUS/CREB3L1 fusion gene. Lab Invest 2005;85(3):408–15.

57. Matsuyama A, Hisaoka M, Shimajiri S, et al. Molecular detection of FUS-CREB3L2 fusion transcripts in low-grade fibromyxoid sarcoma using formalin-fixed, paraffin-embedded tissue specimens. Am J Surg Pathol 2006;30(9):1077–84.

58. Lau PP, Lui PC, Lau GT, et al. EWSR1-CREB3L1 gene fusion: a novel alternative molecular aberration of low-grade fibromyxoid sarcoma. Am J Surg Pathol 2013;37(5):734–8.

59. Lee CH, Marino-Enriquez A, Ou W, et al. The clinicopathologic features of YWHAE-FAM22 endometrial stromal sarcomas: a histologically high-grade and clinically aggressive tumor. Am J Surg Pathol 2012;36(5):641–53.

60. Lewis N, Soslow RA, Delair DF, et al. ZC3H7B-BCOR high-grade endometrial stromal sarcomas: a report of 17 cases of a newly defined entity. Mod Pathol 2018;31(4):674–84.

61. Panagopoulos I, Thorsen J, Gorunova L, et al. Fusion of the ZC3H7B and BCOR genes in endometrial stromal sarcomas carrying an X;22-translocation. Genes Chromosomes Cancer 2013;52(7):610–8.

62. Isphording A, Ali RH, Irving J, et al. YWHAE-FAM22 endometrial stromal sarcoma: diagnosis by reverse transcription-polymerase chain reaction in formalin-fixed, paraffin-embedded tumor. Hum Pathol 2013; 44(5):837–43.

63. Marino-Enriquez A, Lauria A, Przybyl J, et al. BCOR internal tandem duplication in high-grade uterine sarcomas. Am J Surg Pathol 2018;42(3):335–41.

64. Allen AJ, Ali SM, Gowen K, et al. A recurrent endometrial stromal sarcoma harbors the novel fusion JAZF1-BCORL1. Gynecol Oncol Rep 2017;20: 51–3.

65. Croce S, Hostein I, Ribeiro A, et al. YWHAE rearrangement identified by FISH and RT-PCR in endometrial stromal sarcomas: genetic and pathological correlations. Mod Pathol 2013;26(10):1390–400.

66. Jakate K, Azimi F, Ali RH, et al. Endometrial sarcomas: an immunohistochemical and JAZF1 rearrangement study in low-grade and undifferentiated tumors. Mod Pathol 2013;26(1):95–105.

67. Chiang S, Cotzia P, Hyman DM, et al. NTRK fusions define a novel uterine sarcoma subtype with features of fibrosarcoma. Am J Surg Pathol 2018; 42(6):791–8.

68. Lee CH, Ali R, Gilks CB. Molecular genetics of mesenchymal tumors of the female genital tract. Surg Pathol Clin 2009;2(4):823–34.

69. Kolin DL, Dong F, Baltay M, et al. SMARCA4-deficient undifferentiated uterine sarcoma (malignant rhabdoid tumor of the uterus): a clinicopathologic entity distinct from undifferentiated carcinoma. Mod Pathol 2018;31(9):1442–56.

70. Schoolmeester JK, Sciallis AP, Greipp PT, et al. Analysis of MDM2 amplification in 43 endometrial stromal tumors: a potential diagnostic pitfall. Int J Gynecol Pathol 2015;34(6):576–83.

71. Rios I, Rovirosa A, Morales J, et al. Undifferentiated uterine sarcoma: a rare, not well known and aggressive disease: report of 13 cases. Arch Gynecol Obstet 2014;290(5):993–7.

72. Chen E, O'Connell F, Fletcher CD. Dedifferentiated leiomyosarcoma: clinicopathological analysis of 18 cases. Histopathology 2011;59(6):1135–43.

73. Shah VI, McCluggage WG. Cyclin D1 does not distinguish YWHAE-NUTM2 high-grade endometrial stromal sarcoma from undifferentiated endometrial carcinoma. Am J Surg Pathol 2015;39(5): 722–4.

74. Nucci MR. Practical issues related to uterine pathology: endometrial stromal tumors. Mod Pathol 2016;29(Suppl 1):S92–103.

75. Clement PB, Scully RE. Uterine tumors resembling ovarian sex-cord tumors. A clinicopathologic analysis of fourteen cases. Am J Clin Pathol 1976; 66(3):512–25.

76. Irving JA, Carinelli S, Prat J. Uterine tumors resembling ovarian sex cord tumors are polyphenotypic neoplasms with true sex cord differentiation. Mod Pathol 2006;19(1):17–24.

77. Krishnamurthy S, Jungbluth AA, Busam KJ, et al. Uterine tumors resembling ovarian sex-cord tumors have an immunophenotype consistent with true sex-cord differentiation. Am J Surg Pathol 1998; 22(9):1078–82.

78. Kabbani W, Deavers MT, Malpica A, et al. Uterine tumor resembling ovarian sex-cord tumor: report of a case mimicking cervical adenocarcinoma. Int J Gynecol Pathol 2003;22(3):297–302.

79. Hurrell DP, McCluggage WG. Uterine tumour resembling ovarian sex cord tumour is an immunohistochemically polyphenotypic neoplasm which exhibits coexpression of epithelial, myoid and sex cord markers. J Clin Pathol 2007;60(10):1148–54.

80. Staats PN, Garcia JJ, Dias-Santagata DC, et al. Uterine tumors resembling ovarian sex cord tumors (UTROSCT) lack the JAZF1-JJAZ1 translocation frequently seen in endometrial stromal tumors. Am J Surg Pathol 2009;33(8):1206–12.

81. de Leval L, Lim GS, Waltregny D, et al. Diverse phenotypic profile of uterine tumors resembling ovarian sex cord tumors: an immunohistochemical study of 12 cases. Am J Surg Pathol 2010;34(12): 1749–61.

82. Fekete PS, Vellios F, Patterson BD. Uterine tumor resembling an ovarian sex-cord tumor: report of a case of an endometrial stromal tumor with foam cells and ultrastructural evidence of epithelial differentiation. Int J Gynecol Pathol 1985;4(4):378–87.

83. Moore M, McCluggage WG. Uterine tumour resembling ovarian sex cord tumour: first report of a large series with follow-up. Histopathology 2017;71(5):751–9.

84. Oliva E, Young RH, Amin MB, et al. An immunohistochemical analysis of endometrial stromal and smooth muscle tumors of the uterus: a study of 54 cases emphasizing the importance of using a panel because of overlap in immunoreactivity for individual antibodies. Am J Surg Pathol 2002;26(4):403–12.

85. Croce S, de Kock L, Boshari T, et al. Uterine tumor resembling ovarian sex cord tumor (UTROSCT) commonly exhibits positivity with sex cord markers FOXL2 and SF-1 but lacks FOXL2 and DICER1 mutations. Int J Gynecol Pathol 2016;35(4):301–8.

86. Wang J, Blakey GL, Zhang L, et al. Uterine tumor resembling ovarian sex cord tumor: report of a case with t(X;6)(p22.3;q23.1) and t(4;18)(q21.1;q21.3). Diagn Mol Pathol 2003;12(3):174–80.

87. Ou JJ, Tantravahi U, Pepperell JR, et al. Genome-wide copy number analysis of uterine tumors resembling ovarian sex cord tumors (UTROSCT). Mod Pathol 2016;29:301A.

88. Umeda S, Tateno M, Miyagi E, et al. Uterine tumors resembling ovarian sex cord tumors (UTROSCT) with metastasis: clinicopathological study of two cases. Int J Clin Exp Pathol 2014;7(3):1051–9.

89. Nucci MR, Schoolmeester JK, Sukov W, et al. Uterine tumors resembling ovarian sex cord tumor (UTROSCT) lack rearrangement of PHF1 by FISH. Mod Pathol 2014;27:298A.

90. Chiang S, Staats PN, Senz J, et al. FOXL2 mutation is absent in uterine tumors resembling ovarian sex cord tumors. Am J Surg Pathol 2015;39(5):618–23.

91. Dickson BC, Childs TJ, Colgan TJ, et al. Uterine Tumor Resembling Ovarian Sex Cord Tumor: A Distinct Entity Characterized by Recurrent NCOA2/3 Gene Fusions. Am J Surg Pathol 2018, [Epub ahead of print].

92. Lee FY, Wen MC, Wang J. Epithelioid leiomyosarcoma of the uterus containing sex cord-like elements. Int J Gynecol Pathol 2010;29(1):67–8.

93. Oliva E, Clement PB, Young RH. Endometrial stromal tumors: an update on a group of tumors with a protean phenotype. Adv Anat Pathol 2000;7(5): 257–81.

94. Clement PB, Scully RE. Mullerian adenosarcomas of the uterus with sex cord-like elements. A clinicopathologic analysis of eight cases. Am J Clin Pathol 1989;91(6):664–72.

95. Hirschfield L, Kahn LB, Chen S, et al. Mullerian adenosarcoma with ovarian sex cord-like differentiation. A light- and electron-microscopic study. Cancer 1986;57(6):1197–200.

96. Schoolmeester JK, Howitt BE, Hirsch MS, et al. Perivascular epithelioid cell neoplasm (PEComa) of the gynecologic tract: clinicopathologic and immunohistochemical characterization of 16 cases. Am J Surg Pathol 2014;38(2):176–88.

97. Folpe AL, Mentzel T, Lehr HA, et al. Perivascular epithelioid cell neoplasms of soft tissue and gynecologic origin: a clinicopathologic study of 26 cases and review of the literature. Am J Surg Pathol 2005;29(12):1558–75.

98. Vang R, Kempson RL. Perivascular epithelioid cell tumor ('PEComa') of the uterus: a subset of HMB-45-positive epithelioid mesenchymal neoplasms with an uncertain relationship to pure smooth muscle tumors. Am J Surg Pathol 2002;26(1):1–13.

99. Lim GS, Oliva E. The morphologic spectrum of uterine PEC-cell associated tumors in a patient with tuberous sclerosis. Int J Gynecol Pathol 2011;30(2): 121–8.

100. Silva EG, Bodurka DC, Scouros MA, et al. A uterine leiomyosarcoma that became positive for HMB45 in the metastasis. Ann Diagn Pathol 2005;9(1): 43–5.

101. Gyure KA, Hart WR, Kennedy AW. Lymphangiomyomatosis of the uterus associated with tuberous sclerosis and malignant neoplasia of the female genital tract: a report of two cases. Int J Gynecol Pathol 1995;14(4):344–51.

102. Agaram NP, Sung YS, Zhang L, et al. Dichotomy of genetic abnormalities in PEComas with therapeutic implications. Am J Surg Pathol 2015;39(6):813–25.

103. Silva EG, Deavers MT, Bodurka DC, et al. Uterine epithelioid leiomyosarcomas with clear cells: reactivity with HMB-45 and the concept of PEComa. Am J Surg Pathol 2004;28(2):244–9.

104. Bennett JA, Nardi V, Rouzbahman M, et al. Inflammatory myofibroblastic tumor of the uterus: a clinicopathological, immunohistochemical, and molecular analysis of 13 cases highlighting their broad morphologic spectrum. Mod Pathol 2017;30(10):1489–503.

105. Haimes JD, Stewart CJR, Kudlow BA, et al. Uterine inflammatory myofibroblastic tumors frequently harbor ALK fusions with IGFBP5 and THBS1. Am J Surg Pathol 2017;41(6):773–80.

106. Parra-Herran C, Quick CM, Howitt BE, et al. Inflammatory myofibroblastic tumor of the uterus: clinical and pathologic review of 10 cases including a subset with aggressive clinical course. Am J Surg Pathol 2015;39(2):157–68.

107. Rabban JT, Zaloudek CJ, Shekitka KM, et al. Inflammatory myofibroblastic tumor of the uterus: a clinicopathologic study of 6 cases emphasizing distinction from aggressive mesenchymal tumors. Am J Surg Pathol 2005;29(10):1348–55.

108. Coffin CM, Watterson J, Priest JR, et al. Extrapulmonary inflammatory myofibroblastic tumor (inflammatory pseudotumor). A clinicopathologic and immunohistochemical study of 84 cases. Am J Surg Pathol 1995;19(8):859–72.

109. Takahashi A, Kurosawa M, Uemura M, et al. Anaplastic lymphoma kinase-negative uterine inflammatory myofibroblastic tumor containing the ETV6-NTRK3 fusion gene: a case report. J Int Med Res 2018;46(8):3498–503.

110. Parra-Herran C, Schoolmeester JK, Yuan L, et al. Myxoid leiomyosarcoma of the uterus: a clinicopathologic analysis of 30 cases and review of the literature with reappraisal of its distinction from other uterine myxoid mesenchymal neoplasms. Am J Surg Pathol 2016;40(3):285–301.

Radiation-Associated Sarcomas
An Update on Clinical, Histologic, and Molecular Features

Jeffrey K. Mito, MD, PhD[a], Devarati Mitra, MD[b],
Leona A. Doyle, MD[a],*

KEYWORDS

• Soft tissue • Tumor • Sarcoma • Secondary malignancy • Radiation • Radiation-associated
• Immunohistochemistry • Molecular genetics

Key points

- Radiation-associated sarcomas represent approximately 5% of all sarcomas, but the incidence is expected to increase.

- Radiation-associated sarcomas arise in prior radiation fields at least 6 months after radiation therapy and should be histologically distinct from the primary malignancy.

- The most common histologic subtypes are angiosarcoma and unclassified sarcoma. Less common subtypes include leiomyosarcoma, malignant peripheral nerve sheath tumor, and osteosarcoma.

- High histologic grade, deep anatomic location, and positive resection margins are adverse prognostic features.

- Recurrent amplification of *MYC* and corresponding protein overexpression help distinguish atypical postradiation vascular proliferations from radiation-associated angiosarcoma.

ABSTRACT

pproximately half of all cancer patients receive radiation therapy as part of their oncologic treatment. Radiation-associated sarcomas occur in fewer than 1% of patients who receive radiation therapy but account for up to 5% of all sarcomas. As the use of radiation has increased in the past few decades and overall oncologic outcomes are improving, the incidence of radiation-associated sarcomas is also expected to increase. Historically, radiation-associated sarcomas have been associated with poor outcomes but recent data suggest the prognosis is improving. Distinguishing the sarcoma from the primary malignancy is a major diagnostic criterion.

OVERVIEW

Approximately 50% of patients with malignant neoplasms receive radiation therapy as part of their oncologic treatment.[1] Although radiation therapy can be effective at preventing disease recurrence, patients can also experience significant radiation-associated morbidity. One of the

---

The authors have no conflicts of interest to declare.
[a] Department of Pathology, Brigham and Women's Hospital, Harvard Medical School, 75 Francis Street, Boston, MA 02115, USA; [b] Department of Radiation Oncology, Brigham and Women's Hospital, Harvard Medical School, 75 Francis Street, Boston, MA 02115, USA
* Corresponding author.
E-mail address: ladoyle@bwh.harvard.edu

most feared late complications of radiation therapy is the development of secondary malignancies due to the carcinogenic effect of ionizing radiation. Secondary malignancy types include carcinoma (eg, breast and thyroid), mesothelioma, and sarcoma. Radiation-associated sarcomas are rare, occurring in fewer than 1% of patients who receive radiation therapy, but account for up to 5% of all sarcomas.[2–7] As the use of radiation therapy increases and the efficacy of oncologic therapy improves, there is a growing population of radiation-exposed cancer survivors from which the incidence of radiation-associated sarcomas is expected to grow.[8] Although many older studies have reported poor survival rates,[2,3,9] recent work from several groups suggests that this may no longer be the case.[4,10,11]

It can be difficult to determine whether a sarcoma is truly radiation induced or radiation associated rather than a local recurrence of the original malignancy or (less likely) an unrelated sarcoma. Careful clinical correlation and histologic review are required to make a diagnosis of radiation-associated sarcoma. Although precise criteria for defining a radiation-associated sarcoma have varied over time, the authors have adopted criteria similar to those defined by Cahan and Woodard[12] and others, specifically, (1) the tumor must arise within, or adjacent to, a previously irradiated field; (2) the tumor should arise at least 6 months after the cessation of radiation therapy; and (3) histologic confirmation of a sarcoma, distinct from a patient's prior malignancy, is needed.[4,13] The third criterion is often the most difficult to prove.

This article reviews the histologic and molecular features of radiation-associated sarcomas, potential diagnostic challenges, and clinical characteristics of patients with radiation-associated sarcomas, including current radiation therapy approaches, prognostication, and outcome data.

CLINICAL CHARACTERISTICS OF PATIENTS WITH RADIATION-ASSOCIATED SARCOMAS

Recent data show most patients with radiation-associated sarcomas are female (approximately 70%), reflecting the frequency of radiation therapy for the management of breast cancer, a common disease that is frequently cured with standard therapeutic approaches.[2,11,14] The median age of patients with radiation-associated sarcoma is approximately 60, but the range is wide because of the variable latency period between initial and secondary malignancy (months to >50 years) and the diverse patient population who receive radiation therapy. For instance, pediatric patients may develop radiation-associated sarcomas in their 20s, whereas those who receive radiation therapy for malignancies more common in older adults may develop radiation-associated tumors into their 80s or beyond. In a recent study, the median latency from primary malignancy to diagnosis of radiation-associated sarcoma was 11 years, with a significantly shorter median latency for patients with radiation-associated angiosarcoma of breast compared with patients with other types of radiation-associated sarcomas (8 years vs 15 years, respectively).[11]

Currently, the most common primary malignancy for which patients received radiation therapy and subsequently developed radiation-associated sarcoma is carcinoma of the breast.[11,13] This reflects the high incidence of this diagnosis and common use of breast-conserving therapy with lumpectomy followed by breast radiation.[14] The second most common group of patients with radiation-associated sarcomas is those who received radiation therapy for treatment of lymphoma.[11,13] It is likely, however, that the size of this population will diminish with time as treatment paradigms have shifted away from high-dose, large-volume radiation treatment fields, with many patients no longer receiving any radiation therapy due to the use of newer, effective, and well-tolerated chemotherapy agents. The remaining patients include those with primary gynecologic or prostatic primaries, unrelated sarcoma types, head and neck cancers, and colorectal cancer or germ cell tumors, all of which are commonly treated with radiation therapy.

The anatomic sites in which radiation-associated sarcomas arise reflect the initial radiation field, and, therefore, superficial locations on the chest wall or an extremity are most common, followed by deep cavitary body sites (intrathoracic and intra-abdominal/pelvic) and head and neck.[11,13]

CURRENT RADIATION THERAPY APPROACHES

Radiation dose and field are believed to play a significant role in the likelihood of developing a radiation-associated sarcoma. These parameters are affected by disease biology, anatomic location, and the overall oncologic management strategy (including the use of systemic therapy and surgical resection). Most cancer patients receive conventionally fractionated radiation administered 1.8 Gy to 2 Gy per day over the course of 5 weeks to 8 weeks; patients receiving definitive radiation without plans for surgical resection typically receive higher doses of radiation than patients receiving preoperative or postoperative radiation therapy. For example, prostate, head and neck, and cervical carcinomas are frequently managed successfully without surgical resection and, therefore, typically receive radiation doses in the 70-Gy to 80-Gy range. The biology of adjacent normal tissue also influences radiation dose and field. For example, most gastrointestinal malignancies receive 45 Gy to 50.4 Gy, because the surrounding bowel is only able to tolerate radiation doses up to this level before significant enteritis occurs. Analogously, most intrathoracic malignancies receive up 60 Gy to 66 Gy due to the sensitivity of lung parenchyma to large volumes of intermediate radiation dose levels. Another parameter that influences radiation dose and field is the anticipated frequency and site of local-regional recurrence. For example, for breast cancer, 50 Gy was the standard whole-breast radiation dose for many years, but because local-regional recurrence is most frequent at the site of initial disease, a boost dose of 10 Gy to 16 Gy was subsequently added to the lumpectomy cavity/mastectomy scar for a common total dose of 60 Gy to 66 Gy.

The technicalities of radiation therapy are constantly evolving, which complicates the extrapolation of prior radiation-associated malignancy risk factors with future risk. The most obvious example of this can perhaps be seen with mantle field radiation for Hodgkin lymphoma, which involved radiating large regions of the upper torso, including the neck, upper extremities, and mediastinum in typically young and otherwise healthy individuals, and resulted in a high rate of secondary breast cancer. In the modern era, this radiation approach is no longer performed, such that the risk of radiation-associated malignancy from the much smaller involved node, involved site, or involved field is less well characterized. In addition, there has been a recent increase in the use of hypofractionated radiation approaches, frequently with smaller radiation fields, and the resulting risk of secondary malignancy is similarly less understood.

Patient-specific factors also play an important role in the risk of secondary malignancy after radiation therapy. Inherited germline variants, such as deficiencies in the double-strand break repair pathway, result in uniquely high rates of secondary malignancy, such that radiation therapy is rarely used in these patients.[15]

HISTOLOGIC FEATURES OF RADIATION-ASSOCIATED SARCOMAS

The 2 most common histologic subtypes of radiation-associated sarcoma are angiosarcoma

and unclassified sarcoma.[11,16] Less common subtypes are malignant peripheral nerve sheath tumor (MPNST), leiomyosarcoma, osteosarcoma (either arising in soft tissue or bone), and, rarely, chondrosarcoma, dedifferentiated liposarcoma, and pleomorphic liposarcoma.[2,4,6,11,13,16] Unclassified sarcomas may have a predominant spindle cell, pleomorphic, or less often epithelioid cytomorphology (**Fig. 1A–D**). Similar to non–radiation-associated unclassified sarcomas, they lack any identifiable line of differentiation morphologically, immunohistochemically, and molecularly. It can be difficult to make this diagnosis confidently in patients previously radiated for carcinoma, when the differential diagnosis of sarcomatoid carcinoma should be considered. An approach to such cases includes careful evaluation for any areas with residual epithelial differentiation morphologically, for example, squamous or glandular or cohesive clusters or nests of epithelioid cells; evaluation of multiple broad-spectrum keratins, AE1/3, Pan-K, and CAM5.2 (p63 and GATA3 if there is a history of breast carcinoma or PAX8 if renal cell carcinoma); and evaluation of the clinical extent of disease, for example, multiple regional lymph node involvement may favor recurrent carcinoma. The lack of any of these features favors a diagnosis of sarcoma.

Classifiable histologic subtypes of radiation-associated sarcoma, such as MPNST (**Fig. 2**), leiomyosarcoma, and osteosarcoma (**Fig. 1E**), are morphologically and immunohistochemically similar to their non–radiation-associated counterparts. Because most MPNSTs arising after radiation are high grade, loss of H3Kme27 expression is a frequent finding.[17]

Although the mechanisms are uncertain, rare cases of translocation-associated sarcomas have been reported to occur as radiation-associated sarcomas, for example, synovial sarcoma.[18]

Radiation-associated sarcomas, in particular nonangiosarcomas, should be graded histologically where possible, using the French Fédération Nationale des Centres de Lutte Contre le Cancer grading system. Using this system, most radiation-associated sarcomas are morphologically high grade (51%).[11] High tumor grade in unclassified sarcomas is associated with a worse outcome on multivariate analysis.[11] Although less common, low-grade and intermediate-grade radiation-associated sarcomas are correspondingly associated with improved outcomes (**Fig. 1F**).

RADIATION-ASSOCIATED ANGIOSARCOMA

Most radiation-associated angiosarcomas arise in the breast after treatment of breast carcinoma,

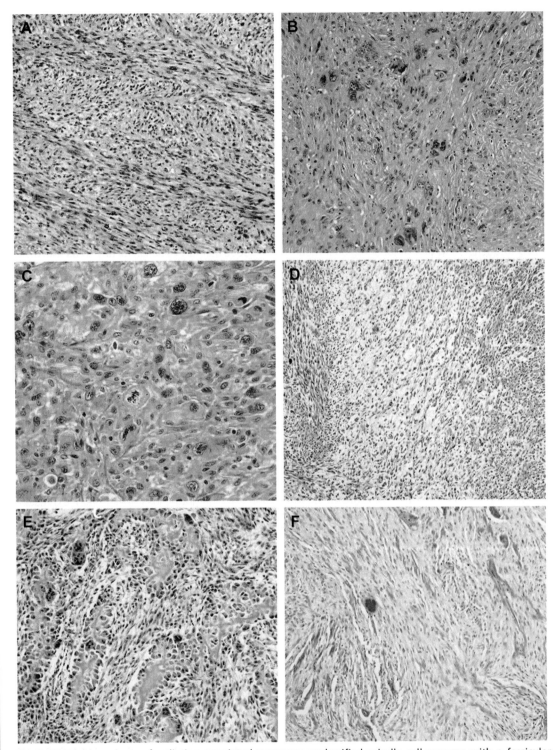

Fig. 1. Histologic variants of radiation-associated sarcomas: unclassified spindle cell sarcoma with a fascicular growth pattern and marked cytologic atypia (*A*). Unclassified pleomorphic sarcoma with numerous large, highly atypical and sometimes multinucleate giant cells (*B*). Some unclassified sarcomas have an epithelioid appearance (*C*) or a prominent myxoid stroma (*D*), mimicking other sarcoma types. Soft tissue osteosarcoma arising postradiation (*E*). Some unclassified radiation-associated sarcomas are morphologically low to intermediate grade, like this unclassified spindle cell sarcoma with mild cytologic atypia and scattered mitotic activity (*F*).

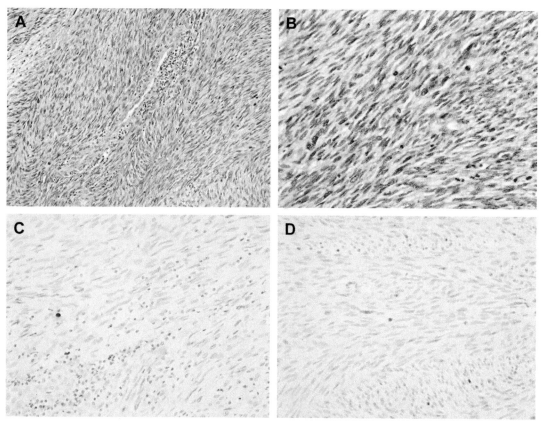

Fig. 2. MPNST showing a characteristic fascicular spindle cell pattern with perivascular accentuation (*A*), conspicuous cytologic atypia, and mitotic activity (*B*). Scattered S100-positive tumor cells are present (*C*), and there is loss of expression of H3Kme27 (*D*).

either for invasive or in situ disease. Radiation-associated angiosarcomas have a similar spectrum of morphologic features to non–radiation-associated angiosarcomas and can show vasoformative or solid areas and epithelioid or spindle cell cytomorphology (**Fig.** 3A–C). Similarly, expression of markers of endothelial differentiation, such as ERG and CD31, is present in greater than 90% of cases and CD34 expression in approximately 50%.

Atypical vascular proliferations/lesions (APRVPs) are relatively common in radiated skin, in the presence or absence of angiosarcoma, and can form a visible erythematous lesion. APRVP consists of dilated round or angulated vessels in the dermis lined by a single layer of endothelium that shows mild cytologic atypia, usually in the form of hyperchromasia or mild enlargement of endothelial cell nuclei (**Fig. 4**).[19] Whether these proliferations represent true precursor lesions or are a marker of increased risk of developing angiosarcoma is unclear, because most such lesions are clinically undetected. Although APRVP is usually readily identified

histologically, worrisome features such as endothelial multilayering, mitoses, or infiltrative growth, should warrant a diagnosis of angiosarcoma.

Amplification of *MYC* by fluorescence in situ hybridization (FISH) and corresponding MYC protein over-expression is detected in nearly 100% of secondary angiosarcomas (radiation-associated and chronic lymphedema-associated [**Fig.** 3D]) but not in APRVP.[20] Detection of MYC expression by immunohistochemistry can be diagnostically useful in 2 settings: (1) to distinguish angiosarcoma from florid APRVP or other benign vascular mimics and (2) to map the extent of disease in resections for angiosarcoma, especially when there has been neoadjuvant chemotherapy and only small amounts of residual angiosarcoma remain.

MYC expression, however, does not confirm that an angiosarcoma has arisen in the setting of radiation therapy: approximately 20% of non–radiation-associated cutaneous angiosarcomas (usually head and neck of elderly patients) show overexpression of MYC by IHC (a subset of which also show amplification by FISH),[21] and non–

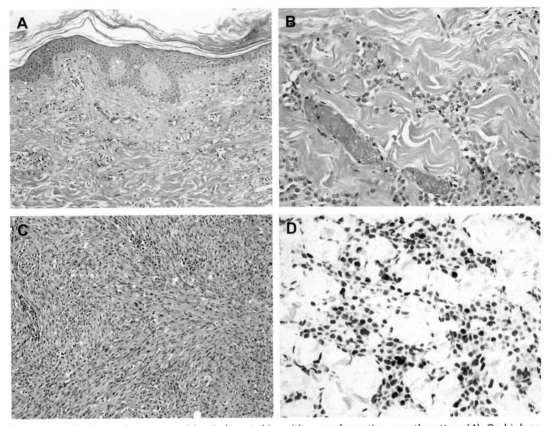

Fig. 3. Postradiation angiosarcoma arising in breast skin, with a vasoformative growth pattern (*A*). On high power, there are endothelial multilayering and atypia (*B*). Postradiation angiosarcoma of breast with a spindle cell morphology and solid growth; red blood cell extravasation and a relatively monotonous appearance to the tumor cells are characteristic (*C*). Nuclear MYC expression is present in almost all postradiation angiosarcomas (*D*).

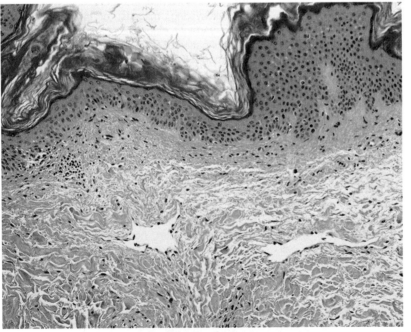

Fig. 4. Atypical postradiation vascular proliferations comprise slightly dilated or angulated thin-walled vessels (usually lymphatic in appearance) in the superficial or deep dermis, with at most mild endothelial cell atypia and without a dissecting architecture.

radiation-associated angiosarcoma of visceral sites (eg, liver and heart) may occasionally show MYC expression by IHC. Therefore, knowledge of the clinical context (history and anatomic location) is required for a diagnosis of radiation-associated angiosarcoma.

Grading of radiation-associated angiosarcomas imparts less prognostic association,[11] because, similar to non–radiation-associated angiosarcomas of breast,[22] many cases that appear morphologically well differentiated due to the presence of a predominantly vasoformative growth pattern pursue clinical courses similar to those with high-grade morphology.

MOLECULAR CHARACTERISTICS OF RADIATION-ASSOCIATED SARCOMAS

Ionizing radiation directly damages DNA, resulting in double-strand breaks, and generates reactive oxygen species that act on DNA to generate a variety of insults, including direct damage to bases, single-strand breaks, and DNA cross-linking. This damage results in a spectrum of molecular alterations from single-base substitutions to catastrophic genomic events. Similar to other environmental carcinogens (tobacco and ultraviolet radiation), a mutational signature characteristic of radiation is emerging. A small number of radiation-associated neoplasms (including 9 sarcomas) analyzed by whole-genome sequencing showed 2 main features.[23] First, compared with radiation-naïve tumors, radiation-associated neoplasms (including carcinomas and sarcomas) show a greater number of small deletions (with proportionately more deletions than insertions), a feature also described in BRCA1-associated and BRCA2-associated breast carcinoma. The second characteristic of this ionizing radiation signature is enrichment of balanced inversions, which are relatively less common in radiation-naïve tumors and are believed to result from chromothripsis and other forms of structural damage.[23] A transcriptome analysis of radiation-induced sarcomas has shown a signature of genes that are differentially expressed compared with non–radiation-induced sarcomas and which suggests a background of chronic oxidative stress based on the function of the genes involved.[24]

Targeted gene analysis has shown that TP53 mutations occur in approximately one-third of radiation-associated sarcomas in patients without hereditary predisposition syndromes and that inactivation of one allele is an early event in tumor formation.[25] The mutation pattern of TP53 in radiation-associated sarcomas differs from radiation-naïve/sporadic sarcomas, in that mutations are usually due to small deletions, with recurrent mutations at codons 135 and 237.[26]

When looking at specific histotypes, radiation-associated angiosarcoma is distinguished genetically by the consistent presence of high-level MYC amplification,[20,27,28] which is rare in sporadic angiosarcomas or other radiation-associated sarcoma types. MYC (chromosome 8q24) is a transcription factor involved in angiogenesis, among other processes, which functions as a proto-oncogene and is aberrantly expressed in numerous tumor types, in particular breast carcinoma, and, therefore, MYC expression does not distinguish sarcomatoid breast carcinoma from sarcoma. Coamplification of FLT4, a gene involved in lymphatic development, with MYC occurs in 25% of secondary angiosarcomas and may be associated with response to tyrosine kinase inhibitor therapy.[27]

There are still relatively few data on the genetics of other radiation-associated sarcoma types. MYC amplification has been reported to occur in unclassified sarcomas and leiomyosarcomas arising postradiation at a greater frequency than in sporadic counterparts, but not as often as in radiation-associated angiosarcomas. Amplification may be high level or low level, unlike postradiation angiosarcoma, which is usually always high level.[29] This finding is likely reflected in the usually low frequency and extent of immunohistochemical protein expression in nonangiosarcoma radiation-associated sarcomas (**Fig. 5**).[30]

PROGNOSTICATION AND CLINICAL MANAGEMENT OF RADIATION-ASSOCIATED SARCOMAS

Radiation-associated sarcomas have generally been considered to have a particularly poor prognosis among sarcomas, predominantly based on older literature reporting 5-year survival rates of 14% to 33%.[2,3] However, 2 recent studies have suggested that outcomes may be improving, with 5-year survival rates of 58% to 68%.[4,11] In the few large studies examining outcomes of patients with radiation-associated sarcomas, the following clinical and histologic features have been significantly associated with worse overall survival: positive margins, deep tumor location (intrathoracic or intra-abdominal), and high grade.[2,4,11,13] Correspondingly, low or intermediate tumor grade, superficial location, and margin-negative excision are associated with improved outcomes. The strongest driver for better outcome is complete surgical excision, and, therefore,

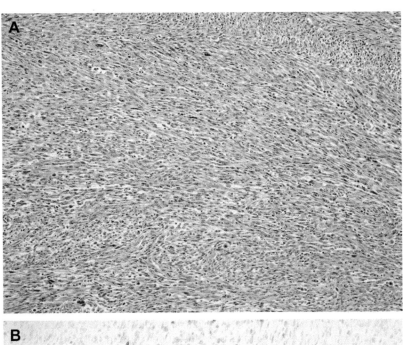

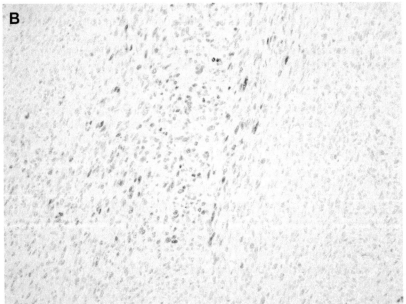

Fig. 5. Unclassified spindle cell sarcoma (*A*) with multifocal weak nuclear MYC expression (*B*). This tumor had low-level *MYC* amplification.

amenability to complete excision is also associated with improved outcome.

Some studies have reported differences in outcome based on histologic type. Radiation-associated MPNST has been shown to have a worse prognosis compared with other radiation-associated sarcomas.[4,7] Radiation-associated unclassified sarcomas have been shown to have a worse prognosis than their nonradiation-associated counterparts.[10] In a recent study, the authors' group found several differences between radiation-associated angiosarcoma of the breast

arising after treatment of breast carcinoma and other radiation-associated sarcomas.[11] Specifically, there is a shorter latency from time of initial radiation therapy to time of development of sarcoma (8 years vs 15 years) and a trend toward improved overall survival, with 3-year overall survival rates of 84% versus 68% and significantly fewer distant metastases.

The cornerstone of treatment is surgery for those patients with localized disease at presentation. Excision with microscopic negative margins results in significant survival differences compared with margin-positive excision. The use of reirradiation for the treatment of radiation-associated sarcoma has been associated with better outcomes in small studies.[7] Larger studies have not seen this association. Contemporary radiation techniques that allow more accurate targeting of the radiation dose may make this modality a more appropriate treatment in the future. Similar to other sarcomas, available chemotherapies include doxorubicin, olaratumab, pazopanib, trabectedin, and eribulin. Contemporary approaches to the management of radiation-associated angiosarcoma of the breast include neoadjuvant chemotherapy with tyrosine kinase inhibitors (usually sorafenib) followed by mastectomy and chest wall resection to include all radiated skin that may be at risk for development of future angiosarcoma.[31,32] In general, patients who receive radiation or chemotherapy for radiation-associated sarcomas often have more advanced disease than those who undergo surgical excision alone or have recurrent disease after surgery, and, therefore, this may act as a confounding factor when evaluating outcomes in this context.

FUTURE DIRECTIONS

Emerging data evaluating the genetic landscape of radiation-associated sarcomas have shown some differences between radiation-associated sarcomas and sporadic sarcomas, and a molecular mutational signature is starting to emerge.[23] Translating this into a clinically useful assay to distinguish true radiation-induced sarcomas from non–radiation-induced sarcomas or sarcomatoid carcinoma would make a significant impact on current diagnostic approaches.

Similar to other sarcomas, chemotherapy has limited efficacy in the management of advanced radiation-associated sarcomas. It is likely that more will be learned about the molecular pathogenesis of this tumor type in the near future, with the hope that effective therapeutic agents will eventually become available. With the approval of immune checkpoint inhibitors across various solid tumor types that are demonstrated to be mismatch-repair deficient, identification of mismatch repair deficiency and mutational burden load patterns in radiation-associated sarcomas will be of interest.[33,34]

Radiation therapy approaches that allow higher-dose conformality to the lesional area and reducing radiation to adjacent normal tissues have already improved the morbidity associated with radiation therapy. Whether this will result in a reduced risk of developing radiation-associated sarcomas is unknown but seems a reasonable hypothesis.

REFERENCES

1. Miller KD, Siegel RL, Lin CC, et al. Cancer treatment and survivorship statistics, 2016. CA Cancer J Clin 2016;66(4):271–89.
2. Bjerkehagen B, Smeland S, Walberg L, et al. Radiation-induced sarcoma: 25-year experience from the Norwegian Radium Hospital. Acta Oncol 2008; 47(8):1475–82.
3. Davidson T, Westbury G, Harmer CL. Radiation-induced soft-tissue sarcoma. Br J Surg 1986;73(4): 308–9.
4. Gladdy RA, Qin LX, Moraco N, et al. Do radiation-associated soft tissue sarcomas have the same prognosis as sporadic soft tissue sarcomas? J Clin Oncol 2010;28(12):2064–9.
5. Mavrogenis AF, Pala E, Guerra G, et al. Post-radiation sarcomas. Clinical outcome of 52 Patients. J Surg Oncol 2012;105(6):570–6.
6. Neuhaus SJ, Pinnock N, Giblin V, et al. Treatment and outcome of radiation-induced soft-tissue sarcomas at a specialist institution. Eur J Surg Oncol 2009;35(6):654–9.
7. Riad S, Biau D, Holt GE, et al. The clinical and functional outcome for patients with radiation-induced soft tissue sarcoma. Cancer 2012;118(10):2682–92.
8. Kim KS, Chang JH, Choi N, et al. Radiation-induced sarcoma: a 15-year experience in a single large tertiary referral center. Cancer Res Treat 2016;48(2):650–7.
9. Laskin WB, Silverman TA, Enzinger FM. Postradiation soft tissue sarcomas. An analysis of 53 cases. Cancer 1988;62(11):2330–40.
10. Dineen SP, Roland CL, Feig R, et al. Radiation-associated undifferentiated pleomorphic sarcoma is associated with worse clinical outcomes than sporadic lesions. Ann Surg Oncol 2015;22(12):3913–20.
11. Mito JKMD, Barysauskas CM, Fletcher CDM, et al. Clinicopathologic and prognostic features of radiation-associated sarcomas: a single institution study of 188 cases (93). Mod Pathol 2018;31(suppl 2):33.
12. Cahan WG, Woodard HQ, Higinbotham NL, et al. Sarcoma arising in irradiated bone; report of 11 cases. Cancer 1948;1(1):3–29.
13. Cha C, Antonescu CR, Quan ML, et al. Long-term results with resection of radiation-induced soft tissue sarcomas. Ann Surg 2004;239(6):903–9, [discussion: 909–10].
14. Bryant AK, Banegas MP, Martinez ME, et al. Trends in Radiation Therapy among Cancer Survivors in the United States, 2000-2030. Cancer Epidemiol Biomarkers Prev 2017;26(6):963–70.
15. Bernstein JL, Haile RW, Stovall M, et al. Radiation exposure, the ATM Gene, and contralateral breast cancer in the women's environmental cancer and

radiation epidemiology study. J Natl Cancer Inst 2010;102(7):475–83.

16. Salminen SH, Sampo MM, Bohling TO, et al. Radiation-associated sarcoma after breast cancer in a nationwide population: Increasing risk of angiosarcoma. Cancer Med 2018;7(9):4825–35.

17. Prieto-Granada CN, Wiesner T, Messina JL, et al. Loss of H3K27me3 expression is a highly sensitive marker for sporadic and radiation-induced MPNST. Am J Surg Pathol 2016;40(4):479–89.

18. Egger JF, Coindre JM, Benhattar J, et al. Radiation-associated synovial sarcoma: clinicopathologic and molecular analysis of two cases. Mod Pathol 2002; 15(9):998–1004.

19. Patton KT, Deyrup AT, Weiss SW. Atypical vascular lesions after surgery and radiation of the breast: a clinicopathologic study of 32 cases analyzing histologic heterogeneity and association with angiosarcoma. Am J Surg Pathol 2008; 32(6):943–50.

20. Mentzel T, Schildhaus HU, Palmedo G, et al. Post-radiation cutaneous angiosarcoma after treatment of breast carcinoma is characterized by MYC amplification in contrast to atypical vascular lesions after radiotherapy and control cases: clinico-pathological, immunohistochemical and molecular analysis of 66 cases. Mod Pathol 2012;25(1): 75–85.

21. Shon W, Sukov WR, Jenkins SM, et al. MYC amplification and overexpression in primary cutaneous angiosarcoma: a fluorescence in-situ hybridization and immunohistochemical study. Mod Pathol 2014;27(4): 509–15.

22. Nascimento AF, Raut CP, Fletcher CD. Primary angiosarcoma of the breast: clinicopathologic analysis of 49 cases, suggesting that grade is not prognostic. Am J Surg Pathol 2008;32(12):1896–904.

23. Behjati S, Gundem G, Wedge DC, et al. Mutational signatures of ionizing radiation in second malignancies. Nat Commun 2016;7:12605.

24. Hadj-Hamou NS, Ugolin N, Ory C, et al. A transcriptome signature distinguished sporadic from postradiotherapy radiation-induced sarcomas. Carcinogenesis 2011;32(6):929–34.

25. Gonin-Laurent N, Hadj-Hamou NS, Vogt N, et al. RB1 and TP53 pathways in radiation-induced sarcomas. Oncogene 2007;26(41):6106–12.

26. Gonin-Laurent N, Gibaud A, Huygue M, et al. Specific TP53 mutation pattern in radiation-induced sarcomas. Carcinogenesis 2006;27(6): 1266–72.

27. Guo T, Zhang L, Chang NE, et al. Consistent MYC and FLT4 gene amplification in radiation-induced angiosarcoma but not in other radiation-associated atypical vascular lesions. Genes Chromosomes Cancer 2011;50(1):25–33.

28. Manner J, Radlwimmer B, Hohenberger P, et al. MYC high level gene amplification is a distinctive feature of angiosarcomas after irradiation or chronic lymphedema. Am J Pathol 2010;176(1):34–9.

29. Kacker C, Marx A, Mossinger K, et al. High frequency of MYC gene amplification is a common feature of radiation-induced sarcomas. Further results from EORTC STBSG TL 01/01. Genes Chromosomes Cancer 2013;52(1):93–8.

30. Mito JK, Jo VY, Doyle LA. MYC expression and loss of histone H3K27 trimethylation are infrequent among unclassified radiation-associated sarcomas (94). Mod Pathol 2018;31(suppl 2):33.

31. Li GZ, Fairweather M, Wang J, et al. Cutaneous radiation-associated breast angiosarcoma: radicality of surgery impacts survival. Ann Surg 2017; 265(4):814–20.

32. Morgan EA, Kozono DE, Wang Q, et al. Cutaneous radiation-associated angiosarcoma of the breast: poor prognosis in a rare secondary malignancy. Ann Surg Oncol 2012;19(12):3801–8.

33. Le DT, Uram JN, Wang H, et al. PD-1 blockade in tumors with mismatch-repair deficiency. N Engl J Med 2015;372(26):2509–20.

34. Nebot-Bral L, Brandao D, Verlingue L, et al. Hypermutated tumours in the era of immunotherapy: The paradigm of personalised medicine. Eur J Cancer 2017;84:290–303.

SWI/SNF Complex-Deficient Soft Tissue Neoplasms

A Pattern-Based Approach to Diagnosis and Differential Diagnosis

Abbas Agaimy, MD

KEYWORDS

- Rhabdoid tumor • Epithelioid sarcoma • Undifferentiated pediatric sarcoma
- Extraskeletal myxoid chondrosarcoma • Myoepithelial carcinoma • SWI/SNF complex • SMARCB1
- INI1 • SMARCA4

Key points

- The family of SWI/SNF-driven neoplasia is expanding rapidly.

- Biologic, prognostic and therapeutic heterogeneity of these neopalsms underline their differential diagnostic complexity.

- Many of SWI/SNF-deficient neoplasms have not much in common other than the SWI/SNF deregulation.

- Considering topographic, demographic and phenotypic chatacteritics is pivotal for correct diagnosis.

ABSTRACT

Loss of different components of the Switch/sucrose nonfermentable (SWI/SNF) chromatin remodeling complex has been increasingly recognized as a central molecular event driving the initiation and/or dedifferentiation of mostly lethal but histogenetically diverse neoplasms in different body organs. This review summarizes and discusses the morphologic and phenotypic diversity of primary soft tissue neoplasms characterized by SWI/SNF complex deficiency with an emphasis on convergent and divergent cytoarchitectural patterns.

OVERVIEW

THE SWI/SNF COMPLEX: STRUCTURE AND FUNCTION

The switch/sucrose nonfermentable (SWI/SNF) complex is a multisubunit system composed of a large group of genes mapping to different chromosomal regions but functioning in a highly coordinated, albeit complex, ATP-ase dependent manner.[1,2] The complex is involved in the process of chromatin remodeling and hence close monitoring of transcriptional regulation.[1,2] Via its enrichment at promoters and enhancers of active genes, the SWI/SNF complex determines which genes are to be expressed and, through this, contributes to the regulation of cell differentiation and cell proliferation processes.[3,4] It is this close regulation of the transcription, and hence the cellular differentiation, that is responsible for the distinctive cytoarchitectural morphology of SWI/SNF-driven neoplasia, which ranges from fully anaplastic to well-differentiated organotypical lesions (Table 1). From a simplified oncopathogenic point of view, the SWI/SNF complex functions collectively as a tumor suppressor.[5] Accordingly, the inactivation of any of its constituent components is frequently associated with tumor initiation and/or progression.[5]

Grant support to this study: none.
Disclosure/Conflict of Interest: The author has no conflicts of interest or NIH finding to disclose.
Institute of Pathology, Friedrich-Alexander University Erlangen-Nürnberg (FAU), University Hospital, Krankenhausstrasse 8-10, 91054 Erlangen, Germany
E-mail address: abbas.agaimy@uk-erlangen.de

Surgical Pathology 12 (2019) 149–163
https://doi.org/10.1016/j.path.2018.10.006

Table 1
Common cytoarchitectural patterns in SWI/SNF-deficient soft tissue neoplasms and their main differential diagnoses

Rhabdoid/large cell pattern	Genetic marker/s
Epithelioid sarcoma, proximal	SMARCB1 loss (very rarely, SMARCA4 loss)
MRT, pediatric	SMARCB1 loss (98%); SMARCA4 loss (2%)
SCCOHT, large cell type	SMARCA4 loss
Epithelioid MPNST	SMARCB1 loss (50%)
Undifferentiated/dedifferentiated carcinomas	Loss of variable SWI/SNF subunits, site dependent
Epithelioid/histiocytoid (bland)	
Epithelioid sarcoma, distal	SMARCB1 loss
Undifferentiated round cell morphology	
SCCOHT, classical type	SMARCA4 loss
Undifferentiated pediatric sarcomas (variant MRT!)	SMARCB1 loss
Chordoma, poorly differentiated, pediatric	SMARCB1 loss
Small cell synovial sarcoma	SS18-SSX fusion + frequent SMARCB1 loss
Myxoid/chordoid (EMC-like)	
Extraskeletal myxoid chondrosarcoma	*EWSR1-NR4A3* fusion; SMARCB1 loss (20%)
Myoepithelial carcinoma	Diverse gene fusions; SMARCB1 loss (40% pediatric; 10% adults cases)
Chordoma, poorly differentiated, pediatric	SMARCB1 loss
Primary intracranial myxoid sarcoma	*EWSR1-CREB* fusions; SMARCB1 loss (likely mutually exclusive with *EWSR1-CREB* fusions)
Primary pulmonary myxoid sarcoma	EWSR1-CREB fusions; SMARCB1 loss (Single case reported; mutually exclusive with *EWSR1-CREB* fusion)
Myxoid epithelioid sarcoma (rare)	SMARCB1 loss

Abbreviations: EMC, extraskeletal myxoid chondrosarcoma; MPNST, malignant peripheral nerve sheath tumor; MRT, malignant rhabdoid tumor; SCCOHT, small cell carcinoma of ovary, hypercalcemic type; SWI/SNF, Switch/sucrose nonfermentable.

Several recent studies reported inactivating mutations in genes encoding different SWI/SNF subunits in a variety of cancers at a surprisingly high overall frequency (>20%), approaching the frequency of *TP53* mutations in cancer.[3–5] The SWI/SNF mutations and other passenger or driver gene mutations such as *TP53* are not mutually exclusive, an observation that might explain the phenotypic heterogeneity of the SWI/SNF-related malignancies.[5,6]

SMARCB1

The SWI/SNF-related, matrix associated, actin-dependent regulator of chromatin, subfamily B, member 1 (SMARCB1; synonyms: integrase interactor 1 [INI1]; BAF47, hSNF5, etc.), is a core subunit of the SWI/SNF complex encoding a 47-Kda protein, mapping to chromosome 22q11.2.[7] SMARCB1 is responsible for the functional integrity of the SWI/SNF complex and is closely involved in the transcriptional processes and in the cell-cycle regulation via interactions with several cell-cycle–regulating molecules, including pRb and HDAC1.[7] Being evolutionarily highly conserved, SMARCB1 is ubiquitously expressed in all types of human normal tissues.[8] Loss of SMARCB1 protein expression results from biallelic inactivation caused by different types of deleterious genetic and/or epigenetic errors.[9,10]

SMARCB1–DEFICIENT SOFT TISSUE NEOPLASMS: MORPHOTYPIC VARIATIONS

With a few exceptions, SMARCB1-deficient soft tissue neoplasms are unified by the presence of a varying component of rhabdoid cells.[6] The "hallmark" rhabdoid cell possesses 1 or 2 large vesicular nuclei containing a very thin rim of marginated chromatin, a centrally located eosinophilic macronucleolus, and a large paranuclear filamentous cytoplasmic inclusion, the "rhabdoid body," which displaces the nucleus to the periphery of the cell. The term rhabdoid was first coined by Beckwith and Palmer for an aggressive variant of Wilms' tumor composed of cells mimicking rhabdomyoblasts but lacking true rhabdomyosarcomatous differentiation.[11] Subsequently, the term "malignant rhabdoid tumor (MRT) of the kidney" has been coined for this distinctive entity.[12] The presence and extent of the rhabdoid cell component in SMARCB1-deficient neoplasms varies greatly within same tumor and among different neoplasms from being totally absent to uniformly present (100%) throughout.[6]

However, with increasing characterization of the SWI/SNF-deficient tumor family, the morphologic landscape of this group of neoplasms has been evolving dynamically thereby highlighting significant morphotypic, immunophenotypic, and molecular–genetic heterogeneity.[6] In brief, SWI/SNF-deficient neoplasms fall into 1 of 5 major morphologic (cytoarchitectural) categories: (1) prototypic rhabdoid, (2) anaplastic nondescript large cell, (3) small round cell, (4) myxoid chordoid, and (5) heterogeneous differentiated organotypical categories or variable combination thereof (Box 1).

SMARCB1–DEFICIENT SOFT TISSUE NEOPLASMS WITH RHABDOID/EPITHELIOID MORPHOLOGY

Pediatric central ([AT/RT] atypical teratoid/rhabdoid tumor) of the central nervous system) and noncentral (renal and extrarenal) MRTs are the prototypes of this category. They are indistinguishable on the basis of morphologic and phenotypic features alone (Box 2). They may occur as single diseases or multifocal (synchronous or metachronous) involving both central and peripheral (eg, kidney or soft tissue) body sites.[13,14] Distinguishing primary multifocal disease in the setting of SMARCB1 germline mutations from oligometastatic disease is rather arbitrary or impossible. Extrarenal MRT may occur at any soft tissue sites or within parenchymal visceral organs such as liver, urinary bladder, and others. Affected are mainly children 3 years of age

---

Box 1
Morphologic categories of SWI/SNF–deficient soft tissue neoplasms

1. Prototypical rhabdoid

2. Anaplastic nondescript large cell

3. Small round cell

4. Myxoid chordoid

5. Heterogeneous differentiated organotypical

Box 2
Key features of pediatric malignant rhabdoid tumors

Affect patients ≤3 years of age

May be unifocal or multifocal, frequently widespread

Poor prognosis

Aside from loss of SMARCB1, immunophenotype is variable and nonspecific

---

or younger. Most patients present with widespread metastatic disease and die within 1 or 2 years.[15,16] MRTs are composed of large monotonous undifferentiated tumor cells that are strikingly rhabdoid in appearance (Fig. 1A, B).[15,16] Others display large anaplastic cells with similar nuclear morphology, but frequently with more conspicuous macronucleoli (Fig. 1C). Other less common patterns include small round cell (Fig. 1D) and spindled (Fig. 1E) morphologies that may represent focal findings in otherwise conventional variants or predominate, thus representing a diagnostic challenge. Distinguishing MRTs of soft tissue from proximal-type (large cell) epithelioid sarcoma on morphologic grounds alone is rather arbitrary as the extent of the rhabdoid differentiation might be the only features that help their distinction (described elsewhere in this article). Other than demonstrating the loss of SMARCB1 in the neoplastic cells, immunohistochemistry is of little help to subtype those predominantly rhabdoid malignancies in childhood because the majority tend to coexpress pancytokeratins and vimentin with variable nonconsistent and nonreproducible coexpression of diverse other primitive markers including CD34 and neural markers (Fig. 1F). However, pediatric MRTs may display nonrhabdoid morphology and, particularly because biopsy material is frequently limited, immunohistochemistry is mandatory to confirm SMARCB1 loss and rule out other differential diagnoses.

The concept of pure extrarenal MRTs as a single disease entity has been later challenged by the observation of similarly rhabdoid cells forming a component in otherwise differentiated neoplasms occurring at a wider age range, leading to the conceptualization of composite extrarenal rhabdoid tumors as a common final pathway of dedifferentiation in a variety of neoplasms.[17] In contrast with earlier studies showing intact SMARCB1 locus in composite extrarenal rhabdoid tumors,[18] several recent studies from different organs confirmed the occurrence of true composite neoplasms composed of a differentiated (organ-specific, SWI/

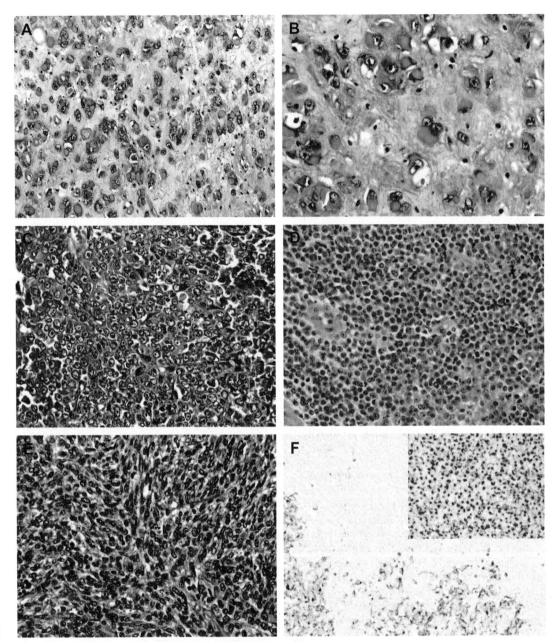

Fig. 1. The morphologic spectrum of pediatric malignant rhabdoid tumors varies greatly from extensively rhabdoid (*A, B*), to large cell anaplastic (*C*), small round cell (*D*) and spindled (*E*). Pankeratin is variably expressed with variable loss (*F*; main image). Diffuse and strong paranuclear vimentin is a consistent feature in nearly all cases (inset) (H&E, original magnification [*A*] ×200; [*B–E*] ×400) (*F*, Pancytokeratin immunostain, original magnification ×100 Inset: Vimentin immunostain, original magnification ×200).

SNF intact) and an SWI/SNF-deficient undifferentiated variably rhabdoid component driven by secondary SWI/SNF gene deletions/inactivation.[19,20]

EPITHELIOID SARCOMA

Epithelioid sarcoma is a distinctive soft tissue neoplasm with predilection for young adult males (**Box 3**). The prototypical (classical)

epithelioid sarcoma occurs predominantly in the subcutaneous or deep soft tissue of the distal parts of the extremities; hence, the designation distal type.[21] The tumor is composed predominantly of relatively bland-looking histiocytoid epithelioid cells with eosinophilic cytoplasm disposed into multiple nodules frequently featuring central palisaded necrosis, imparting a granuloma-like

---

Box 3
Key features of epithelioid sarcoma

Distal type

    Predominately arises in subcutaneous tissue of extremities

    Bland histiocytoid cells with frequent central palisaded necrosis

Proximal type

    Predilection for limb girdles and deep pelviperineal soft tissue

    Large undifferentiated anaplastic cells with high grade nuclear features and prominent nucleoli

    Significant morphologic overlap with pediatric malignant rhabdoid tumor

    Affects adults

    Usually unifocal at presentation

---

appearance (**Fig. 2**A, B).[21–23] This pattern is responsible for epithelioid sarcoma being frequently overlooked as benign granulomatous or reactive lesion.[21]

The proximal-type epithelioid sarcoma occurs mainly more proximally or axially around limb girdles with a striking predilection for deep soft tissues of the pelviperineal area.[24] Infrequently, other sites of the extremities and distal sites similar to the classical type may be observed as well.[24] This variant is characterized by large, undifferentiated, anaplastic-looking cells with high-grade nuclear features, prominent central nucleoli, and a variable rhabdoid cell component (**Fig. 2**C). Proximal-type epithelioid sarcoma may show significant morphologic overlap with pediatric MRT and the undifferentiated rhabdoid or anaplastic carcinoma variants reported in the pancreas and other gastrointestinal sites.[19,20] Accordingly, diagnosis and distinction from metastatic undifferentiated carcinoma (may be SMARCB1-deficient as well) essentially relies on primary soft tissue origin and absence of another visceral primary. On occasion, the rhabdoid component may be as prominent so as to suggest the alternative diagnosis of MRT.[25] As stated elsewhere in this article, distinction of the 2 depends on clinical and demographic features of the 2 diseases rather than morphology alone. In contrast with MRT, proximal-type epithelioid sarcoma usually present as localized, nonmetastatic soft tissue mass involving the proximal extremities or the pelviperineal area in adults with a mean age of 42 years.[24] This finding is in sharp contrast with the clinical presentation of the pediatric MRTs.[15,16]

Epithelioid sarcoma has a high propensity for local recurrences and may eventually metastasize to regional lymph nodes or to distant sites.[21,22] A consistent presence of a rhabdoid component in the large cell (proximal) type and its absence in the classical type is in line with the more aggressive course of the former.

The histopathologic spectrum of epithelioid sarcoma, in particular the proximal variant, varies greatly. Uncommon features include fibroma-like, angiomatoid, hemangiopericytoma-like, signet ring cells, prominent osteoclastic giant cells, spindling, and small round cell-like patterns (**Fig. 2**D–F).[21–26] A subset of cases may show transition to classical areas (mixed type epithelioid sarcoma).[21,22,27] Similar to SWI/SNF-deficient neoplasms in general, immunohistochemistry shows strong coexpression of vimentin, pancytokeratin, and epithelial membrane antigen (EMA) in most cases of epithelioid sarcoma irrespective of the subtype. EMA is valuable in those more challenging keratin-poor tumors. Up to one-half of the cases express also CD34 and variably ERG, although expression of the latter might be influenced by antibody or clone seleection.[28–30] SMARCB1 loss resulting from biallelic deletion of the *SMARCB1* gene locus defines both types of epithelioid sarcoma (see **Fig. 2**F).[31,32] However, the frequency of SMARCB1 loss in epithelioid sarcoma varies depending on the diagnostic criteria applied in different studies and ranges from 80% to 100%.[31] Recent studies suggested involvement of other SWI/SNF members in the pathogenesis of SMARCB1-proficient cases. Loss of SMARCA4, SMARCC1, and SMARCC2 was observed in 2, 1, and 1 of 6 SMARCB1-proficient proximal type epithelioid sarcomas, respectively.[33] Although concurrent loss of additional SWI/SNF subunits such as PBRM1 (seen in 74% of epithelioid sarcomas) did not correlate with morphology, concurrent loss of BRM, PBRM1, and SMARCB1 expression was detected in cases with pure rhabdoid features in same study.[34]

DOES PARENCHYMAL/VISCERAL EPITHELIOID SARCOMA EXIST?

A rare subset of visceral carcinomas may undergo secondary rhabdoid transformation as a consequence of SMARCB1 loss or loss of other SWI/SNF markers during tumor progression. Such neoplasms shave been reported from the gastroenteropancreatic and genitourinary tracts with or without detectable differentiated epithelial component.[6,19,20] Although the anaplastic or rhabdoid component of these composite neoplasms is indistinguishable from the

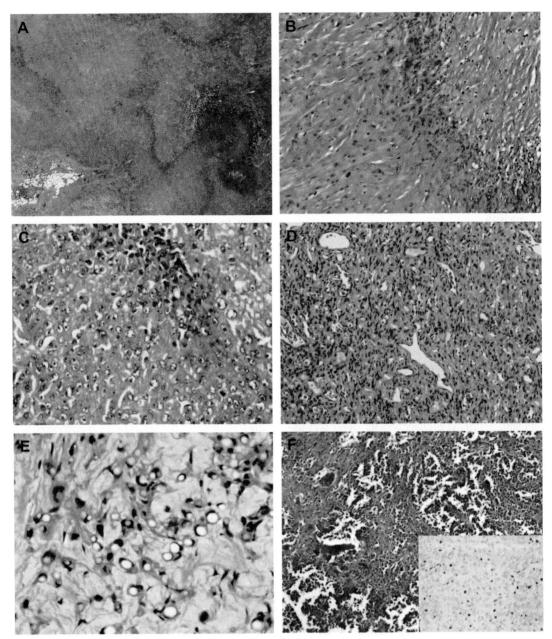

Fig. 2. Histologic variation of epithelioid sarcoma. Prominent hyalinizing or necrotizing "palisaded granuloma"-like pattern is characteristic of distal type epithelioid sarcoma (*A, B*). On the contrary, the proximal type features highly anaplastic large cells with vesicular chromatin and macronucleoli indistinguishable from anaplastic variants of carcinoma and other malignancies (*C*). Uncommon patterns in proximal epithelioid sarcoma include hemangiopericytoma-like (*D*), signet ring cells mimicking carcinoma or epithelioid hemangioendothelioma (*E*) and papillary architecture with prominent osteoclastic giant cells (*F*). SMARCB1 loss (*F*, inset) is a defining feature of both types of epithelioid sarcoma (H&E, original magnification [*A*] ×100; [*B*] ×200; [*C*] ×400; [*D*] ×200; [*E*] ×400; [*F*] ×200, Inset: SMARCB1 immunostain, ×400).

proximal type epithelioid sarcoma of soft tissue, including even aberrant expression of CD34 in some cases, thereby justifying naming them as such in the view of some authors,[35,36] current genetic and demographic evidence indicates their unequivocal epithelial origin from the mucosa (as carcinoma variants) and argues against classifying them as visceral epithelioid sarcomas.[19,20]

A recently reported variant of dedifferentiated (mainly retroperitoneal) liposarcoma is composed predominantly or exclusively of rhabdoid/epithelioid cells indistinguishable from the proximal type of epithelioid sarcoma, MRT, and undifferentiated rhabdoid carcinomas, and showed variable expression of pancytokeratin as well. Fortunately, all these cases were found to have intact SWI/SNF expression and instead are characterized by coexpression and/or amplification of MDM2 and CDK4.[37,38] Other malignancies that may display a prominent rhabdoid morphology include rhabdoid melanoma and epithelioid/rhabdoid rhabdomyosarcoma; both of these retain their defining immunophenotypic features and do not show SWI/SNF loss.

SMARCB1-DEFICIENT PERIPHERAL NERVE SHEATH TUMORS

Loss of SMARCB1 expression is observed in around 50% to 67% of epithelioid malignant peripheral nerve sheath tumors (MPNST).[39,40] Epithelioid MPNSTs are composed of monotonous epithelioid cells with nuclear features not different from the anaplastic-looking large cells of a proximal-type epithelioid sarcoma. In addition, variable but usually less conspicuous rhabdoid cell features and myxoid stromal changes might be seen as well, which would suggest the possibility of MRT or myoepithelial carcinoma (Fig. 3A, B). Fortunately, epithelioid MPNST retains uniform expression of Schwann cell markers (S100, SOX10), a feature highly valuable in distinguishing them from MRT, epithelioid sarcoma, and epithelioid malignant melanoma (epithelioid malignant melanoma frequently retains expression of specific melanocytic markers such as melanoma cocktail and HMB45).[39,40] Rare cases of SMARCB1-deficient epithelioid MPNST developed within neuroblastoma-like schwannoma in patients with the rhabdoid tumor predisposition syndrome type 1 and neuroblastoma-like schwannomatosis caused by a SMARCB1 germline mutation.[41,42] Very recently, loss of SMARCB1 has been reported in 42% of benign epithelioid

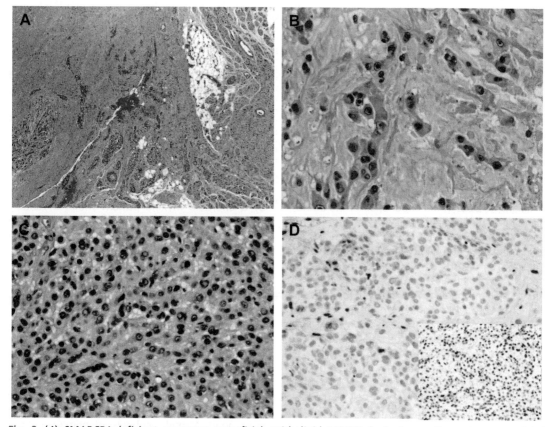

Fig. 3. (A) SMARCB1-deficient recurrent superficial epithelioid MPNST (note traumatic neuroma on right) showing prominent myxoid changes and large epithelioid cells with macronucleoli (B). (C) Cells of this epithelioid schwannoma are not atypical and showed variable nuclear vacuolation, loss of SMARCB1 (D) and retained strong diffuse SOX10 expression (D, inset) (SMARCB1 immunostain, ×200; Inset: SOX10 immunostain, ×200) (H&E, original magnification [A] ×100; [B] x200; [C] x200).

schwannomas, confirming the notion that SMARCB1 loss per se is not indicative of malignancy or aggressiveness (**Fig. 3**C, D).[43]

According to recent studies, 10% and 50% of patients with sporadic and familial schwannomatosis carry germline *SMARCB1* mutations, respectively.[42,44,45] Multiple (usually nonvestibular) schwannomas in this syndromic setting tend to show neuroblastoma-like morphology and to display SMARCB1 mosaic staining pattern.[44,45]

SWI/SNF ALTERATIONS IN SMALL ROUND CELL NEOPLASMS

A nondescript, small, round cell morphology is occasionally encountered in several SWI/SNF-deficient malignancies. Small cell carcinoma of the ovary, hypercalcemic type (SCCOHT) is the prototype of this category.[46] In its classical (name-giving) form, SCCOHT displays diffuse sheets of small hyperchromatic cells frequently interrupted by variably dilated cystic (follicle-like) spaces containing pale secretory material.[46] SCCOHT is uniformly SMARCA4/SMARCA2 deficient, making SMARCA4 loss detected by immunohistochemistry a highly valuable and defining diagnostic marker for this entity.[47,48] In line with their neoplastic nature, the cells lining these pseudofollicular spaces are similarly SMARCA4 deficient (**Fig. 4**A, B). On rare occasions, SMARCA4-deficient malignancies indistinguishable from the large cell variant of SCCOHT do occur in retroperitoneal soft tissues. Such rare lesions might represent predominantly rhabdoid variants of SMARCA4-driven proximal epithelioid sarcomas, extension from a SMARCA4-deficient renal cell carcinoma, or metastasis from SMARCA4-deficient NSCLC. In the experience of the author, almost all patients diagnosed with undifferentiated SMARCA4-deficient soft tissue malignancies are found to have lung primary (Agaimy, unpublished data, 2018). SMARCB1-deficient undifferentiated pediatric malignancies (sarcomas) showing small round cell morphology have been reported as well. They probably represent nonrhabdoid small cell variants of MRT.[49,50] The nosologic classification of similarly undifferentiated small round cell lesions in adults remains unclear (**Fig. 3**E, F).

Small cell synovial sarcoma is an important consideration when encountering SMARCB1-deficient undifferentiated round cell sarcomas, particularly in young adults (**Fig. 3**C, D). Several older and recent studies have suggested close relationship of the *SS18* (SYT) gene to the SWI/SNF complex.[51] Indeed, co-localization and interaction of SMARCA2 with SYT and SYT-SSX proteins in the nucleus in vitro was proposed as explanation of gene transcription activation via the SYT protein.[51]

A distinctive pattern of SMARCB1 expression in synovial sarcoma was reported in several studies with the majority (up to 100%) showing reduced expression and up to 21% complete loss.[52–55] While no correlation was seen with the histologic subtype or presence or absence of rhabdoid cells, complete loss of SMARCB1 seems to be much frequent among poorly differentiated small cell synovial sarcomas. This feature is in sharp contrast with retained expression of SMARCB1 in other histologically comparable sarcoma types such as fibrosarcoma and conventional MPNST and might be of differential diagnostic relevance but this remains to be verified. While the mechanisms leading to SMARCB1 loss in synovial sarcoma remains obscure, a recent study suggested post-transcriptional mechanisms as the most likely cause of the altered SMARCB1 expression in synovial sarcoma.[56]

MYXOID PATTERN SMARCB1–DEFICIENT SOFT TISSUE NEOPLASMS

Although rare in pediatric MRT (**Fig. 5**A–C), variable myxoid features are not uncommon in proximal type epithelioid sarcoma (**Fig. 5**D, E) and many other SWI/SNF-deficient neoplasms. SMARCB1 loss has been demonstrated in subsets of soft tissue myoepithelial carcinomas (40% of pediatric and 10% of adult cases), extraskeletal myxoid chondrosarcomas (20%) and poorly differentiated chordomas, the latter particularly in pediatric patients.[39,57–60] Notably, all these entities are characterized morphologically by a chordoid myxoid pattern within a variably myxoid background and they coexpress vimentin and variably pancytokeratin. Furthermore, some if not most of them have to some extent myoepithelial-like immunophenotypic features. However, irrespective of the SMARCB1 status, the exact diagnosis of these entities is based mainly on phenotypic (brachyury in chordoma), genotypic (*EWSR1-NR4A3* gene fusion in extraskeletal myxoid chondrosarcoma) or a combination of both (as in cases of myoepithelial carcinomas).

Moreover, recent observations pointed to SMARCB1 loss as the likely alternative event in neoplasms known to be *EWSR1-CREB* rearranged. Namely, subsets of primary pulmonary myxoid sarcoma and intracranial myxoid sarcoma, both known to be driven by *EWSR1-CREB* gene rearrangements,[61,62] harbored no detectable *EWSR1* aberrations and, instead,

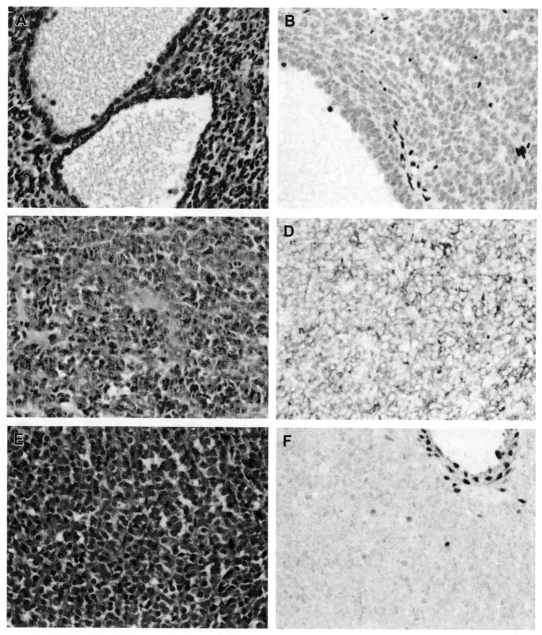

Fig. 4. Nondescript small round cell morphology is uncommon but characteristic feature in a subset of SWI/SNF-deficient neoplasms. (*A*) Classic variant of small cell carcinoma of ovary, hypercalcemic type. (*B*) SMARCA4 is lost both in the diffuse sheets and the cells lining the pseudofollicular cystic spaces (the faint nuclear staining in some cells is nonspecific). (*C*) This primary soft tissue malignancy of distal extremity showed small round cell morphology, expressed only vimentin and EMA (H&E, original magnification ×400) (*D*) and showed SMARCB1 loss, suggesting variant of epithelioid sarcoma or analogous to pediatric undifferentiated SMARCB1-lost round cell sarcomas) (EMA immunostain, ×400). Small cell synovial sarcoma (H&E, original magnification ×400) (*E*) frequently shows total loss of SMARCB1 (*F*) in contrast with the reduced or heterogeneous pattern in other variants (SMARCB1 immunostain, ×400).

were SMARCB1-deficient (**Fig. 5**F).[63,64] The subject became even more complicated by the recent study by Huang and colleagues[65] demonstrating simultaneous *EWSR1* involvement detectable by

FISH in the context of 22q11.2 regional alterations in *SMARCB1*-deleted neoplasms. Accordingly, and as stated above, diagnosis of these biologically distinctive but morphologically

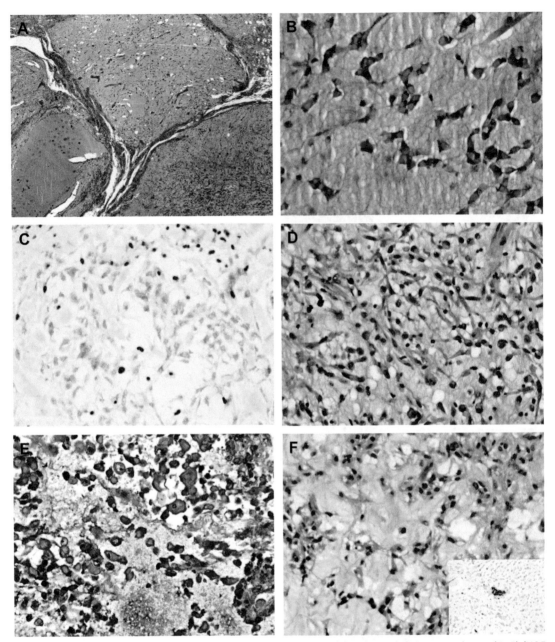

Fig. 5. Prominent myxoid chordoid pattern can be seen in a variety of SWI/SNF-deficient neoplasms. (*A*, *B*) (H&E, original magnification [*A*] ×100; [*B*] ×200) dermal/subcutaneous malignant rhabdoid tumor with close resemblance to pediatric myoepithelial carcinoma but lacking any myoepithelial phenotypic features (note uniformly rhabdoid cytology). (*C*) SMARCB1 is lost in the neoplastic cells (faint cytoplasmic staining of the rhabdoid inclusions is frequent) (SMARCB1 immunostain, ×200). (*D*) highly myxoid vulvoperineal proximal type epithelioid sarcoma with bland spindled cells and few scattered rhabdoid cells (H&E, original magnification ×200). In other areas, rhabdoid cells predominate (*E*). (*F*) This primary intracranial myxoid sarcoma (PIMS) lacked *EWSR1* gene rearrangement but showed SMARCB1 loss instead (*F*, inset) (H&E, original magnification ×200).

and phenotypically highly overlapping entities needs careful clinicopathologic correlation. Thus, any *EWSR1* alterations detected in the context of SMARCB1 deficiency should be verified by more specific supplementary molecular methods.[65] On rare occasions, MRT my closely mimic myxoid myoepithelial carcinoma and, on the other hand, myoepithelial carcinoma and its mimics may display frankly rhabdoid cell features as well, underlining the need for careful interpretation of histologic and immunophenotypic features.[65,66]

MOSAIC SMARCB1 LOSS

As stated in the section on nerve sheath tumors above, loss of SMARCB1 restricted to a subpopulation of the neoplastic cells has been characteristically observed in cases of schwannomatosis related to germline SMARCB1 mutations.[44,45] Similar observations were made in rare soft tissue neoplasms developing post-MRT in a background of germline SMARCB1 mutations including one case of uterine leiomyoma.[67] Other tumors developing in same setting showed complete loss of SMARCB1.[68,69] In one study, 74% of ossifying fibromyxoid tumors of soft parts showed mosaic SMARCB1 loss.[70]

IMMUNOPHENOTYPIC HETEROGENEITY OF SWI/SNF–DEFICIENT SOFT TISSUE TUMORS

Traditionally, MRT of childhood were shown to express multilineage markers including consistent coexpression of pancytokeratin and vimentin in addition to other epithelial (epithelial membrane antigen) and neural (glial fibrillary acidic protein, neurofilament, synaptophysin) markers. As the role of SMARCB1 loss in different neoplasms has been better defined, it became evident that many of these neoplasms have not much in common other than the unifying loss of the SMARCB1 expression.[71] Indeed, the phenotype and the clinicopathologic and demographic features remain central factors for diagnostic categorization.[71] A subset of these malignancies are keratin-poor (either totally negative or showing limited focal expression that may be missed on biopsy) and could be challenging if this is not thought of. EMA is a valuable adjunct if keratins were negative.

RECENTLY DESCRIBED SMARCA4-DEFICIENT MALIGNANCIES

Since the recent characterization of the role of SMARCA4 inactivation as the driver event in subsets of SMARCB1-proficient MRT[72] and in the vast majority of small cell carcinoma of the ovary, hypercalcemic type (SCCOHT),[73] SMARCA4 loss has been increasingly recognized in diverse neoplasms of either unequivocal epithelial origin (such as NSCLC),[74] of definite mesenchymal origin (epithelioid sarcoma subsets[33]) or of uncertain histogenesis (**Box 4**). The latter encompasses in particular a rare subset of unique, highly lethal thoracopulmonary (mainly mediastinal) malignancies reported recently as SMARCA4-deficient thoracic malignancies closely related to BAF-deficient sarcomas.[75]

Since then, the term "sarcoma" has been used rather loosely and uncritically to refer to any undifferentiated SMARCA4-deficient malignancy with many reports documenting this disease in parenchymatous visceral organs such as the lung,[76] and most recently the uterine body.[77] Comparative transcriptomic profiling analyses suggested distinctness from lung carcinomas and instead relationship to MRT and SCCOHT.[75]

Based on the increasing evidence that inactivation of the SWI/SNF chromatin remodeling complex is a feature shared by subsets of carcinomas and sarcomas with frequently epithelioid and/or rhabdoid morphology and variable coexpression of cytokeratin and vimentin, distinction between carcinoma and sarcoma with the aforementioned phenotype became more challenging. Recently, expression of the tight junction-associated protein claudin-4 has been proposed as promising adjunct of epithelial differentiation in this context.[78] Notably, claudin-4 was expressed in a variety of SWI/SNF deficient carcinomas with the exception of SCCOHT, but was absent in sarcomas other than synovial sarcoma.[78] However, given the fact that undifferentiated carcinomas in general can be completely devoid of any cytokeratin expression, the same might apply for claudin-4 reactivity which may be lost in the least differentiated variants of the SMARCA4-deficient carcinomas. Current evidence suggests that, at least a subset of these highly aggressive thoracopulmonary malignancies are more akin to carcinomas than sarcomas, based on their intrapulmonary localization, and frequent association with heavy smoking exposure and pulmonary emphysema/bullae.[75,76] Cases of SMARCA4-deficient non–small cell lung cancer with demonstrable transition from differentiated

---

Box 4
SMARCA4-deficient malignancies

Small cell carcinoma of the ovary, hypercalcemic type (100%)

SMARCA4-deficient thoracic malignancy related to BAF-deficient sarcoma (100%)

Subset of malignant rhabdoid tumors (~2%)

Subset of epithelioid sarcoma (<1%)

Subset of non–small cell lung carcinoma (5%–10%)

Subsets of dedifferentiated and undifferentiated carcinomas of endometrium, digestive tract, urogenital system, and head and neck

carcinoma to undifferentiated (sarcoma-like) component were reported.[74]

THERAPEUTIC IMPLICATIONS OF SWI/SNF DEFICIENCY

To date, treatment of MRT and epithelioid sarcoma as the main SWI/SNF-driven soft tissue malignancies has been a combination of surgery and radiochemotherapy in a stage-based oncological intent. Unfortunately, small molecule inhibitors targeting the SWI/SNF alteration as the central genetic event in these frequently highly lethal neoplasms are not available yet. However, with emergence of the genetic landscape of SWI/SNF-driven malignancies, therapeutic opportunities targeting some of the pathways upregulated as a consequence of the SWI/SNF complex disruption are emerging.[79] More recently, inactivation of an SWI/SNF component (PBRM1) was found as the most powerful biomarker predicting response to immune-oncological therapy via checkpoint inhibition in renal cell carcinoma.[80] Based on recent studies showing frequent concurrent loss of PBRM1 in epithelioid sarcoma (74%),[34] it is not excluded that similar concepts be established for those soft tissue malignancies with disrupted PBRM1 and other components of the SWI/SNF complex.

REFERENCES

1. Peterson CL, Dingwall A, Scott MP. Five SWI/SNF gene products are components of a large multisubunit complex required for transcriptional enhancement. Proc Natl Acad Sci U S A 1994;91:2905–8.
2. Reisman D, Glaros S, Thompson EA. The SWI/SNF complex and cancer. Oncogene 2009;28:1653–68.
3. Wang X, Haswell JR, Roberts CW. Molecular pathways: SWI/SNF (BAF) complexes are frequently mutated in cancer–mechanisms and potential therapeutic insights. Clin Cancer Res 2014;20:21–7.
4. Wilson BG, Roberts CW. SWI/SNF nucleosome remodellers and cancer. Nat Rev Cancer 2011;11:481–92.
5. Oike T, Ogiwara H, Nakano T, et al. Inactivating mutations in SWI/SNF chromatin remodeling genes in human cancer. Jpn J Clin Oncol 2013;43:849–55.
6. Agaimy A. The expanding family of SMARCB1(INI1)-deficient neoplasia: implications of phenotypic, biological, and molecular heterogeneity. Adv Anat Pathol 2014;21:394–410.
7. Betz BL, Strobeck MW, Reisman DN, et al. Re-expression of hSNF5/INI1/BAF47 in pediatric tumor cells leads to G1 arrest associated with induction of p16ink4a and activation of RB. Oncogene 2002;21:5193–203.
8. Judkins AR. Immunohistochemistry of INI1 expression: a new tool for old challenges in CNS and soft tissue pathology. Adv Anat Pathol 2007;14:335–9.
9. Biegel JA, Rorke LB, Packer RJ, et al. Monosomy 22 in rhabdoid or atypical tumors of the brain. J Neurosurg 1990;73:710–4.
10. Versteege I, Sévenet N, Lange J, et al. Truncating mutations of hSNF5/INI1 in aggressive paediatric cancer. Nature 1998;394:203–6.
11. Beckwith JB, Palmer NF. Histopathology and prognosis of Wilms tumors: results from the First National Wilms' Tumor Study. Cancer 1978;41:1937–48.
12. Weeks DA, Beckwith JB, Mierau GW, et al. Rhabdoid tumor of kidney. A report of 111 cases from the National Wilms' tumor study pathology center. Am J Surg Pathol 1989;13:439–58.
13. Biegel JA, Fogelgren B, Wainwright LM, et al. Germline INI1 mutation in a patient with a central nervous system atypical teratoid tumor and renal rhabdoid tumor. Genes Chromosomes Cancer 2000;28:31–7.
14. Savla J, Chen TT, Schneider NR, et al. Mutations of the hSNF5/INI1 gene in renal rhabdoid tumors with second primary brain tumors. J Natl Cancer Inst 2000;92:648–50.
15. Parham DM, Weeks DA, Beckwith JB. The clinicopathologic spectrum of putative extrarenal rhabdoid tumors. An analysis of 42 cases studied with immunohistochemistry or electron microscopy. Am J Surg Pathol 1994;18:1010–29.
16. Fanburg-Smith JC, Hengge M, Hengge UR, et al. Extrarenal rhabdoid tumors of soft tissue: a clinicopathologic and immunohistochemical study of 18 cases. Ann Diagn Pathol 1998;2:351–62.
17. Wick MR, Ritter JH, Dehner LP. Malignant rhabdoid tumors: a clinicopathologic review and conceptual discussion. Semin Diagn Pathol 1995;12:233–48.
18. Fuller CE, Pfeifer J, Humphrey P, et al. Chromosome 22q dosage in composite extrarenal rhabdoid tumors: clonal evolution or a phenotypic mimic? Hum Pathol 2001;32:1102–8.
19. Agaimy A, Daum O, Märkl B, et al. SWI/SNF complex-deficient undifferentiated/rhabdoid carcinomas of the gastrointestinal tract: a series of 13 cases highlighting mutually exclusive loss of SMARCA4 and SMARCA2 and frequent co-inactivation of SMARCB1 and SMARCA2. Am J Surg Pathol 2016;40:544–53.
20. Agaimy A, Cheng L, Egevad L, et al. Rhabdoid and undifferentiated phenotype in renal cell carcinoma: analysis of 32 cases indicating a distinctive common pathway of dedifferentiation frequently associated with SWI/SNF complex deficiency. Am J Surg Pathol 2017;41:253–62.
21. Enzinger FM. Epithelioid sarcoma. A sarcoma simulating a granuloma or a carcinoma. Cancer 1970;26:1029–41.

22. Fisher C. Epithelioid sarcoma of Enzinger. Adv Anat Pathol 2006;13:114–21.

23. Chbani L, Guillou L, Terrier P, et al. Epithelioid sarcoma: a clinicopathologic and immunohistochemical analysis of 106 cases from the French sarcoma group. Am J Clin Pathol 2009;131:222–7.

24. Guillou L, Wadden C, Coindre JM, et al. "Proximal-type" epithelioid sarcoma, a distinctive aggressive neoplasm showing rhabdoid features. Clinicopathologic, immunohistochemical, and ultrastructural study of a series. Am J Surg Pathol 1997;21:130–46.

25. Brand A, Covert A. Malignant rhabdoid tumor of the vulva: case report and review of the literature with emphasis on clinical management and outcome. Gynecol Oncol 2001;80:99–103.

26. Mills SE, Fechner RE, Bruns DE, et al. Intermediate filaments in eosinophilic cells of epithelioid sarcoma: a light-microscopic, ultrastructural, and electrophoretic study. Am J Surg Pathol 1981;5:195–202.

27. Kosemehmetoglu K, Kaygusuz G, Bahrami A, et al. Intra-articular epithelioid sarcoma showing mixed classic and proximal-type features: report of 2 cases, with immunohistochemical and molecular cytogenetic INI-1 study. Am J Surg Pathol 2011;35: 891–7.

28. Miettinen M, Wang Z, Sarlomo-Rikala M, et al. ERG expression in epithelioid sarcoma: a diagnostic pitfall. Am J Surg Pathol 2013;37:1580–5.

29. Stockman DL, Hornick JL, Deavers MT, et al. ERG and FLI1 protein expression in epithelioid sarcoma. Mod Pathol 2014;27:496–501.

30. Machado I, Mayordomo-Aranda E, Scotlandi K, et al. Immunoreactivity using anti-ERG monoclonal antibodies in sarcomas is influenced by clone selection. Pathol Res Pract 2014;210:508–13.

31. Hornick JL, Dal Cin P, Fletcher CD. Loss of INI1 expression is characteristic of both conventional and proximal-type epithelioid sarcoma. Am J Surg Pathol 2009;33:542–50.

32. Sullivan LM, Folpe AL, Pawel BR, et al. Epithelioid sarcoma is associated with a high percentage of SMARCB1 deletions. Mod Pathol 2013;26:385–92.

33. Kohashi K, Yamamoto H, Yamada Y, et al. SWI/SNF chromatin-remodeling complex status in SMARCB1/INI1-preserved epithelioid sarcoma. Am J Surg Pathol 2018;42:312–8.

34. Li L, Fan XS, Xia QY, et al. Concurrent loss of INI1, PBRM1, and BRM expression in epithelioid sarcoma: implications for the cocontritions of multiple SWI/SNF complex members to pathogenesis. Hum Pathol 2014;45:2247–54.

35. Maggiani F, Debiec-Rychter M, Ectors N, et al. Primary epithelioid sarcoma of the oesophagus. Virchows Arch 2007;451:835–8.

36. Venizelos I, Anagnostou E, Papathomas TG, et al. Proximal-type epithelioid sarcoma of the uterine corpus. Histopathology 2011;58:321–3.

37. Makise N, Yoshida A, Komiyama M, et al. Dedifferentiated liposarcoma with epithelioid/epithelial features. Am J Surg Pathol 2017;41:1523–31.

38. Agaimy A, Michal M, Hadravsky L, et al. Dedifferentiated liposarcoma composed predominantly of rhabdoid/epithelioid cells: a frequently misdiagnosed highly aggressive variant. Hum Pathol 2018; 77:20–7.

39. Hollmann TJ, Hornick JL. INI1-deficient tumors: diagnostic features and molecular genetics. Am J Surg Pathol 2011;35:e47–63.

40. Jo VY, Fletcher CD. Epithelioid malignant peripheral nerve sheath tumor: clinicopathologic analysis of 63 cases. Am J Surg Pathol 2015;39:673–82.

41. Carter JM, O'Hara C, Dundas G, et al. Epithelioid malignant peripheral nerve sheath tumor arising in a schwannoma, in a patient with "neuroblastoma-like" schwannomatosis and a novel germline SMARCB1 mutation. Am J Surg Pathol 2012;36: 154–60.

42. Agaimy A, Foulkes WD. Hereditary SWI/SNF complex deficiency syndromes. Semin Diagn Pathol 2018;35:193–8.

43. Jo VY, Fletcher CDM. SMARCB1/INI1 loss in epithelioid schwannoma: a clinicopathologic and immunohistochemical study of 65 cases. Am J Surg Pathol 2017;41:1013–22.

44. Hulsebos TJ, Plomp AS, Wolterman RA, et al. Germline mutation of INI1/SMARCB1 in familial schwannomatosis. Am J Hum Genet 2007;80: 805–10.

45. Hulsebos TJ, Kenter S, Verhagen WI, et al. Premature termination of SMARCB1 translation may be followed by reinitiation in schwannomatosis-associated schwannomas, but results in absence of SMARCB1 expression in rhabdoid tumors. Acta Neuropathol 2014;128:439–48.

46. Young RH, Oliva E, Scully RE. Small cell carcinoma of the ovary, hypercalcemic type. A clinicopathological analysis of 150 cases. Am J Surg Pathol 1994; 18:1102–16.

47. Karanian-Philippe M, Velasco V, Longy M, et al. SMARCA4 (BRG1) loss of expression is a useful marker for the diagnosis of ovarian small cell carcinoma of the hypercalcemic type (ovarian rhabdoid tumor): a comprehensive analysis of 116 rare gynecologic tumors, 9 soft tissue tumors, and 9 melanomas. Am J Surg Pathol 2015;39: 1197–205.

48. Conlon N, Silva A, Guerra E, et al. Loss of SMARCA4 expression is both sensitive and specific for the diagnosis of small cell carcinoma of ovary, hypercalcemic type. Am J Surg Pathol 2016;40:395–403.

49. Kreiger PA, Judkins AR, Russo PA, et al. Loss of INI1 expression defines a unique subset of pediatric undifferentiated soft tissue sarcomas. Mod Pathol 2009;22:142–50.

50. Machado I, Yoshida A, Morales MGN, et al. Review with novel markers facilitates precise categorization of 41 cases of diagnostically challenging, "undifferentiated small round cell tumors". A clinicopathologic, immunophenotypic and molecular analysis. Ann Diagn Pathol 2018;34:1–12.

51. Thaete C, Brett D, Monaghan P, et al. Functional domains of the SYT and SYT-SSX synovial sarcoma translocation proteins and co-localization with the SNF protein BRM in the nucleus. Hum Mol Genet 1999;8:585–91.

52. Kohashi K, Oda Y, Yamamoto H, et al. Reduced expression of SMARCB1/INI1 protein in synovial sarcoma. Mod Pathol 2010;23:981–90.

53. Mularz K, Harazin-Lechowska A, Ambicka A, et al. Specificity and sensitivity of INI-1 labeling in epithelioid sarcoma. Loss of INI1 expression as a frequent immunohistochemical event in synovial sarcoma. Pol J Pathol 2012;63:179–83.

54. Arnold MA, Arnold CA, Li G, et al. A unique pattern of INI1 immunohistochemistry distinguishes synovial sarcoma from its histologic mimics. Hum Pathol 2013;44:881–7.

55. Rekhi B, Jambhekar AN. Immunohistochemical validation of INI1/SMARCB1 in a spectrum of musculoskeletal tumors: an experience at a Tertiary Cancer Referral Centre. Pathol Res Pract 2013;209:758–66.

56. Kadoch C, Crabtree GR. Reversible disruption of mSWI/SNF (BAF) complexes by the SS18-SSX oncogenic fusion in synovial sarcoma. Cell 2013;153:71–85.

57. Kohashi K, Oda Y, Yamamoto H, et al. SMARCB1/INI1 protein expression in round cell soft tissue sarcomas associated with chromosomal translocations involving EWS: a special reference to SMARCB1/INI1 negative variant extraskeletal myxoid chondrosarcoma. Am J Surg Pathol 2008;32:1168–74.

58. Le Loarer F, Zhang L, Fletcher CD, et al. Consistent SMARCB1 homozygous deletions in epithelioid sarcoma and in a subset of myoepithelial carcinomas can be reliably detected by FISH in archival material. Genes Chromosomes Cancer 2014;53:475–86.

59. Mobley BC, McKenney JK, Bangs CD, et al. Loss of SMARCB1/INI1 expression in poorly differentiated chordomas. Acta Neuropathol 2010;120:745–53.

60. Antonelli M, Raso A, Mascelli S, et al. SMARCB1/INI1 involvement in pediatric chordoma: a mutational and immunohistochemical analysis. Am J Surg Pathol 2017;41:56–61.

61. Thway K, Nicholson AG, Lawson K, et al. Primary pulmonary myxoid sarcoma with EWSR1-CREB1 fusion: a new tumor entity. Am J Surg Pathol 2011;35:1722–32.

62. Kao YC, Sung YS, Zhang L, et al. EWSR1 fusions with CREB family transcription factors define a novel myxoid mesenchymal tumor with predilection for intracranial location. Am J Surg Pathol 2017;41:482–90.

63. Agaimy A, Duell T, Morresi-Hauf AT. EWSR1-fusion-negative, SMARCB1-deficient primary pulmonary myxoid sarcoma. Pol J Pathol 2017;68:261–7.

64. Velz J, Agaimy A, Frontzek K, et al. Molecular and clinicopathologic heterogeneity of intracranial tumors mimicking extraskeletal myxoid chondrosarcoma. J Neuropathol Exp Neurol 2018;77:727–35.

65. Huang SC, Zhang L, Sung YS, et al. Secondary EWSR1 gene abnormalities in SMARCB1-deficient tumors with 22q11-12 regional deletions: potential pitfalls in interpreting EWSR1 FISH results. Genes Chromosomes Cancer 2016;55:767–76.

66. Thway K, Bown N, Miah A, et al. Rhabdoid variant of myoepithelial carcinoma, with ewsr1 rearrangement: expanding the spectrum of EWSR1-rearranged myoepithelial tumors. Head Neck Pathol 2015;9:273–9.

67. Hulsebos TJ, Kenter S, Siebers-Renelt U, et al. SMARCB1 involvement in the development of leiomyoma in a patient with schwannomatosis. Am J Surg Pathol 2014;38:421–5.

68. Ammerlaan AC, Ararou A, Houben MP, et al. Long-term survival and transmission of INI1-mutation via nonpenetrant males in a family with rhabdoid tumour predisposition syndrome. Br J Cancer 2008;98:474–9.

69. Forest F, David A, Arrufat S, et al. Conventional chondrosarcoma in a survivor of rhabdoid tumor: enlarging the spectrum of tumors associated with SMARCB1 germline mutations. Am J Surg Pathol 2012;36:1892–6.

70. Graham RP, Dry S, Li X, et al. Ossifying fibromyxoid tumor of soft parts: a clinicopathologic, proteomic, and genomic study. Am J Surg Pathol 2011;35:1615–25.

71. Bourdeaut F, Fréneaux P, Thuille B, et al. hSNF5/INI1-deficient tumours and rhabdoid tumours are convergent but not fully overlapping entities. J Pathol 2007;211:323–30.

72. Hasselblatt M, Gesk S, Oyen F, et al. Nonsense mutation and inactivation of SMARCA4 (BRG1) in an atypical teratoid/rhabdoid tumor showing retained SMARCB1 (INI1) expression. Am J Surg Pathol 2011;35:933–5.

73. Witkowski L, Carrot-Zhang J, Albrecht S, et al. Germline and somatic SMARCA4 mutations characterize small cell carcinoma of the ovary, hypercalcemic type. Nat Genet 2014 May;46(5):438–43.

74. Agaimy A, Fuchs F, Moskalev EA, et al. SMARCA4-deficient pulmonary adenocarcinoma: clinicopathological, immunohistochemical, and molecular characteristics of a novel aggressive neoplasm with a consistent TTF1neg/CK7pos/HepPar-1pos immunophenotype. Virchows Arch 2017;471:599–609.

75. Le Loarer F, Watson S, Pierron G, et al. SMARCA4 inactivation defines a group of undifferentiated thoracic malignancies transcriptionally related to BAF-deficient sarcomas. Nat Genet 2015;47: 1200–5.

76. Yoshida A, Kobayashi E, Kubo T, et al. Clinico-pathological and molecular characterization of SMARCA4-deficient thoracic sarcomas with comparison to potentially related entities. Mod Pathol 2017;30:797–809.

77. Kolin DL, Dong F, Baltay M, et al. SMARCA4-deficient undifferentiated uterine sarcoma (malignant rhabdoid tumor of the uterus): a clinicopathologic entity distinct from undifferentiated carcinoma. Mod Pathol 2018;31(9):1442–56.

78. Schaefer IM, Agaimy A, Fletcher CD, et al. Claudin-4 expression distinguishes SWI/SNF complex-deficient undifferentiated carcinomas from sarcomas. Mod Pathol 2017;30:539–48.

79. St Pierre R, Kadoch C. Mammalian SWI/SNF complexes in cancer: emerging therapeutic opportunities. Curr Opin Genet Dev 2017;42:56–67.

80. Miao D, Margolis CA, Gao W, et al. Genomic correlates of response to immune checkpoint therapies in clear cell renal cell carcinoma. Science 2018;359: 801–6.

Mesenchymal Tumors with *EWSR1* Gene Rearrangements

Khin Thway, MD, FRCPath[a],*, Cyril Fisher, MD, DSc, FRCPath[b]

KEYWORDS

- *EWSR1* • Sarcoma • Angiomatoid fibrous histiocytoma • Clear cell sarcoma
- Desmoplastic small round cell tumor • Myxoid liposarcoma • Myoepithelial tumor
- *EWSR1*–NFATC2

Key points

- *EWSR1* is the most common gene involved in recurrent, characteristic gene fusions in soft tissue tumors.

- *EWSR1* can partner with a large variety of partner genes, resulting in a variety of different mesenchymal and non-mesenchymal tumor types.

- Fusions of *EWSR1* with different partner genes can generate genetically different but phenotypically identical neoplasms (e.g. in Ewing sarcoma). Alternatively, *EWSR1* can fuse with the same gene in clinically and histologically different tumors.

- The finding of an *EWSR1* gene rearrangement in isolation by FISH is non-specific. The use of RT-PCR or sequencing techniques can help to identify specific fusion transcripts, but these themselves may not be specific.

- Interpretation of molecular findings requires careful interpretation in view of the complete clinico-pathological picture.

ABSTRACT

Among the various genes that can be rearranged in soft tissue neoplasms associated with nonrandom chromosomal translocations, *EWSR1* is the most frequent one to partner with other genes to generate recurrent fusion genes. This leads to a spectrum of clinically and pathologically diverse mesenchymal and nonmesenchymal neoplasms, variably manifesting as small round cell, spindle cell, clear cell or adipocytic tumors, or tumors with distinctive myxoid stroma. This review summarizes the growing list of mesenchymal neoplasms that are associated with *EWSR1* gene rearrangements.

OVERVIEW

Approximately one-third of soft tissue sarcomas harbor characteristic, recurrent, chromosomal translocations. These translocations are usually balanced and reciprocal and mostly associated with simple karyotypes. Chromosomal translocations involve the exchange of genetic material between 2, usually nonhomologous, chromosomes and lead to tumorigenesis via a variety of mechanisms, generating neoplasms with distinct clinical and pathologic features.[1] Pathogenic translocations are usually initial or early steps in tumor formation; chimeric gene fusions can result in novel, tumor-specific transcription factors that lead to dysregulated gene expression, such as in Ewing

Disclosures: The authors have no conflicts of interest or funding to disclose.
[a] Sarcoma Unit, Royal Marsden Hospital, The Royal Marsden NHS Foundation Trust, 203 Fulham Road, London SW3 6JJ, UK; [b] Department of Musculoskeletal Pathology, Royal Orthopaedic Hospital NHS Foundation Trust, Robert Aitken Institute for Clinical Research, University of Birmingham, Birmingham B15 2TT, UK
* Corresponding author.
E-mail address: khin.thway@rmh.nhs.uk

Surgical Pathology 12 (2019) 165–190
https://doi.org/10.1016/j.path.2018.10.007

sarcoma (ES), or by juxtaposition of promoter regions that drive expression of oncogenes, for example, *MYC* overexpression in leukemia/lymphoma. Secondary genetic or epigenetic events are required for expression of particular tumoral phenotypes, because there are significant differences in gene expression patterns between different neoplasms harboring the same fusion. Identical gene fusions can generate clinically and pathologically different neoplasms through the instigation of novel differentiation programs characteristic of the properties of their specific target cells. Although the reasons for specific gene rearrangements are not clear, a factor may be the spatial proximity between 2 given genes within the 3-dimensional chromosomal arrangement in the nucleus.[2,3]

The Ewing sarcoma breakpoint region 1 gene (*EWSR1*) is a partner in a large, diverse range of mesenchymal (and some nonmesenchymal) tumors (**Tables 1** and **2**). As the 5′ partner, *EWSR1* is able to fuse with an array of genes. These fusions can generate genetically different but phenotypically identical neoplasms. Alternatively, *EWSR1* can fuse with the same gene in clinically and histologically different tumors. Mesenchymal neoplasms harboring *EWSR1* gene rearrangements include ES,[4] myxoid liposarcoma (MLPS),[5–9] clear cell sarcoma of soft tissue (CCS), and clear cell sarcoma-like tumors of gastrointestinal tract (CCSLTGT),[10–12] angiomatoid fibrous histiocytoma (AFH),[13–16] desmoplastic small round cell tumor (DSRCT),[17–19] extraskeletal myxoid chondrosarcoma (EMC),[20–27] primary pulmonary myxoid sarcoma (PPMS),[28] myoepithelial tumors of skin, soft tissue and bone,[29,30] some sclerosing epithelioid fibrosarcomas (SEF),[31] and low-grade fibromyxoid

sarcomas (LGFMS)[32] and newly described myxoid neoplasms harboring *EWSR1-CREM* fusions, which predominate in intracranial sites of young patients.[33] This article reviews the spectrum of mesenchymal neoplasms that harbor *EWSR1* gene rearrangements.

THE *EWSR1* GENE

The *EWSR1* gene is a member of the TET (translocated in liposarcoma [TLS]/fused in sarcoma [FUS], *EWSR1*, TATA-binding protein-associated factor 15 [TAF15]) family,[34] a group of genes involved in several translocation-associated sarcomas.[35–39] *EWSR1*, sited between base-pairs 29,663,998 and 29,696,515 on chromosome 22q12, was first noted to be rearranged in ES[40] and encodes a multifunctional protein involved in a variety of cellular mechanisms, including gene expression, meiotic and mitotic cell division, cell signaling, DNA repair, and cellular aging.[38,41,42] *EWSR1* has a 17-exon coding sequence,[43,44] which encodes a 656-amino-acid nuclear protein,[45] which includes a carboxy-terminus 87-amino-acid RNA-binding domain (exons 11–13) involved in protein-RNA binding, transcription, and RNA metabolism.[43,46] *EWSR1* and *FUS* are highly homologous and can variably serve as alternative binding partners in several translocation-associated tumors,[47] including AFH, MLPS, LGFMS, and SEF. Other TET family gene members may function as alternatives to *EWSR1* in genetic rearrangements, such as *TAF15*, which can act as a partner in some examples of EMC.[48] *EWSR1* fusion sites vary for different neoplasms; exon 7 is the most frequent site in ES,[49,50] in *EWSR1-WT1* of DSRCT, in *EWSR1-DDIT3* of

---

Table 1
Ewing sarcoma and small round cell neoplasms with *EWSR1* rearrangements resembling Ewing sarcoma

	Translocation	Fusion Gene
EWSR1/ETS fusions	t(11;22)(q24;q12)	*EWSR1-FLI1* (85%)
	t(21;22)(q22;q12)	*EWSR1-ERG* (10%)
	t(19;der(ins.inv(21;22))	*EWSR1-ERG*
	t(7;22)(p22;q12)	*EWSR1-ETV1*
	t(17;22) (q12;q12)	*EWSR1-ETV4*
	t(2;22)(q33;q12)	*EWSR1-FEV*
TET/ETS fusions	t(16;21)(p11;q22)	*FUS-ERG*
	t(2;16)(q36;p11)	*FUS-FEV*
Non-TET/ETS fusions	t(20;22)(q13;q12)	*EWSR1-NFATC2*
	t(6;22)(p21;q12)	*EWSR1-POU5F1*
	t(4;22)(q31;q12)	*EWSR1-SMARCA5*
	t(1;22)(q36.1;q12)	*EWSR1-PATZ1*
	t(2;22)(q31;q12)	*EWSR1-SP3*

Table 2
Other tumors with *EWSR1* fusions

	Translocation	Fusion Gene	Histology	Immunohistochemistry
Tumors with *WT1* fusion				
DSRCT	t(11;22)(p13;q12)	*EWSR1-WT1*	Small round cells, cellular fibrous stroma	CD99−, desmin+, CK+
Tumors with *DDIT3* fusion				
MLPS	t(12;22)(q13;q12)	*EWSR1-DDIT3* FUS-DDIT3 (90%)	Spindle/polygonal cells myxoid stroma	S100pr+
Tumors with *NR4A3* fusion				
EMC	t(9;22)(q22;q12)	*EWSR1-NR4A3* TAF15-NR4A3	Polygonal cells, myxoid stroma	S100pr+
Tumors with CREB1 or ATF1 fusion				
AFH	t(2;22) (q33;q12) t(12;22)(q13;q12) t(12;16)(q13;p11)	*EWSR1-CREB1* EWSR1-ATF1 FUS-ATF1	Sheets of ovoid cells, hemorrhage, fibrous and lymphoid cuff	Desmin+, CD99+, EMA+
CCS	t(12;22)(q13;q12)	*EWSR1-ATF1*	Clear cells	S100pr+, Melan-A+, HMB45+
Clear-cell sarcoma-like tumor of gastrointestinal tract	t(2;22)(q33;q12)	*EWSR1-CREB1*	Clear cells, osteoclast-like giant cells	S100pr+, melan-A−HMB45−
PPMS	t(2;22)(q33;q12)	*EWSR1-CREB1*	Spindle cells myxoid stroma	No specific markers
Myoepithelial tumor	t(12;22)(q13;q12)	*EWSR1-ATF1*	Epithelioid cell cords, chondromyxoid stroma	S100pr+, EMA+
HCCC of salivary gland	t(12;22)(q13;q12)	*EWSR1-ATF1*	Clear cells, hyalinized stroma	S100pr+
Angiosarcoma	t(12;22)(q13;q12)	*EWSR1-ATF1*	Epithelioid and spindle cells	CD31, FVIIIRAg, D2-40

(continued on next page)

Table 2
(continued)

	Translocation	Fusion Gene	Histology	Immunohistochemistry
Tumors with other fusions				
Myoepithelial tumors	t(6;22)(p21;q12) t(1;22)(q23;q12)	ESWR1-POU5F1 EWSR1-PBX1	Clear cells in nests Spindle or clear cells, fibrous stroma	S100pr+, EMA+, CK±, GFAP± S100pr+, EMA+
	t(19;22)(q13;q12)	EWSR1-ZNF444	Epithelioid/clear cells, sclerotic stroma	CK+, S100pr+, EMA±, GFAP±
LGFMS and SEF	t(16;22)(p11;q12) t(7;16)(q33;p11) t(11;16)(p13;p11)	EWSR1-CREB3L1 FUS-CREB3L2 FUS-CREB3L1 (rare)	Spindle or epithelioid cells, fibromyxoid or sclerosing stroma	MUC4+
Mesothelioma	t(14;22)(q23;q12) t(12;22)(q13;q12) t(12;16)(q13;p11)	EWSR1-YY1 EWSR1-ATF1 FUS-ATF1	Epithelioid cells	BAP1-retained
Acral fibroblastic spindle cell tumor	(t(15;22)(15q22;q12)	EWSR1-SMAD3	Bland spindle cells, peripheral hypercellular areas, hypocellular hyalinized central areas	ERG+ (of uncertain significance); negative for all other markers
Epithelioid or spindle cell rhabdomyosarcomas	t(12;22)(12q13;q12) t(12;16)(12q13;p11)	EWSR1-TFCP2 FUS-TFCP2	Monotonous epithelioid cells, sheets and short fascicles, fibrous stroma with focal sclerosis	Desmin+, myogenin+, MyoD1+, epithelial markers+, ALK+, TERT+
	t(12;16)(12q13;p11)	FUS-TFCP2	Relatively monomorphic spindle to epithelioid cells, short fascicles, sclerosis	Diffuse desmin and MyoD1+, more limited myogenin+, ALK+, variable AE1/AE3 and CAM5.2+
Benign hemangioma of bone	t(18;22)(q23;q12)	EWSR1-NFATC1	Lobular proliferations of vessels of varying caliber, lined by bland endothelial cells	CD31+, CD34+, WT1+

MLPS,[5,6,51,52] and in *EWSR1-CREB1* of PPMS.[28] However, in CCS, the most frequent *EWSR1* fusion site is exon 8[53] and for *EWSR1-NR4A3* in EMC it is exon 12.

TUMORS WITH *EWSR1-ETS* FAMILY FUSIONS

EWING SARCOMA

ES is an aggressive bone and soft tissue tumor predominantly occurring in children and young adults. ES comprises a group of round cell neoplasms with common morphologic, immunohistochemical, and molecular features, including balanced reciprocal translocations between *EWSR1* and, most frequently, genes encoding various members of the *ETS* family of transcription factors (most commonly *FLI1* and *ERG*). ES is now considered a single disease entity,[54] encompassing neoplasms previously described as primitive peripheral neuroectodermal tumors, and those arising within the bone and soft tissues, the paravertebral region, thoracopulmonary region[55] (Askin tumor), skin, and in rarer sites including the viscera and retroperitoneum. ES occurs mostly in the first 3 decades of life, although it can occur in much older adults. With current treatments, the 5-year survival can reach 70% for patients with localized disease,[56] but is less than 35% in patients who have metastatic disease at presentation.[57] ES does not correspond to any known normal counterpart cell; neuroectodermal/neural differentiation can be present to a variable degree, although this does not correlate with clinical behavior.[58]

ES are typically composed of sheets or nests of very uniform cells with ovoid or rounded vesicular nuclei with even, finely granular chromatin, often small nucleoli and small amounts of cytoplasm (**Fig. 1**), which may show prominent glycogen deposits. According to the degree of neural differentiation, ES can contain Homer-Wright rosettes with central fibrillary cores (**Fig. 2**). Tumor necrosis is relatively frequent, with tumor preservation around vessels. Large cell (atypical) (**Fig. 3**), spindle cell, clear cell (due to glycogen), adamantinoma-like (cytokeratin positive), and sclerosing variants are well described.[58–61] More than 90% of ES diffusely and strongly express CD99 in a membranous pattern, and two-thirds express nuclear FLI1. Neural/neuroendocrine markers neurofilament, chromogranin, synaptophysin, and neuron-specific enolase are variably expressed. NKX2.2 (a downstream target of *EWSR1-ETS* fusion genes) is a sensitive (although not wholly specific) marker,[62] whereas caveolin-1 expression may be contributory to the diagnosis of CD99-negative cases.[61] There is variable expression of S100 protein, keratins (although CK20 is negative), and CD117. Although desmin can be rarely expressed,[63] myogenin is negative. TLE1 and CD56 are also typically negative. ES with *ERG* rearrangements are positive for ERG immunohistochemically.[64]

Genetically, ES harbor characteristic chromosomal translocations, which most frequently generate chimeric *EWSR1*-ETS family oncoproteins.[65] Approximately 85% of ES harbor *EWSR1-FLI1* fusions arising from t(11;22)(q24;q12),[35] and about 5% to 10% contain *EWSR1-ERG* fusions

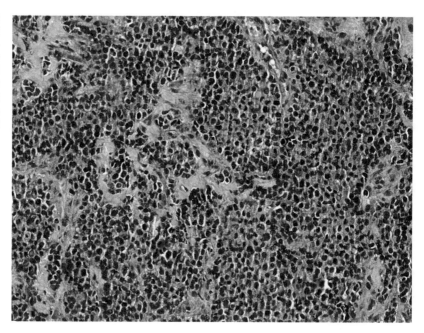

Fig. 1. ES. These tumors are typically composed of sheets or nests of very uniform cells with ovoid or rounded vesicular nuclei with even, finely granular chromatin, often small nucleoli and small amounts of cytoplasm (H&E, original magnification ×100).

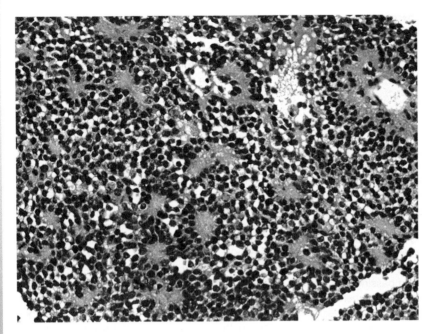

Fig. 2. ES. There can be variable degrees of neural differentiation. This neoplasm has cells arranged in Homer-Wright rosettes with central fibrillary cores (H&E, original magnification ×200).

from t(21;22)(q22;q12).[64,66,67] Exon 7, the most common ES fusion site, fuses with the segment encoding the DNA-binding domain of a variety of *ETS* family genes.[49,50] Most diagnostic laboratories use either or both ancillary techniques of fluorescence in situ hybridization (FISH) with an *EWSR1*-specific break-apart probe to identify *EWSR1* rearrangements, or reverse transcription-polymerase chain reaction (RT-PCR) to detect specific fusion transcripts involving *EWSR1*, in formalin-fixed, paraffin-embedded tissues. A minority of ES (<1%), usually showing typical morphologic and immunohistochemical features, harbors variant fusions, such that standard molecular investigations are negative. These ES include *EWRSR1/ETS* fusions *EWSR1-ETV1*,[68] *EWSR1-ETV4*,[69] and *EWSR1-FEV*,[70] and *TET/ETS* fusions *FUS-FEV*[71] and *FUS-ERG*.[72,73] These variants are usually similar morphologically and clinically, although some differences have been described (albeit in

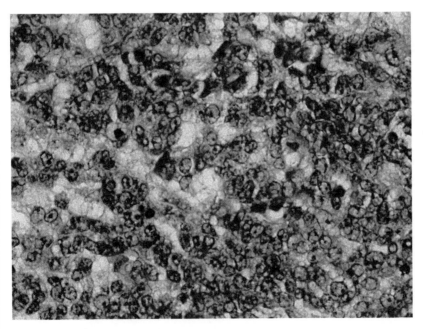

Fig. 3. ES. This can show atypical features. Here, the cells are larger and less uniform than usual and can resemble other tumors such as carcinoma (H&E, original magnification ×400).

small series), such as the suggestion of propensity for women and children in a younger age group and the occurrence in extraosseous sites in the t(7;22)(*EWSR1-ETV1*) variant.[74] Non-*TET*, non-*ETS* fusions are also rare and include *EWSR1-NFATC2*,[75] *EWSR1-POU5F1*[76] (CD99 negative; also present in some myoepithelial tumors), *EWSR1-PATZ1*[77] (CD99 negative), *EWSR1-SMARCA5*,[78] and *EWSR1-SP3*.[79] *PAX7* has been shown to be one of the most differentially expressed genes in ES relative to other small round cell sarcomas.[80,81] Its expression by immunohistochemistry has been noted in *EWSR1*-rearranged tumors with *FLI1*, *ERG*, and *NFATC2* partner genes.[82] It is still uncertain whether these neoplasms with variant fusions should be considered subgroups of ES or classified separately as undifferentiated small round cell sarcomas, but currently they are treated similarly.[83,84]

The *FLI1* gene normally encodes a protein with involvement in hemopoiesis and neural crest development. In ES the 5' (amino-terminal) transactivation domain of *EWSR1* fuses with the 3' (carboxy-terminal) ETS domain of *FLI1*. The resulting fusion protein acts as an aberrant transcriptional activator[85,86] or suppressor.[87] Multiple target genes are involved in oncogenesis and cell proliferation and include *ERG*,[88] *CAV*,[89] cyclin D1,[90] *EZH2*,[91] *FOXM1*,[92] *GLI1*,[93] *NKX2.2*,[62] and *NR0B1(DAX1)*.[94] Alternative splicing of *EWSR1* generates several variant transcripts. In type 1 fusions, exons 1 to 7 of *EWSR1* fuse with exons 6 to 10 of *FLI1*, whereas exon 7 fuses to exon 5 in type 2. Although type 1 fusion has been thought to confer a prognostic advantage, the findings are not clear.[95]

Tumors in the differential diagnosis of ES include *CIC-DUX4* and *BCOR*-rearranged undifferentiated round cell sarcomas.[96] In contrast to ES, these tumors often contain myxoid areas and a spindle cell (or epithelioid) component.[96] *CIC-DUX4* gene fusions, resulting from t(4;19)(q35;q13) or t(10;19)(q26.3;q13) appear to be the most frequent recurrent genetic abnormality in small round cell neoplasms lacking *EWSR1* rearrangement in pediatric and young adult patients and are aggressive tumors occurring predominantly in the extremities of young adult men.[97–100] *BCOR*-rearranged tumors arise largely in bones or less frequently in the deep soft tissues of adolescents or young adults, again with a male predominance.[101,102] These tumors show a range of morphologic features but most show at least a focal undifferentiated component of rounded cells with similarity to ES. The round cell component of mesenchymal chondrosarcoma also mimics ES, and is CD99 positive; this can be particularly difficult to distinguish from ES in small

biopsy material in which the cartilaginous islands may be absent. However, mesenchymal chondrosarcoma does not harbor *EWSR1* rearrangement and is characterized by *HEY1-NCOA2* gene fusions.[103]

TUMORS WITH *EWSR1-WT1* FUSION

DESMOPLASTIC SMALL ROUND CELL TUMOR

DSRCT is an aggressive small round cell neoplasm predominantly arising within the abdominal cavity (including the pelvis, retroperitoneum, omentum, and mesentery,[54,104] often with widespread serosal involvement) in adolescents and young adults with a male predisposition. DSRCT can more rarely arise in older (including elderly) patients[105] and occur as a primary tumor in rarer sites, including intrascrotally/paratesticularly, intrathoracically,[106] and within the head and neck (including the brain, salivary glands, and sinonasal cavity),[106–108] and visceral organs such as kidney, ovary, and bowel.[109–113] Histologically, DSRCT is composed of sharply demarcated nests and islands of uniform small cells with rounded or ovoid hyperchromatic or vesicular nuclei, inconspicuous nucleoli, scanty cytoplasm, and indistinct cell borders, associated with frequent mitoses and necrosis. There is a characteristic, marked desmoplastic stromal reaction around the tumor islands, comprising spindled fibroblasts and myofibroblasts in a collagenous extracellular matrix (**Fig. 4**).[54] DSRCT classically shows a polyphenotypic immunohistochemical profile, with variable coexpression of epithelial markers (epithelial membrane antigen [EMA] and cytokeratins, although not CK5/6 or CK20) and desmin (often with a dot pattern) in most cases,[114] neural markers such as neuron-specific enolase and CD57, and WT1. However, antigen expression varies between tumors, and not all antigens (including desmin and cytokeratins) may be expressed.[115] About 65% to 90% are immunoreactive toward antibodies selectively directed toward the carboxy-terminus of the Wilms tumor (WT1) protein.[114,116] There can be variable S100 protein and actin expression,[104,114] although CD99 is usually negative.

DSRCT is associated with a characteristic reciprocal translocation, t(11;22)(p13;q12),[117] in which the Wilms tumor gene (*WT1*) is fused with *EWSR1*, generating a chimeric transcription factor that causes aberrant regulation of several genes,[118] including platelet-derived growth factor alpha (*PDGFA*). *PDGFA* codes for a potent fibroblast growth factor,[119] and its induction may contribute to the prominent stromal proliferation. Because ES can also arise intra-abdominally and be associated with a nested pattern and stromal desmoplasia, RT-

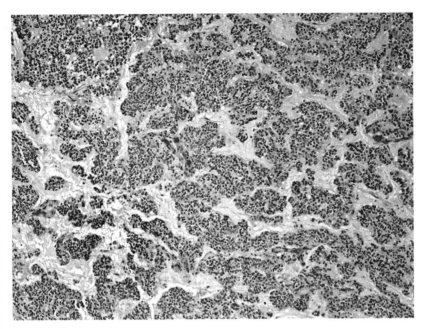

Fig. 4. DSRCT. There are prominent rounded to angulated nests of small cells with round to ovoid nuclei, distributed in cellular fibrous stroma (H&E, original magnification ×40).

PCR with confirmation of *EWSR1-WT1* fusion transcripts, which are not found in ES, is diagnostically optimal. Although most tumors with *EWSR1-WT1* fusions represent DSRCT, this fusion is not wholly specific for it, as *EWSR1-WT1* fusion transcripts have been described in 2 cases of pediatric intra-abdominal spindle cell neoplasms resembling leiomyosarcomas, but which have shown a favorable outcome.[120] *EWSR1-WT1* transcripts have also been found in a low-grade small round cell tumor of the cauda equina,[121] which was clinically indolent and comprised nests and cords of small round cells with some rosettelike structures, infrequent mitotic figures, immunophenotypic features of smooth muscle differentiation, and focal CD99 and Neu-N expression.[121] It is therefore crucial to correlate the finding of *EWSR1-WT1* fusion transcripts with the clinical and pathologic findings for a correct diagnosis of DSRCT.

TUMORS WITH *EWSR1-DDIT3* FUSION

MYXOID LIPOSARCOMA

MLPS most frequently occurs within the deep soft tissues of proximal extremities and trunk in young to middle-aged adults, with rare cases arising in children. MLPS is exceptional within the retroperitoneum or abdominal cavity, and metastatic disease should first be excluded at these sites. Metastases occur in up to one-third of patients, typically to other soft tissue sites, the lungs, or bones,[122] and metastatic risk is related to the proportion of round cell change present.[123] Histologically, MLPS comprises moderately cellular

proliferations of small, ovoid to spindle cells in patternless distributions, clusters and cords in myxoid stroma, with prominent interspersed small to medium-sized, thin-walled curvilinear vessels (**Fig. 5**). The amount of adipocytic differentiation varies, with relatively small lipoblasts with single or multiple vacuoles, or sometimes areas of differentiated mature fat.[124] Areas with round cell change show greater cellularity and loss of the interspersed fine vascular pattern. However, pure round cell morphology is very rare, with most tumors with round cell features also harboring myxoid areas with transitional foci.[122,123,125,126] MLPS is negative for most immunohistochemical markers other than S100 protein, which is variably expressed within lesional cells.[127]

MLPS is characteristically associated with rearrangements of the *DDIT3* (DNA damage inducible transcript 3) gene on 12q13, a member of the CCAAT/enhancer-binding family of transcription factors, which has multiple roles including involvement in erythropoiesis and adipogenesis.[125,128] The *DDIT3* gene induces adipogenesis in cell lines[129] and helps in growth arrest; after gene rearrangement, this function is lost, aiding proliferation.[130] Although *DDIT3* most frequently partners with *FUS* on 16p11 [t(12;16)(q13;p11)] (in approximately 90% of MLPS), more rarely it fuses with *EWSR1* [t(12;22)(q13;q12)],[5] described in approximately 5% to 10% of tumors.[131] No histologic differences are evident between genetic subtypes of MLPS. Four fusion types are identified, respectively, involving exon 7 to 2, exon 10 to 2, exon 13 to 2, and exon 13 to 3. It has been noted that MLPS with type 1 fusions, whereby

Fig. 5. MLPS. This shows a patternless distribution of small cells with short spindled nuclei in prominent myxoid stroma. There is variable adipocytic differentiation, with interspersed small lipoblasts. Thin-walled curvilinear vessels are interspersed (H&E, original magnification ×400).

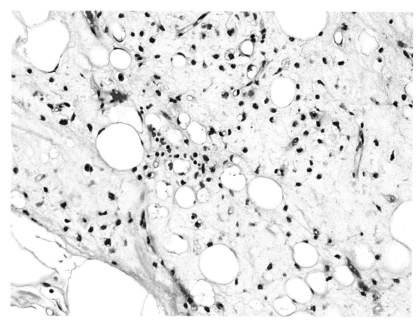

EWSR1 exon 7 is fused in-frame to *DDIT3* exon 2, may be associated with a more favorable outcome.

TUMORS WITH *EWSR1-NR4A3* (*CHN*) FUSION

EXTRASKELETAL MYXOID CHONDROSARCOMA

This neoplasm arises most frequently in extremity deep soft tissues of adults, particularly the limbs and limb girdles, as well as the head and neck, the abdomen, retroperitoneum and pelvic cavity, and rarely, primarily in the bone (osseous myxochondroid sarcoma).[132–135] EMC is associated with high rates of both local recurrence and distant metastases, with overall 5-, 10-, and 15-year survival rates of 90%, 70%, and 60%, respectively.[134] Metastases often occur many years after initial presentation and prolonged survival may occur in the presence of metastasis.[136] Despite its name, EMC does not show cartilaginous differentiation,[137] and histologically, these are lobulated, variably cellular neoplasms, comprising relatively small, rounded to ovoid cells with variable amounts of eosinophilic cytoplasm, present as single cells, files, cords, or reticular distributions in extensive hypovascular myxoid stroma (**Fig. 6**), sometimes showing features of hemorrhage. More rarely, EMC can show higher-grade morphology, with more pronounced cellularity and less stromal component, with cells showing epithelioid morphology and mitotic activity.[138] Very occasionally, EMC can

undergo dedifferentiation to pleomorphic sarcoma.[139] EMC shows variable, focal, often weak S100 protein expression, and some cases are variably immunoreactive for neuroendocrine markers (synaptophysin and sometimes chromogranin).

EMC most frequently harbor the t(9;22)(q22;q12) in which *EWSR1* fuses with *NR4A3* (formerly *CHN*).[53,140] Rarer translocations are t(9;17)(q22;q11), t(3;9)(q12;q22), and t(9;15)(q22;q21) in which *NR4A3* fuses with *TAF15* (associated with some EMC with neuroendocrine differentiation),[141] *TFG* and *TCF12*, as well as a variant *FUS-NR4A3* t(9;16)(q22;p11.2).[142] The chimeric *EWSR1*-NR4A3 protein may activate the nuclear receptor gene *PPARG*, a potential treatment target.[143] A single case of a tumor with morphologic features of both EMC and synovial sarcoma has been described,[144] which genetically harbored both *EWSR1-NR4A3* and *SS18-SSX2* fusion transcripts. In terms of *EWSR1*-rearranged neoplasms, EMC can closely mimic myoepithelial tumors, particularly when cellular, but myoepithelial neoplasms do not harbor *NR4A3* rearrangements.[145]

TUMORS WITH *EWSR1-CREB1* OR *EWSR1-ATF1* FUSIONS

The *ATF1* gene encodes the cyclic AMP-dependent transcription factor ATF1. This gene is a member of the cyclic-AMP response element binding protein (CREB)-ATF transcription factor family, which binds to cyclic adenosine monophosphate (cAMP)-inducible promoters. CREB proteins are related in functional terms to ATF,

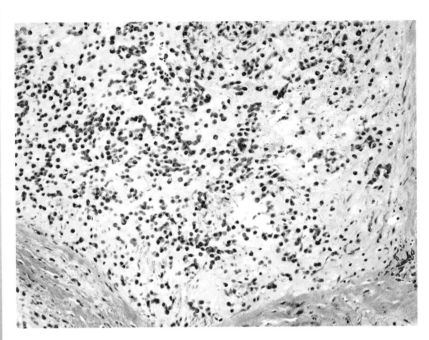

Fig. 6. EMC. This is composed of cords and files of cells with small nuclei and small to moderate amounts of eosinophilic cytoplasm in extensive myxoid stroma. The stroma is typically hypovascular (H&E, original magnification ×100).

with *CREB1* serving as an alternative gene to *ATF1* in AFH and CCS.[16] *EWSR1-ATF1* and/or *EWSR1-CREB1* gene fusions are characteristically associated with 5 clinically and pathologically different tumors: AFH, CCS (of tendons and aponeuroses), CCSLTGT, PPMS, and hyalinizing clear cell carcinoma (HCCC) of the salivary gland.[146] *EWSR1-ATF1* fusion has also been reported in a soft tissue myoepithelial tumor[147] as well as in a parotid gland angiosarcoma.[148] The soft tissue neoplasms of this group of tumors do not resemble any normal cellular counterpart. CCS and CCSLTGT show variable melanocytic differentiation, whereas AFH can variably show myoid features and PPMS does not show a detectable lineage. Identical gene fusions might generate phenotypically different neoplasms because of the influences of different anatomic sites on similar progenitor cells,[149] or because they occur in different progenitor cells (possibly mesenchymal stem cells), which activate specific sets of transcription factors. *EWSR1-ATF1* fusion transcripts are characteristic of HCCC, a low-grade carcinoma typically occurring in intraoral minor salivary glands in adult women[150–153] and its odontogenic counterpart clear cell odontogenic carcinoma (CCOC); these tumors are composed of infiltrative nests of uniform cells with granular to clear cytoplasm in myxohyaline stroma and express cytokeratins and EMA, but lack myoepithelial differentiation and are negative for actin, calponin, and S100 protein.[150,151,154,155] *EWSR1-CREB1* is now also described in CCOC,[156] and these genetics demonstrate that this fusion can generate

neoplasms with epithelial differentiation. Salivary glandular carcinomas, which can mimic HCCC such as epithelial-myoepithelial carcinoma, lack *EWSR1* rearrangements.[155]

Angiomatoid fibrous histiocytoma (originally described as angiomatoid malignant fibrous histiocytoma)[157] is a soft tissue tumor of intermediate biologic potential. AFH typically arises within extremity deep dermis and subcutis in children and young adults,[157–159] but can arise in older adults and in a variety of sites, including the head and neck and trunk, and more rarely other soft tissue sites or in viscera,[14,160–168] and is sometimes associated with systemic symptoms.[169] Most AFHs behave in a relatively indolent manner, although local recurrence occurs in up to 15%. Metastases are rare, occurring in between approximately 2% and 5%, sometimes after multiple recurrences,[159] and most frequently to regional nodes and exceptionally to the lungs.[170,171]

AFH are circumscribed, lobulated neoplasms that are often surrounded by a thick, frequently incomplete, fibrous pseudocapsule. Most also have a surrounding, although variably dense lymphoplasmacytic infiltrate or cuff of B and T cells, often with germinal centers. There is a wide spectrum of morphology, with the only constant finding being sheets or short fascicles of ovoid, spindled, or epithelioid cells with bland, vesicular nuclei and moderate amounts of eosinophilic cytoplasm (**Figs. 7** and **8**). Mitoses are usually rare, although there may be atypical forms, and small numbers of tumors exhibit focal or more marked pleomorphism, but none of these features has been

Fig. 7. AFH. This tumor is composed of cellular sheets of relatively uniform cells with ovoid nuclei, with a surrounding thick fibrous capsule and lymphoplasmacytic cuff with prominent hemosiderin deposition (H&E, original magnification ×200).

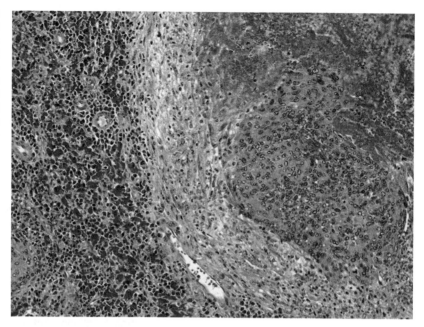

associated with a worse clinical outcome.[157,172–178] Multifocal hemorrhage with blood-filled cysts lined by lesional cells is typical. Rarer findings include the presence of rhabdomyoblast-like or clear cells[14] or reticulated cellular patterns in myxoid stroma.[14,163,179] Extension of AFH into the deep fascia or muscle has been described to show correlation with local recurrence and distant metastasis.[180] Desmin is variably positive in about 50% (and potential origin of AFH from fibroblastic reticulum cells has been postulated, with a subset of these cells expressing desmin),[181] and smooth muscle actin (SMA) and h-caldesmon may sometimes be expressed, but myogenin and MyoD1 are consistently negative. AFH can also express EMA, CD99, and CD68.[159,169]

Most AFH harbor *EWSR1* (rather than *FUS*) rearrangements, and AFH has 3 characteristic translocations: t(2;22)(q33;q12) generating *EWSR1-CREB1* fusion,[15,16] t(12;22)(q13;q12) with *EWSR1-ATF*,[13,15,164,182] and t(12;16)(q13;p11) with *FUS-ATF1*.[182] *FUS* encodes a multifunctional RNA binding protein component of the heterogeneous nuclear ribonucleoprotein complex. *EWSR1* and

Fig. 8. AFH. The neoplasm contains many blood-filled, pseudoangiomatoid spaces of varying sizes. These lack an endothelial lining. The tumor cells have ovoid nuclei and lack pleomorphism (H&E, original magnification ×400).

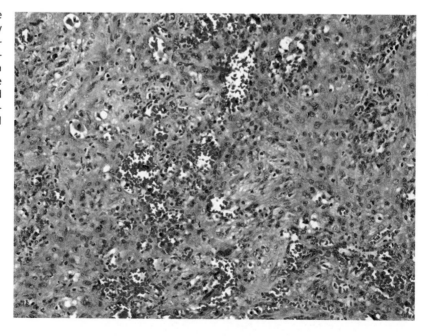

FUS can both act as 5′ partners for *ATF1*,[13] and *FUS* can act as an alternative to *EWSR1*[20] in other sarcomas[36,65,72] and acute myeloid leukemia.[183] The most common fusion is *EWSR1-CREB1*,[15,16] whereas *EWSR1-ATF1* has been described more frequently in AFH occurring within viscera[14]; however, individual fusions have not been related to specific anatomic sites, and the type of fusion is not related to behavior. Multiple copies of the *EWSR1-CREB1* fusion gene have been described in AFH with pleomorphism.[173] Performing RT-PCR for specific fusion transcripts and FISH using break-apart probes in conjunction is recommended, because the presence of *EWSR1* rearrangement alone may not reliably differentiate AFH from other *EWSR1*-rearranged neoplasms.[184]

CLEAR CELL SARCOMA (OF TENDONS AND APONEUROSES; OF SOFT PARTS; CONVENTIONAL CLEAR CELL SARCOMA)

CCS (of tendons and aponeuroses; of soft parts; conventional clear cell sarcoma) is a malignant mesenchymal neoplasm that exhibits melanocytic differentiation and arises predominantly in younger to middle-aged adults with an equal gender distribution.[185,186] CCS typically occurs in the foot or ankle region, often associated with tendons or aponeuroses, but can occur in other sites, such as the gastrointestinal tract and the head and neck.[187] CCS are aggressive neoplasms with frequent local recurrence, and propensity for metastases to lymph nodes, lungs, liver, brain, and bone. The 5-year survival with current management strategies varies between approximately 40% and 65%.[188–192]

Histologically, CCS is composed of nests of uniform ovoid to spindle cells with small ovoid or rounded vesicular nuclei, small single nucleoli, and relatively abundant clear to eosinophilic granular cytoplasm. Tumor nests are characteristically intersected by thin connective tissue septa (**Fig. 9**),[186] and variable numbers of Touton-like multinucleated tumor cells may be interspersed. Melanin pigment is present in up to 65%.[193] Rarer features include a microcystic pattern, small numbers of rhabdoid cells, myxoid change, or a pattern resembling seminoma with lymphoid infiltrate.[11] Immunohistochemically, CCS resembles melanoma, with diffuse and strong expression of S100 protein, HMB45, MelanA,[193] SOX10,[194] and microphthalmia transcription factor (MiTF). Neuroendocrine or neural markers may be focally expressed.[11]

Most CCS harbor reciprocal t(12;22)(q13;q12) translocations that generate *EWSR1-ATF1* fusions, whereas smaller numbers harbor *EWSR1-CREB1* gene fusions,[11,12] although clinical behavior has not been associated with fusion variant.[195] There are several different *EWSR1-ATF1* fusions transcripts,[12,186,196,197] most frequently fusion of *EWSR1* exon 8 to exon 4 of *ATF1*.[12,53] In the fusion protein, the *EWSR1* N-terminal domain is linked to the *ATF1* basic leucine zipper domain.[10] Phosphorylation of the kinase-inducible domain of *ATF1* usually regulates its activity,[198] but this is replaced by the *EWSR1* domain in CCS to produce a cAMP-independent transcriptional activator[198–200]; this fusion product is

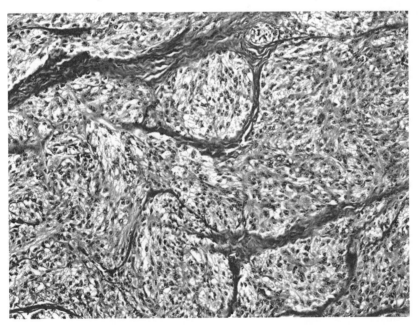

Fig. 9. CCS. This comprises nests of uniform ovoid to spindle cells with small ovoid or rounded vesicular nuclei, small single nucleoli, and relatively abundant clear to eosinophilic granular cytoplasm. Tumor nests are characteristically intersected by thin connective tissue septa (H&E, original magnification ×200).

thought to dysregulate several genes regulated by *CREB1/ATF1*,[198] such as *MiTF*.[198] *MiTF* has various splice forms, including the *MiTF-M* isoform, which is characteristic for melanocytes, cells of melanoma,[201–203] and CCS (and whose transcript is not expressed in AFH with *EWSR1-ATF1* fusion),[13,204] suggesting significant differences in downstream factors activated, according to the specific target cell of the *EWSR1-ATF1* fusion. In normal melanocytes, CREB1 and ATF1 drive the expression of *MiTF*, along with other factors, including SOX10, a transcription factor active in neural crest and neural cells. In CCS, the chimeric *EWSR1-ATF1* product causes constitutive *MiTF* expression,[198] which in the presence of SOX10 promotes proliferation and expression of the melanocytic phenotype. CCS has been shown to cluster with melanoma on gene expression profiling. The differential diagnosis of CCS includes melanoma, CCSLTGT, epithelioid malignant peripheral nerve sheath tumor (MPNST), perivascular epithelioid cell tumor, and melanotic schwannoma. However, other than CCSLTGT, these other neoplasms lack *EWSR1-ATF1* and *EWSR1-CREB1* fusions.

CLEAR CELL SARCOMA-LIKE TUMOR OF THE GASTROINTESTINAL TRACT

CCSLTGT tumor (also described as osteoclast-rich tumor of the gastrointestinal tract with features resembling clear cell sarcoma of soft parts or malignant gastrointestinal tract neuroectodermal tumor) is a very rare, highly aggressive neoplasm arising in the wall of the stomach, small or large intestines, predominantly in children or young adults.[205,206] Although CCSLTGT can show some morphologic resemblance to CCS, it differs from CCS in that it rarely shows melanocytic differentiation and is more aggressive, with high local recurrence rates, as well as high rates of nodal and visceral metastases and early death from disease. CCSLTGT can show a relatively heterogeneous morphology, but most neoplasms are composed of monomorphic, medium-sized to large rounded to ovoid cells with amphophilic, eosinophilic or clear cytoplasm, small nucleoli and frequent mitotic figures, arranged in sheets, or sometimes alveolar or pseudopapillary patterns. Usually, the nested architecture of CCS is lacking (**Fig. 10**). Tumors can show marked pleomorphism or oncocytic change.[207,208] Necrosis is typically prominent. CD68-positive osteoclast-like giant cells may be present, but the tumor giant cells of CCS are lacking. Immunohistochemically, CCSLTGT shows at least focal S100 protein and SOX10 positivity, but typically lacks HMB45 and MelanA. It is variably associated with focal neural/neuroendocrine marker expression. Electron microscopy studies have shown CCSLTGT to lack melanosomes, although dense core granules have been observed in some cases.[209] Genetically, CCSLTGT have been shown to harbor *EWSR1-CREB1* or sometimes *EWSR1-ATF1* fusions, with cases with *EWSR1-ATF1* sometimes more closely resembling conventional CCS. However, CCS with typical features of those of soft tissue sites can also occur within the gastrointestinal tract, with most of these containing *EWSR1-ATF1* fusions.[186,210]

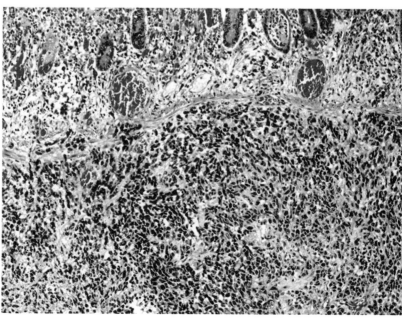

Fig. 10. CCS-like tumor of gastrointestinal tract. This neoplasm has a more heterogeneous morphology than conventional CCS. Most are composed of monomorphic, medium-sized to large rounded to ovoid cells with amphophilic, eosinophilic, or clear cytoplasm, small nucleoli and frequent mitotic figures, arranged in sheets, or sometimes alveolar or pseudopapillary patterns, and typically lack the nested architecture of CCS (H&E, original magnification ×200).

PRIMARY PULMONARY MYXOID SARCOMA

PPMS is a rare lung neoplasm that predominantly arises endobronchially in young to middle-aged adult women and is characterized by *EWSR1-CREB1* gene fusion. It tends to behave as a low-grade sarcoma; in the largest series of 10 cases, 2 of 6 patients with follow-up had distant metastasis (to kidney and brain, with the latter leading to death).[27] Morphologically, PPMS has a lobulated architecture and comprises cords and clusters of relatively small, ovoid, polygonal, or slender spindle cells, dispersed in extensive myxoid, hyaluronidase-sensitive matrix (**Figs. 11** and **12**). Often, the cells show a prominent reticular pattern that closely resembles EMC. Focally, the cells can show a more solid pattern. Although the cells are predominantly bland, there can be some variable focal cellular atypia, although pleomorphism is not marked. There may be focal necrosis, although the mitotic index is low, and there is no apparent correlation between morphologic features with behavior. Most tumors show areas of chronic inflammatory infiltrate, including lymphoid aggregates with germinal centers that can be present peripherally or mixed within the neoplasm. PPMS is negative for almost all immunohistochemical markers, expressing only vimentin and sometimes weak focal EMA. PPMS harbors *EWSR1-CREB1* fusions, with *EWSR1* exon 7 fusion site, and usually a breakpoint involving exon 7 for *CREB1*. The differential diagnosis includes EMC, soft tissue myoepithelial tumor,[211,212] and myxoid AFH.[179] The reticulated

cellular distribution in myxoid stroma is highly reminiscent of EMC, but PPMS lacks the translocations of EMC in which *NR4A3* on chromosome 9q22 fuses with a variety of partners. Soft tissue myoepithelial neoplasms can show similar features to PPMS and approximately half are associated with *EWSR1* rearrangements, but *CREB1* has not so far been reported as a partner gene. AFH is rarely documented within the lung and has been associated with both *EWSR1-CREB1*[14] and *EWSR1-ATF1*[162] fusions, but the cases described have shown the typical features of AFH, without the prominent myxoid stroma and reticular cell morphology of PPMS. AFH can rarely exhibit a reticular pattern[177] and myxoid stroma, but the reticular architecture is a predominant feature of PPMS. In addition, in contrast to AFH, PPMS always lacks desmin expression.[28]

TUMORS WITH OTHER CREB FAMILY TRANSCRIPTION FACTOR FUSIONS

EWSR1-CREM FUSIONS

Recently, a novel group of myxoid mesenchymal neoplasms has been described,[33] predominantly at intracranial sites in children or young adults with equal gender distribution, although one case has been described in perirectal soft tissues. These tumors are circumscribed and lobulated, typically comprising cords or reticular distributions of bland, uniform ovoid cells dispersed in a prominent myxoid/microcystic matrix. Mitoses are

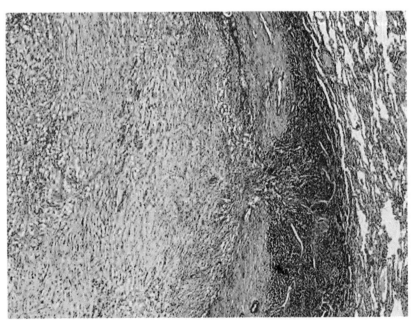

Fig. 11. PPMS. This is a nodular tumor composed of cords and clusters of relatively small, ovoid, polygonal, or slender spindle cells, dispersed in extensive myxoid matrix. Most tumors show areas of chronic inflammatory infiltrate, including lymphoid aggregates with germinal centers that can be present peripherally or mixed within the neoplasm (H&E, original magnification ×100).

Fig. 12. PPMS. Although there can be occasional pleomorphism, typically, lesional cells are uniform, disposed in cordlike patterns or as single cells within extensive myxoid stroma, reminiscent of EMC (H&E, original magnification ×400).

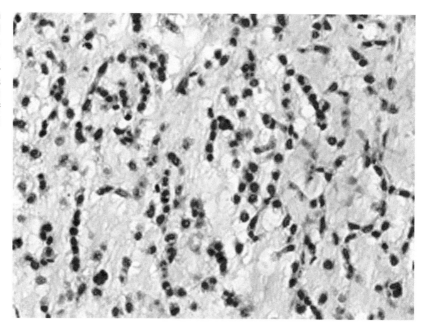

infrequent, and necrosis is absent.[213] Most are associated with sunburst amianthoid fibers. These neoplasms variably express desmin, EMA, GLUT1, and CD99. They are associated with either *EWSR1-CREM* or *EWSR1-CREB1* fusions.[33,213] Although these tumors[213] somewhat resemble the myxoid variant of AFH and can be associated with a fibrous pseudocapsule, other features of AFH such as lymphoid cuffing are lacking, suggesting that these represent a novel entity.[33] *EWSR1-CREM* has also been found in some clear cell carcinomas in the tongue, lung, and nasopharynx with the morphology of HCCC.[214]

SCLEROSING EPITHELIOID FIBROSARCOMA AND LOW-GRADE FIBROMYXOID SARCOMA

Most pure SEFs harbor rearrangements of *EWSR1*, with fusion to *CREB3L1* or more rarely *CREB3L2*, whereas only occasional cases show *FUS* rearrangement.[215] This is in contrast to most LGFMS, which harbor *FUS-CREB3L2* fusions, with *FUS-CREB3L1* fusions in smaller numbers and rare cases with *EWSR1-CREB3L1* fusions, whereas hybrid SEF/LGFMS neoplasms most frequently show *FUS-CREB3L2* rearrangements.[215] Pure SEF with *EWSR1-CREB3L1* fusion has been noted to present with intra-abdominal sarcomatosis, as a large mesenteric-based mass with extensive peritoneal and omental disease with ascites, and comprising uniform cords and nests of epithelioid cells within dense collagenous matrix, highlighting that other *EWSR1*-rearranged tumors than DSRCT need consideration in this clinical picture.[216]

TUMORS WITH OTHER *EWSR1*-NON-*ETS* FUSIONS

MYOEPITHELIAL TUMORS WITH *EWSR1* REARRANGEMENTS

Myoepithelial neoplasms are a heterogeneous group that shows morphologic, immunohistochemical, and ultrastructural features suggestive of myoepithelial differentiation. These tumors are well characterized within the salivary glands, but are also described in soft tissue, bone, and visceral locations. Mixed tumors have similar features but in addition show apocrine or eccrine ductular or tubular differentiation and are associated with recurrent *PLAG1* rearrangements, similar to those occurring in salivary glands (pleomorphic adenomas).[217,218] Because of their variation in morphology and immunophenotype, myoepithelial tumors can be difficult to characterize and are often confused with other tumors. Myoepithelial tumors of soft tissue arise most frequently in patients in the fourth decade, but there is a wide age distribution ranging from children to elderly patients. They occur most frequently in extremities, followed by the head and neck and trunk, arising within subcutaneous or deep soft tissues (including the retroperitoneum).[219] Although macroscopically typically circumscribed and lobulated, histologically they are often infiltrative, with heterogeneous morphology, and comprise epithelioid, spindled, plasmacytoid, or clear cells in variable proportions, arranged in small nests, strands, or files (**Figs. 13** and **14**).

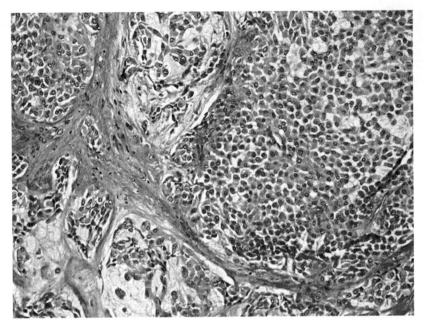

Fig. 13. Myoepithelial tumor. These neoplasms are morphologically heterogeneous and are composed of epithelioid, spindled, plasmacytoid, or clear cells in variable proportions, arranged in small nests, strands, or files. Here, many cells have a somewhat plasmacytoid appearance and are arranged in cords, trabeculae, or more solid distributions, with relatively prominent amounts of myxoid stroma (H&E, original magnification ×200).

The surrounding matrix varies from collagenous to myxoid or chondromyxoid, sometimes with areas of chondroid or bone. The mitotic index is typically less than 5 per 10 high-power fields. Histologic features of malignancy include pleomorphism, prominent nucleoli, necrosis, and atypical mitotic figures.[211] Cases with histologically "benign" morphology may recur but usually do not metastasize, whereas recurrence occurs in approximately 40% of malignant myoepithelial tumors, with metastases in approximately one-third, to lymph nodes, soft tissues, or lungs.[211] Malignant myoepithelial neoplasms of the soft tissue in children and teenagers (up to age 17) are aggressive, with metastases in approximately half.[220] Myoepithelial tumors at cutaneous sites are typically circumscribed with similar features to those of soft tissue, sometimes displaying solid syncytial growth patterns of spindle, ovoid, or histiocytoid cells,[30,221] or are mixed tumors (chondroid syringomas).[222–225] Cutaneous myoepithelial tumors are rarely pleomorphic but can show focal necrosis; recurrence or metastasis has not been described.

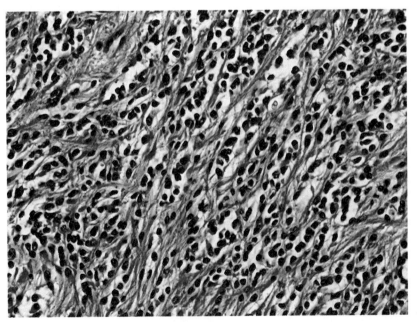

Fig. 14. Myoepithelial tumor. Here, the cells are arranged in a packeted distribution and are epithelioid and relatively uniform, with rounded hyperchromatic nuclei and small amounts of amphophilic cytoplasm (H&E, original magnification ×200).

There is a highly variable immunophenotypic spectrum, including expression of S100 protein, cytokeratins, EMA, SMA, calponin, CD10, and glial fibrillary acidic protein (GFAP), and the expression of S100 protein and an epithelial marker might be considered minimal requirements. Cutaneous myoepithelial tumors express S100 protein and EMA, with variable actins, cytokeratins, and GFAP.[30,224,225] Nuclear p63 occurs in about one-quarter of cases, and desmin expression is infrequent. There is nuclear INI1 loss in approximately 10% of adult soft tissue myoepithelial carcinomas, and 40% of childhood myoepithelial tumors.[226,227]

EWSR1 (or more rarely *FUS*) rearrangements have been documented in approximately 50% of myoepithelial neoplasms of soft tissue and bone, and about 45% of cutaneous tumors.[228–230] This includes most of those arising in the bones and lung, and in a proportion of cutaneous neoplasms.[29] *EWSR1*-rearranged deep soft tissue and bone myoepitheliomas are not associated with ductal or glandular differentiation, or with cartilaginous or bony matrix,[29] in keeping with *EWSR1*-rearranged myoepithelial tumors representing genetically distinct entities from those with PLAG1-rearrangements. *EWSR1* rearrangements in soft tissue myoepithelial neoplasms most frequently involve one of 3 partners. *EWSR1-PBX1* fusion resulting from t(1;22)(q23;q12) is reported in those occurring within soft tissue, bone, and lungs, and composed of clear or spindle cells without atypia, within a collagenous matrix.[231] *EWSR1-POU5F1* gene fusion resulting from t(6;22)(p21;q12) has been described in soft tissue tumors with nested patterns of clear cells as well as in a malignant neoplasm in bone[76] (although has also been reported in ES, a mucoepidermoid carcinoma of salivary glands and in *CRTC1-MAML2*-negative cutaneous hidradenomas).[232] *POU5F1* encodes the protein OCT3/4, although *POU5F1*-rearranged myoepithelial neoplasms do not typically express this immunohistochemically.[29] *EWSR1-ZNF44* resulting from t(19:22)(q13;q12) is rare and is reported in a primary myoepithelial neoplasm of lung[29] and in a myoepithelial carcinoma of the occiput, which metastasized to the lung.[233] These neoplasms were positive for cytokeratins and S100 protein but negative for EMA. *FUS-KLF17* and rarely *EWSR1-KLF17* fusions are also described in myoepithelial tumors, with *KLF17*-rearranged myoepithelial tumors tending to arise in younger patients and showing a trabecular pattern within myxohyaline matrix.[234] *EWSR1-ATF1* fusion has been reported within a pelvic myoepithelial tumor expressing EMA and S100 protein.[147] Myoepithelial tumors have a wide differential diagnosis, which includes carcinoma, EMC, epithelioid sarcoma, MPNST, and ossifying fibromyxoid tumor.[235,236] Sometimes there is a predominant round cell morphology, mimicking small round cell neoplasms such as ES and DSRCT, both of which harbor *EWSR1* gene rearrangements, although myoepithelial neoplasms have not yet been associated with classical fusion transcripts of ES or *EWSR1-WT1* of DSRCT.[237]

OTHER *EWSR1*-REARRANGED TUMORS:

EWSR1-SMAD3 fusions have been shown in 3 locally recurrent superficial acral tumors, in 2 adult women and congenitally in an infant boy.[238] These neoplasms showed low-grade spindle cell/"fibroblastic" morphology, with a nodular growth pattern with zonation, with peripheral hypercellular areas in short fascicles, and hypocellular central areas of hyalinization and infarction in the adult cases, and all showed a nonspecific immunoprofile, with negative SMA, S100 protein, CD31, and CD34, but with consistent ERG expression of uncertain significance.[238] *EWSR1-NFATC1* from t(18;22)(q23;q12) has been described in a benign bony hemangioma located in the clavicle.[239] Fusion of *EWSR1* to the *YY1* gene has been described in 2 peritoneal mesotheliomas and was the first specific fusion gene detected in this neoplasm.[240] *EWSR1/FUS-ATF1* fusions have been subsequently reported in a group of malignant mesotheliomas arising in young adults under the age of 40, lacking a history of asbestos exposure, and occurring within the peritoneum or thorax. These tumors have shown conventional epithelioid morphology with retained expression of BAP1, suggesting a novel subtype.[241] Recently, *EWSR1/FUS–TFCP2* fusions have been shown in an aggressive group of epithelioid rhabdomyosarcomas, predominantly in young adult women, in the pelvic region, the chest wall, and the sphenoid bone.[80] These neoplasms were composed of sheets and short fascicles of cells with monotonous rounded nuclei and prominent nucleoli, with variable fibrous stroma and focal sclerosis. They expressed myogenic markers, including MyoD1 and myogenin, and have been shown to express epithelial markers as well as ALK and TERT, the latter being potential therapeutic targets, and did not cluster with other rhabdomyosarcomas, or with other *EWSR1/FUS*-fused tumors on expression profiling. In addition, *FUS-TFCP2* is reported in a mandibular spindle cell/sclerosing rhabdomyosarcoma of a 72-year-old man.[242]

SUMMARY

The *EWSR1* gene is notable for its ability to rearrange with a wide variety of fusion partners to generate an array of distinct, mostly mesenchymal tumors that show a variety of morphologic features and clinical behaviors. It is evident that the finding of an *EWSR1* gene rearrangement in isolation by FISH is nonspecific, and although the use of RT-PCR in conjunction may identify specific fusion transcripts, even this may not be a diagnostic finding. Both of these routine ancillary molecular techniques need interpretation in correlation with the clinical picture and histologic and immunohisto-chemical findings. The reasons for the propensity of *EWSR1* to partner with many different genes leading to oncogenesis remain to be clarified, as do the mechanisms by which such histologically and clinically diverse neoplasms are generated. Further insight into the secondary genetic and epigenetic factors and the downstream pathways involved in each tumor type will ultimately help to direct targeted approaches to therapy. It is also likely that further novel *EWSR1*-rearranged neoplasms will be detected with the incorporation of more sophisticated sequencing techniques into the routine diagnostic setting.

REFERENCES

1. Mitelman F, Johansson B, Mertens F. The impact of translocations and gene fusions on cancer causation. Nat Rev Cancer 2007;7:233–45.
2. Mani RS, Chinnaiyan AM. Triggers for genomic rearrangements: insights into genomic, cellular and environmental influences. Nat Rev Genet 2010;11:819–29.
3. Soutoglou E, Misteli T. On the contribution of spatial genome organization to cancerous chromosome translocations. J Natl Cancer Inst Monogr 2008;(39):16–9.
4. Arvand A, Denny CT. Biology of EWS/ETS fusions in Ewing's family tumors. Oncogene 2001;20:5747–54.
5. Panagopoulos I, Hoglund M, Mertens F, et al. Fusion of the EWS and CHOP genes in myxoid liposarcoma. Oncogene 1996;12:489–94.
6. Dal Cin P, Sciot R, Panagopoulos I, et al. Additional evidence of a variant translocation t(12;22) with EWS/CHOP fusion in myxoid liposarcoma: clinicopathological features. J Pathol 1997;182:437–41.
7. Hosaka T, Nakashima Y, Kusuzaki K, et al. A novel type of EWS-CHOP fusion gene in two cases of myxoid liposarcoma. J Mol Diagn 2002;4:164–71.
8. Matsui Y, Ueda T, Kubo T, et al. A novel type of EWS-CHOP fusion gene in myxoid liposarcoma. Biochem Biophys Res Commun 2006;348:437–40.
9. Suzuki K, Matsui Y, Endo K, et al. Myxoid liposarcoma with EWS-CHOP type 1 fusion gene. Anticancer Res 2011;30:4679–83.
10. Zucman J, Delattre O, Desmaze C, et al. EWS and ATF-1 gene fusion induced by t(12;22) translocation in malignant melanoma of soft parts. Nat Genet 1993;4:341–5.
11. Hisaoka M, Ishida T, Kuo TT, et al. Clear cell sarcoma of soft tissue: a clinicopathologic, immuno-histochemical, and molecular analysis of 33 cases. Am J Surg Pathol 2008;32:452–60.
12. Wang WL, Mayordomo E, Zhang W, et al. Detection and characterization of EWSR1/ATF1 and EWSR1/CREB1 chimeric transcripts in clear cell sarcoma (melanoma of soft parts). Mod Pathol 2009;22:1201–9.
13. Hallor KH, Mertens F, Jin Y, et al. Fusion of the EWSR1 and ATF1 genes without expression of the MITF-M transcript in angiomatoid fibrous histiocytoma. Genes Chromosomes Cancer 2005;44:97–102.
14. Chen G, Folpe AL, Colby TV, et al. Angiomatoid fibrous histiocytoma: unusual sites and unusual morphology. Mod Pathol 2011;24:1560–70.
15. Rossi S, Szuhai K, Ijszenga M, et al. EWSR1-CREB1 and EWSR1-ATF1 fusion genes in angiomatoid fibrous histiocytoma. Clin Cancer Res 2007;13:7322–8.
16. Antonescu CR, Dal Cin P, Nafa K, et al. EWSR1-CREB1 is the predominant gene fusion in angiomatoid fibrous histiocytoma. Genes Chromosomes Cancer 2007;46:1051–60.
17. Ladanyi M, Gerald W. Fusion of the EWS and WT1 genes in the desmoplastic small round cell tumor. Cancer Res 1994;54:2837–40.
18. Gerald WL, Rosai J, Ladanyi M. Characterization of the genomic breakpoint and chimeric transcripts in the EWS-WT1 gene fusion of desmoplastic small round cell tumor. Proc Natl Acad Sci U S A 1995;92:1028–32.
19. Antonescu CR, Gerald WL, Magid MS, et al. Molecular variants of the EWS-WT1 gene fusion in desmoplastic small round cell tumor. Diagn Mol Pathol 1998;7:24–8.
20. Clark J, Benjamin H, Gill S, et al. Fusion of the EWS gene to CHN, a member of the steroid/thyroid receptor gene superfamily, in a human myxoid chondrosarcoma. Oncogene 1996;12:229–35.
21. Labelle Y, Zucman J, Stenman G, et al. Oncogenic conversion of a novel orphan nuclear receptor by chromosome translocation. Hum Mol Genet 1995;4:2219–26.
22. Sciot R, Dal Cin P, Fletcher C, et al. t(9;22)(q22-31;q11-12) is a consistent marker of extraskeletal myxoid chondrosarcoma: evaluation of three cases. Mod Pathol 1995;8:765–8.
23. Stenman G, Andersson H, Mandahl N, et al. Translocation t(9;22)(q22;q12) is a primary cytogenetic abnormality in extraskeletal myxoid chondrosarcoma. Int J Cancer 1995;62:398–402.

24. Attwooll C, Tariq M, Harris M, et al. Identification of a novel fusion gene involving hTAFII68 and CHN from a t(9;17)(q22;q11.2) translocation in an extra-skeletal myxoid chondrosarcoma. Oncogene 1999; 18:7599–601.

25. Panagopoulos I, Mencinger M, Dietrich CU, et al. Fusion of the RBP56 and CHN genes in extraskele-tal myxoid chondrosarcomas with translocation t(9;17)(q22;q11). Oncogene 1999;18:7594–8.

26. Sjogren H, Meis-Kindblom J, Kindblom LG, et al. Fusion of the EWS-related gene TAF2N to TEC in extraskeletal myxoid chondrosarcoma. Cancer Res 1999;59:5064–7.

27. Sjogren H, Wedell B, Meis-Kindblom JM, et al. Fusion of the NH2-terminal domain of the basic helix-loop-helix protein TCF12 to TEC in extraskeletal myxoid chondrosarcoma with translocation t(9;15)(q22;q21). Cancer Res 2000;60:6832–5.

28. Thway K, Nicholson AG, Lawson K, et al. Primary pulmonary myxoid sarcoma with EWSR1-CREB1 fusion: a new tumor entity. Am J Surg Pathol 2011;35:1722–32.

29. Antonescu CR, Zhang L, Chang NE, et al. EWSR1-POU5F1 fusion in soft tissue myoepithelial tumors. A molecular analysis of sixty-six cases, including soft tissue, bone, and visceral lesions, showing common involvement of the EWSR1 gene. Genes Chromosomes Cancer 2010;49:1114–24.

30. Jo VY, Antonescu CR, Zhang L, et al. Cutaneous syncytial myoepithelioma: clinicopathologic char-acterization in a series of 38 cases. Am J Surg Pathol 2013;37:710–8.

31. Doyle LA, Wang WL, Dal Cin P, et al. MUC4 is a sensitive and extremely useful marker for scle-rosing epithelioid fibrosarcoma: association with FUS gene rearrangement. Am J Surg Pathol 2012;36:1444–51.

32. Lau PP, Lui PC, Lau GT, et al. EWSR1-CREB3L1 Gene fusion: a novel alternative molecular aberra-tion of low-grade fibromyxoid sarcoma. Am J Surg Pathol 2013;37:734–8.

33. Kao YC, Sung YS, Zhang L, et al. EWSR1 fusions with CREB family transcription factors define a novel myx-oid mesenchymal tumor with predilection for intracra-nial location. Am J Surg Pathol 2017;41:482–90.

34. Bertolotti A, Lutz Y, Heard DJ, et al. hTAF(II)68, a novel RNA/ssDNA-binding protein with homology to the pro-oncoproteins TLS/FUS and EWS is asso-ciated with both TFIID and RNA polymerase II. EMBO J 1996;15:5022–31.

35. Delattre O, Zucman J, Plougastel B, et al. Gene fusion with ETS DNA-binding domain caused by chromosome translocation in human tumours. Nature 1992;359:162–5.

36. Crozat A, Aman P, Mandahl N, et al. Fusion of CHOP to a novel RNA-binding protein in human myxoid liposarcoma. Nature 1993;363:640–4.

37. Morohoshi F, Arai K, Takahashi EI, et al. Cloning and mapping of a human RBP56 gene encoding a putative RNA binding protein similar to FUS/TLS and EWS proteins. Genomics 1996;38:51–7.

38. Azuma M, Embree LJ, Sabaawy H, et al. Ewing sar-coma protein ewsr1 maintains mitotic integrity and proneural cell survival in the zebrafish embryo. PLoS One 2007;2:e979.

39. Stolow DT, Haynes SR. Cabeza, a Drosophila gene encoding a novel RNA binding protein, shares ho-mology with EWS and TLS, two genes involved in human sarcoma formation. Nucleic Acids Res 1995;23:835–43.

40. Aurias A, Rimbaut C, Buffe D, et al. Translocation of chromosome 22 in Ewing's sarcoma. C R Seances Acad Sci III 1983;296:1105–7, [in French].

41. Leemann-Zakaryan RP, Pahlich S, Sedda MJ, et al. Dy-namic subcellular localization of the Ewing sarcoma proto-oncoprotein and its association with and stabili-zation of microtubules. J Mol Biol 2009;386:1–13.

42. Li H, Watford W, Li C, et al. Ewing sarcoma gene EWS is essential for meiosis and B lymphocyte development. J Clin Invest 2007;117:1314–23.

43. Plougastel B, Zucman J, Peter M, et al. Genomic structure of the EWS gene and its relationship to EWSR1, a site of tumor-associated chromosome translocation. Genomics 1993;18:609–15.

44. Bovee JV, Devilee P, Cornelisse CJ, et al. Identifica-tion of an EWS-pseudogene using translocation detection by RT-PCR in Ewing's sarcoma. Biochem Biophys Res Commun 1995;213:1051–60.

45. Zakaryan RP, Gehring H. Identification and charac-terization of the nuclear localization/retention signal in the EWS proto-oncoprotein. J Mol Biol 2006;363: 27–38.

46. Fisher C. The diversity of soft tissue tumours with EWSR1 gene rearrangements: a review. Histopa-thology 2014;64:134–50.

47. Aman P, Panagopoulos I, Lassen C, et al. Expres-sion patterns of the human sarcoma-associated genes FUS and EWS and the genomic structure of FUS. Genomics 1996;37:1–8.

48. Riggi N, Cironi L, Suva ML, et al. Sarcomas: ge-netics, signalling, and cellular origins. Part 1: the fellowship of TET. J Pathol 2007;213:4–20.

49. Kim J, Pelletier J. Molecular genetics of chromo-some translocations involving EWS and related family members. Physiol Genomics 1999;1:127–38.

50. Sandberg A, Bridge J. Updates on the cytoge-netics and molecular genetics of bone and soft tis-sue tumors: alveolar soft part sarcoma. Cancer Genet Cytogenet 2002;136:1–9.

51. Sandberg AA, Bridge JA. Updates on cytogenetics and molecular genetics of bone and soft tissue tu-mors: ewing sarcoma and peripheral primitive neu-roectodermal tumors. Cancer Genet Cytogenet 2000;123:1–26.

52. Antonescu CR, Elahi A, Humphrey M, et al. Specificity of TLS-CHOP rearrangement for classic myxoid/round cell liposarcoma. Absence in predominantly myxoid well-differentiated liposarcoma. J Mol Diag 2000;2:132–8.

53. Panagopoulos I, Mertens F, Debiec-Rychter M, et al. Molecular genetic characterization of the EWS/ATF1 fusion gene in clear cell sarcoma of tendons and aponeuroses. Int J Cancer 2002;99: 560–7.

54. Fletcher CDM, Bridge JA, Hogendoorn PCW, et al. WHO classification of tumours of soft tissue and bone. Lyon (France): World Health Organization Classification of Tumours; 2013.

55. Askin FB, Rosai J, Sibley RK, et al. Malignant small cell tumor of the thoracopulmonary region in childhood: a distinctive clinicopathologic entity of uncertain histogenesis. Cancer 1979;43:2438–51.

56. Applebaum MA, Worch J, Matthay KK, et al. Clinical features and outcomes in patients with extraskeletal Ewing sarcoma. Cancer 2011;117:3027–32.

57. Potratz J, Dirksen U, Jurgens H, et al. Ewing sarcoma: clinical state-of-the-art. Pediatr Hematol Oncol 2012;29:1–11.

58. Folpe AL, Goldblum JR, Rubin BP, et al. Morphologic and immunophenotypic diversity in Ewing family tumors: a study of 66 genetically confirmed cases. Am J Surg Pathol 2005;29:1025–33.

59. Bridge JA, Fidler ME, Neff JR, et al. Adamantinoma-like Ewing's sarcoma: genomic confirmation, phenotypic drift. Am J Surg Pathol 1999;23: 159–65.

60. Llombart-Bosch A, Pellin A, Carda C, et al. Soft tissue Ewing sarcoma–peripheral primitive neuroectodermal tumor with atypical clear cell pattern shows a new type of EWS-FEV fusion transcript. Diagn Mol Pathol 2000;9:137–44.

61. Llombart-Bosch A, Machado I, Navarro S, et al. Histological heterogeneity of Ewing's sarcoma/ PNET: an immunohistochemical analysis of 415 genetically confirmed cases with clinical support. Virchows Arch 2009;455:397–411.

62. Yoshida A, Sekine S, Tsuta K, et al. NKX2.2 is a useful immunohistochemical marker for ewing sarcoma. Am J Surg Pathol 2012;36:993–9.

63. Parham DM, Dias P, Kelly DR, et al. Desmin positivity in primitive neuroectodermal tumors of childhood. Am J Surg Pathol 1992;16:483–92.

64. Wang WL, Patel NR, Caragea M, et al. Expression of ERG, an Ets family transcription factor, identifies ERG-rearranged Ewing sarcoma. Mod Pathol 2012; 25:1378–83.

65. Ordonez JL, Osuna D, Herrero D, et al. Advances in Ewing's sarcoma research: where are we now and what lies ahead? Cancer Res 2009;69:7140–50.

66. Sorensen PHB LS, Lopez-Terrada D, Liu XF, et al. A second Ewing's sarcoma translocation t(21;22) fuses the EWS gene to another ETS-family transcription factor ERG. Nat Genet 1994;6:146–51.

67. Maire G, Brown CW, Bayani J, et al. Complex rearrangement of chromosomes 19, 21, and 22 in Ewing sarcoma involving a novel reciprocal inversion-insertion mechanism of EWS-ERG fusion gene formation: a case analysis and literature review. Cancer Genet Cytogenet 2008;181:81–92.

68. Jeon IS, Davis JN, Braun BS, et al. A variant Ewing's sarcoma translocation (7;22) fuses the EWS gene to the ETS gene ETV1. Oncogene 1995;10:1229–34.

69. Kaneko Y, Yoshida K, Handa M, et al. Fusion of an ETS-family gene, EIAF, to EWS by t(17;22)(q12;q12) chromosome translocation in an undifferentiated sarcoma of infancy. Genes Chromosomes Cancer 1996; 15:115–21.

70. Peter M, Couturier J, Pacquement H, et al. A new member of the ETS family fused to EWS in Ewing tumors. Oncogene 1997;14:1159–64.

71. Ng TL, O'Sullivan MJ, Pallen CJ, et al. Ewing sarcoma with novel translocation t(2;16) producing an in-frame fusion of FUS and FEV. J Mol Diagn 2007;9:459–63.

72. Ichikawa H, Shimizu K, Hayashi Y, et al. An RNA-binding protein gene, TLS/FUS, is fused to ERG in human myeloid leukemia with t(16;21) chromosomal translocation. Cancer Res 1994;54:2865–8.

73. Berg T, Kalsaas AH, Buechner J, et al. Ewing sarcoma-peripheral neuroectodermal tumor of the kidney with a FUS-ERG fusion transcript. Cancer Genet Cytogenet 2009;194:53–7.

74. Shulman SC, Katzenstein H, Bridge J, et al. Ewing sarcoma with 7;22 translocation: three new cases and clinicopathological characterization. Fetal Pediatr Pathol 2012;31:341–8.

75. Szuhai K, Ijszenga M, de Jong D, et al. The NFATc2 gene is involved in a novel cloned translocation in a Ewing sarcoma variant that couples its function in immunology to oncology. Clin Cancer Res 2009; 15:2259–68.

76. Yamaguchi S, Yamazaki Y, Ishikawa Y, et al. EWSR1 is fused to POU5F1 in a bone tumor with translocation t(6;22)(p21;q12). Genes Chromosomes Cancer 2005;43:217–22.

77. Mastrangelo T, Modena P, Tornielli S, et al. A novel zinc finger gene is fused to EWS in small round cell tumor. Oncogene 2000;19:3799–804.

78. Sumegi J, Nishio J, Nelson M, et al. A novel t(4;22)(q31;q12) produces an EWSR1-SMARCA5 fusion in extraskeletal Ewing sarcoma/primitive neuroectodermal tumor. Mod Pathol 2011;24:333–42.

79. Wang L, Bhargava R, Zheng T, et al. Undifferentiated small round cell sarcomas with rare EWS gene fusions: identification of a novel EWS-SP3 fusion and of additional cases with the EWS-ETV1 and EWS-FEV fusions. J Mol Diagn 2007;9: 498–509.

80. Watson S, Perrin V, Guillemot D, et al. Transcriptomic definition of molecular subgroups of small round cell sarcomas. J Pathol 2018;245:29–40.

81. Charville GW, Wang WL, Ingram DR, et al. PAX7 expression in sarcomas bearing the EWSR1-NFATC2 translocation. Mod Pathol 2018, [Epub ahead of print].

82. Charville GW, Wang WL, Ingram DR, et al. EWSR1 fusion proteins mediate PAX7 expression in Ewing sarcoma. Mod Pathol 2017;30:1312–20.

83. Fletcher C, Bridge JA, Hogendoorn PCW, et al, editors. WHO classification of tumours of soft tissue and bone. Lyon (France): IARC; 2013. p. 305–10.

84. Sankar S, Lessnick SL. Promiscuous partnerships in Ewing's sarcoma. Cancer Genet 2011;204: 351–65.

85. Ohno T, Rao VN, Reddy ES. EWS/Fli-1 chimeric protein is a transcriptional activator. Cancer Res 1993;53:5859–63.

86. May WA, Lessnick SL, Braun BS, et al. The Ewing's sarcoma EWS/FLI-1 fusion gene encodes a more potent transcriptional activator and is a more powerful transforming gene than FLI-1. Mol Cell Biol 1993;13:7393–8.

87. Hahm KB, Cho K, Lee C, et al. Repression of the gene encoding the TGF-beta type II receptor is a major target of the EWS-FLI1 oncoprotein. Nat Genet 1999;23:222–7.

88. Camoes MJ, Paulo P, Ribeiro FR, et al. Potential downstream target genes of aberrant ETS transcription factors are differentially affected in ewing's sarcoma and prostate carcinoma. PLoS One 2012;7:e49819.

89. Tirado OM, Mateo-Lozano S, Villar J, et al. Caveolin-1 (CAV1) is a target of EWS/FLI-1 and a key determinant of the oncogenic phenotype and tumorigenicity of Ewing's sarcoma cells. Cancer Res 2006;66:9937–47.

90. Matsumoto Y, Tanaka K, Nakatani F, et al. Downregulation and forced expression of EWS-Fli1 fusion gene results in changes in the expression of G(1) regulatory genes. Br J Cancer 2001;84:768–75.

91. Richter GH, Plehm S, Fasan A, et al. EZH2 is a mediator of EWS/FLI1 driven tumor growth and metastasis blocking endothelial and neuroectodermal differentiation. Proc Natl Acad Sci U S A 2009;106:5324–9.

92. Christensen L, Joo J, Lee S, et al. FOXM1 is an oncogenic mediator in ewing sarcoma. PLoS One 2013;8:e54556.

93. Beauchamp E, Bulut G, Abaan O, et al. GLI1 is a direct transcriptional target of EWS-FLI1 oncoprotein. J Biol Chem 2009;284:9074–82.

94. Garcia-Aragoncillo E, Carrillo J, Lalli E, et al. DAX1, a direct target of EWS/FLI1 oncoprotein, is a principal regulator of cell-cycle progression in Ewing's tumor cells. Oncogene 2008;27:6034–43.

95. de Alava E, Kawai A, Healey JH, et al. EWS-FLI1 fusion transcript structure is an independent determinant of prognosis in Ewing's sarcoma. J Clin Oncol 1998;16:1248–55.

96. Yamada Y, Kuda M, Kohashi K, et al. Histological and immunohistochemical characteristics of undifferentiated small round cell sarcomas associated with CIC-DUX4 and BCOR-CCNB3 fusion genes. Virchows Arch 2017;470:373–80.

97. Italiano A, Sung YS, Zhang L, et al. High prevalence of CIC fusion with double-homeobox (DUX4) transcription factors in EWSR1-negative undifferentiated small blue round cell sarcomas. Genes Chromosomes Cancer 2012;51:207–18.

98. Graham C, Chilton-MacNeill S, Zielenska M, et al. The CIC-DUX4 fusion transcript is present in a subgroup of pediatric primitive round cell sarcomas. Hum Pathol 2012;43:180–9.

99. Kawamura-Saito M, Yamazaki Y, Kaneko K, et al. Fusion between CIC and DUX4 up-regulates PEA3 family genes in Ewing-like sarcomas with t(4;19)(q35;q13) translocation. Hum Mol Genet 2006;15:2125–37.

100. Yoshimoto M, Graham C, Chilton-MacNeill S, et al. Detailed cytogenetic and array analysis of pediatric primitive sarcomas reveals a recurrent CIC-DUX4 fusion gene event. Cancer Genet Cytogenet 2009;195:1–11.

101. Pierron G, Tirode F, Lucchesi C, et al. A new subtype of bone sarcoma defined by BCOR-CCNB3 gene fusion. Nat Genet 2012;44:461–6.

102. Puls F, Niblett A, Marland G, et al. BCOR-CCNB3 (Ewing-like) sarcoma: a clinicopathologic analysis of 10 cases, in comparison with conventional Ewing sarcoma. Am J Surg Pathol 2014;38:1307–18.

103. Wang L, Motoi T, Khanin R, et al. Identification of a novel, recurrent HEY1-NCOA2 fusion in mesenchymal chondrosarcoma based on a genome-wide screen of exon-level expression data. Genes Chromosomes Cancer 2012;51:127–39.

104. Ordonez NG. Desmoplastic small round cell tumor: I: a histopathologic study of 39 cases with emphasis on unusual histological patterns. Am J Surg Pathol 1998;22:1303–13.

105. Heikkila AJ, Prebtani AP. Desmoplastic small round cell tumour in a 74 year old man: an uncommon cause of ascites (case report). Diagn Pathol 2011;6:55.

106. Gerald WL, Ladanyi M, de Alava E, et al. Clinical, pathologic, and molecular spectrum of tumors associated with t(11;22)(p13;q12): desmoplastic small round-cell tumor and its variants. J Clin Oncol 1998;16:3028–36.

107. Lopez F, Costales M, Vivanco B, et al. Sinonasal desmoplastic small round cell tumor. Auris Nasus Larynx 2013;40:573–6.

108. Yin WH, Guo SP, Yang HY, et al. Desmoplastic small round cell tumor of the submandibular

gland–a rare but distinctive primary salivary gland neoplasm. Hum Pathol 2010;41:438–42.

109. Yaren A, Degirmencioglu S, Calli Demirkan N, et al. Primary mesenchymal tumors of the colon: a report of three cases. Turk J Gastroenterol 2014;25:314–8.

110. Liu Q, Liu N, Chen D. Primary desmoplastic small round cell tumor of the duodenum. Eur J Med Res 2014;19:38.

111. Thway K. Primitive round cell neoplasms. Surg Pathol Clin 2011;4:799–818.

112. da Silva RC, Medeiros Filho P, Chioato L, et al. Desmoplastic small round cell tumor of the kidney mimicking Wilms tumor: a case report and review of the literature. Appl Immunohistochem Mol Morphol 2009;17:557–62.

113. Rao P, Tamboli P, Fillman EP, et al. Primary intrarenal desmoplastic small round cell tumor: expanding the histologic spectrum, with special emphasis on the differential diagnostic considerations. Pathol Res Pract 2014;210:1130–3.

114. Ordonez NG. Desmoplastic small round cell tumor: II: an ultrastructural and immunohistochemical study with emphasis on new immunohistochemical markers. Am J Surg Pathol 1998;22:1314–27.

115. Trupiano JK, Machen SK, Barr FG, et al. Cytokeratin-negative desmoplastic small round cell tumor: a report of two cases emphasizing the utility of reverse transcriptase-polymerase chain reaction. Mod Pathol 1999;12:849–53.

116. Zhang PJ, Goldblum JR, Pawel BR, et al. Immunophenotype of desmoplastic small round cell tumors as detected in cases with EWS-WT1 gene fusion product. Mod Pathol 2003;16:229–35.

117. Sawyer JRTA, Lewis JM. A novel reciprocal chromosome translocation t(11;22)(p13;q12) in an intraabdominal desmoplastic small round-cell tumor. Am J Surg Pathol 1992;16:411–6.

118. Gerald WL, Haber DA. The EWS-WT1 gene fusion in desmoplastic small round cell tumor. Semin Cancer Biol 2005;15:197–205.

119. Lee SB, Kolquist KA, Nichols K, et al. The EWS-WT1 translocation product induces PDGFA in desmoplastic small round-cell tumour. Nat Genet 1997; 17:309–13.

120. Alaggio R, Rosolen A, Sartori F, et al. Spindle cell tumor with EWS-WT1 transcript and a favorable clinical course: a variant of DSCT, a variant of leiomyosarcoma, or a new entity? Report of 2 pediatric cases. Am J Surg Pathol 2007;31:454–9.

121. Ud Din N, Pekmezci M, Javed G, et al. Low-grade small round cell tumor of the cauda equina with EWSR1-WT1 fusion and indolent clinical course. Hum Pathol 2015;46:153–8.

122. Spillane AJ, Fisher C, Thomas JM. Myxoid liposarcoma–the frequency and the natural history of nonpulmonary soft tissue metastases. Ann Surg Oncol 1999;6:389–94.

123. Smith TA, Easley KA, Goldblum JR. Myxoid/round cell liposarcoma of the extremities. A clinicopathologic study of 29 cases with particular attention to extent of round cell liposarcoma. Am J Surg Pathol 1996;20:171–80.

124. Fritchie KJ, Goldblum JR, Tubbs RR, et al. The expanded histologic spectrum of myxoid liposarcoma with an emphasis on newly described patterns: implications for diagnosis on small biopsy specimens. Am J Clin Pathol 2012;137:229–39.

125. Tallini G, Akerman M, Dal Cin P, et al. Combined morphologic and karyotypic study of 28 myxoid liposarcomas. Implications for a revised morphologic typing, (a report from the CHAMP Group). Am J Surg Pathol 1996;20:1047–55.

126. Kilpatrick SE, Doyon J, Choong PF, et al. The clinicopathologic spectrum of myxoid and round cell liposarcoma. A study of 95 cases. Cancer 1996; 77:1450–8.

127. Hashimoto H, Daimaru Y, Enjoji M, et al. S-100 protein distribution in liposarcoma. An immunoperoxidase study with special reference to the distinction of liposarcoma from myxoid malignant fibrous histiocytoma. Virchows Arch A Pathol Anat Histopathol 1984;405:1–10.

128. Knight JC, Renwick PJ, Cin PD, et al. Translocation t(12;16)(q13;p11) in myxoid liposarcoma and round cell liposarcoma: molecular and cytogenetic analysis. Cancer Res 1995;55:24–7.

129. Antonescu CR, Tschernyavsky SJ, Decuseara R, et al. Prognostic impact of P53 status, TLS-CHOP fusion transcript structure, and histological grade in myxoid liposarcoma: a molecular and clinicopathologic study of 82 cases. Clin Cancer Res 2001;7:3977–87.

130. Engstrom K, Willen H, Kabjorn-Gustafsson C, et al. The myxoid/round cell liposarcoma fusion oncogene FUS-DDIT3 and the normal DDIT3 induce a liposarcoma phenotype in transfected human fibrosarcoma cells. Am J Pathol 2006;168:1642–53.

131. Kubo T, Matsui Y, Naka N, et al. Specificity of fusion genes in adipocytic tumors. Anticancer Res 2010; 30:661–4.

132. Antonescu CR, Argani P, Erlandson RA, et al. Skeletal and extraskeletal myxoid chondrosarcoma. A comparative clinicopathologic, ultrastructural, and molecular study. Cancer 1998;83:1504–21.

133. Enzinger FM, Shiraki M. Extraskeletal myxoid chondrosarcoma. An analysis of 34 cases. Hum Pathol 1972;3:421–35.

134. Meis-Kindblom JM, Bergh P, Gunterberg B, et al. Extraskeletal myxoid chondrosarcoma: a reappraisal of its morphologic spectrum and prognostic factors based on 117 cases. Am J Surg Pathol 1999;23:636–50.

135. Demicco EG, Wang WL, Madewell JE, et al. Osseous myxochondroid sarcoma: a detailed study of 5

cases of extraskeletal myxoid chondrosarcoma of the bone. Am J Surg Pathol 2013;37:752–62.

136. Kawaguchi S, Wada T, Nagoya S, et al. Extraskeletal myxoid chondrosarcoma: a multi-institutional study of 42 cases in Japan. Cancer 2003;97:1285–92.

137. Wehrli BM, Huang W, De Crombrugghe B, et al. Sox9, a master regulator of chondrogenesis, distinguishes mesenchymal chondrosarcoma from other small blue round cell tumors. Hum Pathol 2003;34:263–9.

138. Lucas DR, Fletcher CD, Adsay NV, et al. High-grade extraskeletal myxoid chondrosarcoma: a high-grade epithelioid malignancy. Histopathology 1999;35:201–8.

139. Ramesh K, Gahukamble L, Sarma NH, et al. Extraskeletal myxoid chondrosarcoma with dedifferentiation. Histopathology 1995;27:381–2.

140. Turc-Carel C, Dal Cin P, Rao U, et al. Recurrent breakpoints at 9q31 and 22q12.2 in extraskeletal myxoid chondrosarcoma. Cancer Genet Cytogenet 1988;30:145–50.

141. Harris M, Coyne J, Tariq M, et al. Extraskeletal myxoid chondrosarcoma with neuroendocrine differentiation: a pathologic, cytogenetic, and molecular study of a case with a novel translocation t(9;17)(q22;q11.2). Am J Surg Pathol 2000;24:1020–6.

142. Broehm CJ, Wu J, Gullapalli RR, et al. Extraskeletal myxoid chondrosarcoma with a t(9;16)(q22;p11.2) resulting in a NR4A3-FUS fusion. Cancer Genet 2014;207:276–80.

143. Filion C, Motoi T, Olshen AB, et al. The EWSR1/NR4A3 fusion protein of extraskeletal myxoid chondrosarcoma activates the PPARG nuclear receptor gene. J Pathol 2009;217:83–93.

144. Vergara-Lluri ME, Stohr BA, Puligandla B, et al. A novel sarcoma with dual differentiation: clinicopathologic and molecular characterization of a combined synovial sarcoma and extraskeletal myxoid chondrosarcoma. Am J Surg Pathol 2012;36:1093–8.

145. Flucke U, Tops BB, Verdijk MA, et al. NR4A3 rearrangement reliably distinguishes between the clinicopathologically overlapping entities myoepithelial carcinoma of soft tissue and cellular extraskeletal myxoid chondrosarcoma. Virchows Arch 2012;460:621–8.

146. Thway K, Fisher C. Tumors with EWSR1-CREB1 and EWSR1-ATF1 fusions: the current status. Am J Surg Pathol 2012;36:e1–11.

147. Flucke U, Mentzel T, Verdijk MA, et al. EWSR1-ATF1 chimeric transcript in a myoepithelial tumor of soft tissue: a case report. Hum Pathol 2012;43:764–8.

148. Tanguay J, Weinreb I. What the EWSR1-ATF1 fusion has taught us about hyalinizing clear cell carcinoma. Head Neck Pathol 2013;7:28–34.

149. Taylor BS, Barretina J, Maki RG, et al. Advances in sarcoma genomics and new therapeutic targets. Nat Rev Cancer 2011;11:541–57.

150. Milchgrub S, Gnepp DR, Vuitch F, et al. Hyalinizing clear cell carcinoma of salivary gland. Am J Surg Pathol 1994;18:74–82.

151. Shah AA, Legallo RD, van Zante A, et al. EWSR1 genetic rearrangements in salivary gland tumors: a specific and very common feature of hyalinizing clear cell carcinoma. Am J Surg Pathol 2013;37(4):571–8.

152. Hernandez-Prera JC, Kwan R, Tripodi J, et al. Reappraising hyalinizing clear cell carcinoma: a population-based study with molecular confirmation. Head Neck 2017;39:503–11.

153. Nakano T, Yamamoto H, Nishijima T, et al. Hyalinizing clear cell carcinoma with EWSR1-ATF1 fusion gene: report of three cases with molecular analyses. Virchows Arch 2015;466:37–43.

154. O'Sullivan-Mejia ED, Massey HD, Faquin WC, et al. Hyalinizing clear cell carcinoma: report of eight cases and a review of literature. Head Neck Pathol 2009;3:179–85.

155. Antonescu CR, Katabi N, Zhang L, et al. EWSR1-ATF1 fusion is a novel and consistent finding in hyalinizing clear-cell carcinoma of salivary gland. Genes Chromosomes Cancer 2011;50:559–70.

156. Vogels R, Baumhoer D, van Gorp J, et al. Clear cell odontogenic carcinoma: occurrence of EWSR1-CREB1 as alternative fusion gene to EWSR1-ATF1. Head Neck Pathol 2018, [Epub ahead of print].

157. Enzinger FM. Angiomatoid malignant fibrous histiocytoma: a distinct fibrohistiocytic tumor of children and young adults simulating a vascular neoplasm. Cancer 1979;44:2147–57.

158. Pettinato G, Manivel JC, De Rosa G, et al. Angiomatoid malignant fibrous histiocytoma: cytologic, immunohistochemical, ultrastructural, and flow cytometric study of 20 cases. Mod Pathol 1990;3:479–87.

159. Fanburg-Smith JC, Miettinen M. Angiomatoid "malignant" fibrous histiocytoma: a clinicopathologic study of 158 cases and further exploration of the myoid phenotype. Hum Pathol 1999;30:1336–43.

160. Davies KA, Cope AP, Schofield JB, et al. A rare mediastinal tumour presenting with systemic effects due to IL-6 and tumour necrosis factor (TNF) production. Clin Exp Immunol 1995;99:117–23.

161. Asakura S, Tezuka N, Inoue S, et al. Angiomatoid fibrous histiocytoma in mediastinum. Ann Thorac Surg 2001;72:283–5.

162. Ren L, Guo SP, Zhou XG, et al. Angiomatoid fibrous histiocytoma: first report of primary pulmonary origin. Am J Surg Pathol 2009;33:1570–4.

163. Moura RD, Wang X, Lonzo ML, et al. Reticular angiomatoid "malignant" fibrous histiocytoma–a case

report with cytogenetics and molecular genetic analyses. Hum Pathol 2011;42:1359–63.

164. Dunham C, Hussong J, Seiff M, et al. Primary intracerebral angiomatoid fibrous histiocytoma: report of a case with a t(12;22)(q13;q12) causing type 1 fusion of the EWS and ATF-1 genes. Am J Surg Pathol 2008;32:478–84.

165. Ochalski PG, Edinger JT, Horowitz MB, et al. Intracranial angiomatoid fibrous histiocytoma presenting as recurrent multifocal intraparenchymal hemorrhage. J Neurosurg 2010;112:978–82.

166. Mangham DC, Williams A, Lalam RK, et al. Angiomatoid fibrous histiocytoma of bone: a calcifying sclerosing variant mimicking osteosarcoma. Am J Surg Pathol 2010;34:279–85.

167. Petrey WB, LeGallo RD, Fox MG, et al. Imaging characteristics of angiomatoid fibrous histiocytoma of bone. Skeletal Radiol 2011;40:233–7.

168. Thway K, Fisher C. Angiomatoid fibrous histiocytoma: the current status of pathology and genetics. Arch Pathol Lab Med 2015;139:674–82.

169. Fletcher CD. Angiomatoid "malignant fibrous histiocytoma": an immunohistochemical study indicative of myoid differentiation. Hum Pathol 1991;22:563–8.

170. Thway K, Stefanaki K, Papadakis V, et al. Metastatic angiomatoid fibrous histiocytoma of the scalp, with EWSR1-CREB1 gene fusions in primary tumor and nodal metastasis. Hum Pathol 2013;44:289–93.

171. Tay CK, Koh MS, Takano A, et al. Primary angiomatoid fibrous histiocytoma of the lung with mediastinal lymph node metastasis. Hum Pathol 2016;58:134–7.

172. Costa MJ, Weiss SW. Angiomatoid malignant fibrous histiocytoma. A follow-up study of 108 cases with evaluation of possible histologic predictors of outcome. Am J Surg Pathol 1990;14:1126–32.

173. Tornoczky T, Bogner B, Krausz T, et al. Angiomatoid fibrous histiocytoma: pleomorphic variant associated with multiplication of EWSR1-CREB1 fusion gene. Pathol Oncol Res 2012;18:545–8.

174. Weinreb I, Rubin BP, Goldblum JR. Pleomorphic angiomatoid fibrous histiocytoma: a case confirmed by fluorescence in situ hybridization analysis for EWSR1 rearrangement. J Cutan Pathol 2008;35:855–60.

175. Qian X, Hornick JL, Cibas ES, et al. Angiomatoid fibrous histiocytoma a series of five cytologic cases with literature review and emphasis on diagnostic pitfalls. Diagn Cytopathol 2012;40(Suppl 2):E86–93.

176. Bohman SL, Goldblum JR, Rubin BP, et al. Angiomatoid fibrous histiocytoma: an expansion of the clinical and histological spectrum. Pathology 2014;46:199–204.

177. Kao YC, Lan J, Tai HC, et al. Angiomatoid fibrous histiocytoma: clinicopathological and molecular characterisation with emphasis on variant histomorphology. J Clin Pathol 2014;67(3):210–5.

178. Matsumura T, Yamaguchi T, Tochigi N, et al. Angiomatoid fibrous histiocytoma including cases with pleomorphic features analysed by fluorescence in situ hybridisation. J Clin Pathol 2010;63:124–8.

179. Schaefer IM, Fletcher CD. Myxoid variant of so-called angiomatoid "malignant fibrous histiocytoma": clinicopathologic characterization in a series of 21 cases. Am J Surg Pathol 2014;38(6):816–23.

180. Costa MA, Silva I, Carvalhido L, et al. Angiomatoid fibrous histiocytoma of the arm treated by radiotherapy for local recurrence–case report. Med Pediatr Oncol 1997;28:373–6.

181. Toccanier-Pelte MF, Skalli O, Kapanci Y, et al. Characterization of stromal cells with myoid features in lymph nodes and spleen in normal and pathologic conditions. Am J Pathol 1987;129:109–18.

182. Hallor KH, Micci F, Meis-Kindblom JM, et al. Fusion genes in angiomatoid fibrous histiocytoma. Cancer Lett 2007;251:158–63.

183. Panagopoulos I, Aman P, Fioretos T, et al. Fusion of the FUS gene with ERG in acute myeloid leukemia with t(16;21)(p11;q22). Genes Chromosomes Cancer 1994;11:256–62.

184. Thway K, Gonzalez D, Wren D, et al. Angiomatoid fibrous histiocytoma: comparison of fluorescence in situ hybridization and reverse transcription polymerase chain reaction as adjunct diagnostic modalities. Ann Diagn Pathol 2015;19:137–42.

185. Enzinger FM. Clear-cell sarcoma of tendons and aponeuroses. An Analysis of 21 Cases. Cancer 1965;18:1163–74.

186. Kosemehmetoglu K, Folpe AL. Clear cell sarcoma of tendons and aponeuroses, and osteoclast-rich tumour of the gastrointestinal tract with features resembling clear cell sarcoma of soft parts: a review and update. J Clin Pathol 2010;63:416–23.

187. Feasel PC, Cheah AL, Fritchie K, et al. Primary clear cell sarcoma of the head and neck: a case series with review of the literature. J Cutan Pathol 2016;43:838–46.

188. Sara AS, Evans HL, Benjamin RS. Malignant melanoma of soft parts (clear cell sarcoma). A study of 17 cases, with emphasis on prognostic factors. Cancer 1990;65:367–74.

189. Lucas DR, Nascimento AG, Sim FH. Clear cell sarcoma of soft tissues. Mayo Clinic experience with 35 cases. Am J Surg Pathol 1992;16:1197–204.

190. Deenik W, Mooi WJ, Rutgers EJ, et al. Clear cell sarcoma (malignant melanoma) of soft parts: a clinicopathologic study of 30 cases. Cancer 1999;86:969–75.

191. Finley JW, Hanypsiak B, McGrath B, et al. Clear cell sarcoma: the Roswell Park experience. J Surg Oncol 2001;77:16–20.

192. Dim DC, Cooley LD, Miranda RN. Clear cell sarcoma of tendons and aponeuroses: a review. Arch Pathol Lab Med 2007;131:152–6.

193. Clark MA, Fisher C, Judson I, et al. Soft-tissue sarcomas in adults. N Engl J Med 2005;353:701–11.

194. Karamchandani JR, Nielsen TO, van de Rijn M, et al. Sox10 and S100 in the diagnosis of soft-tissue neoplasms. Appl Immunohistochem Mol Morphol 2012;20:445–50.

195. Coindre JM, Hostein I, Terrier P, et al. Diagnosis of clear cell sarcoma by real-time reverse transcriptase-polymerase chain reaction analysis of paraffin embedded tissues: clinicopathologic and molecular analysis of 44 patients from the French sarcoma group. Cancer 2006;107:1055–64.

196. Jakubauskas A, Valceckiene V, Andrekute K, et al. Discovery of two novel EWSR1/ATF1 transcripts in four chimerical transcripts-expressing clear cell sarcoma and their quantitative evaluation. Exp Mol Pathol 2011;90:194–200.

197. Gineikiene E, Seinin D, Brasiuniene B, et al. Clear cell sarcoma expressing a novel chimerical transcript EWSR1 exon 7/ATF1 exon 6. Virchows Arch 2012;461:339–43.

198. Davis IJ, Kim JJ, Ozsolak F, et al. Oncogenic MITF dysregulation in clear cell sarcoma: defining the MiT family of human cancers. Cancer Cell 2006;9:473–84.

199. Brown AD, Lopez-Terrada D, Denny C, et al. Promoters containing ATF-binding sites are deregulated in cells that express the EWS/ATF1 oncogene. Oncogene 1995;10:1749–56.

200. Fujimura Y, Ohno T, Siddique H, et al. The EWS-ATF-1 gene involved in malignant melanoma of soft parts with t(12;22) chromosome translocation, encodes a constitutive transcriptional activator. Oncogene 1996;12:159–67.

201. Fuse N, Yasumoto K, Suzuki H, et al. Identification of a melanocyte-type promoter of the microphthalmia-associated transcription factor gene. Biochem Biophys Res Commun 1996;219:702–7.

202. Tachibana M, Takeda K, Nobukuni Y, et al. Ectopic expression of MITF, a gene for Waardenburg syndrome type 2, converts fibroblasts to cells with melanocyte characteristics. Nat Genet 1996;14:50–4.

203. Amae S, Fuse N, Yasumoto K, et al. Identification of a novel isoform of microphthalmia-associated transcription factor that is enriched in retinal pigment epithelium. Biochem Biophys Res Commun 1998;247:710–5.

204. Li KK, Goodall J, Goding CR, et al. The melanocyte inducing factor MITF is stably expressed in cell lines from human clear cell sarcoma. Br J Cancer 2003;89:1072–8.

205. Zambrano E, Reyes-Mugica M, Franchi A, et al. An osteoclast-rich tumor of the gastrointestinal tract with features resembling clear cell sarcoma of soft parts: reports of 6 cases of a GIST simulator. Int J Surg Pathol 2003;11:75–81.

206. Huang W, Zhang X, Li D, et al. Osteoclast-rich tumor of the gastrointestinal tract with features resembling those of clear cell sarcoma of soft parts. Virchows Arch 2006;448:200–3.

207. Libertini M, Thway K, Noujaim J, et al. Clear cell sarcoma-like tumor of the gastrointestinal tract: clinical outcome and pathologic features of a molecularly characterized tertiary center case series. Anticancer Res 2018;38:1479–83.

208. Boland JM, Folpe AL. Oncocytic variant of malignant gastrointestinal neuroectodermal tumor: a potential diagnostic pitfall. Hum Pathol 2016;57:13–6.

209. Antonescu CR, Nafa K, Segal NH, et al. EWS-CREB1: a recurrent variant fusion in clear cell sarcoma–association with gastrointestinal location and absence of melanocytic differentiation. Clin Cancer Res 2006;12:5356–62.

210. Covinsky M, Gong S, Rajaram V, et al. EWS-ATF1 fusion transcripts in gastrointestinal tumors previously diagnosed as malignant melanoma. Hum Pathol 2005;36:74–81.

211. Hornick JL, Fletcher CD. Myoepithelial tumors of soft tissue: a clinicopathologic and immunohistochemical study of 101 cases with evaluation of prognostic parameters. Am J Surg Pathol 2003;27:1183–96.

212. Thway K, Fisher C. Myoepithelial tumor of soft tissue: histology and genetics of an evolving entity. Adv Anat Pathol 2014;21:411–9.

213. Bale TA, Oviedo A, Kozakewich H, et al. Intracranial myxoid mesenchymal tumors with EWSR1-CREB family gene fusions: myxoid variant of angiomatoid fibrous histiocytoma or novel entity? Brain Pathol 2018;28:183–91.

214. Chapman E, Skalova A, Ptakova N, et al. Molecular profiling of hyalinizing clear cell carcinomas revealed a subset of tumors harboring a novel EWSR1-CREM fusion: report of 3 cases. Am J Surg Pathol 2018;42(9):1182–9.

215. Prieto-Granada C, Zhang L, Chen HW, et al. A genetic dichotomy between pure sclerosing epithelioid fibrosarcoma (SEF) and hybrid SEF/low-grade fibromyxoid sarcoma: a pathologic and molecular study of 18 cases. Genes Chromosomes Cancer 2015;54:28–38.

216. Stockman DL, Ali SM, He J, et al. Sclerosing epithelioid fibrosarcoma presenting as intraabdominal sarcomatosis with a novel EWSR1-CREB3L1 gene fusion. Hum Pathol 2014;45:2173–8.

217. Bahrami A, Dalton JD, Krane JF, et al. A subset of cutaneous and soft tissue mixed tumors are genetically linked to their salivary gland counterpart. Genes Chromosomes Cancer 2012;51:140–8.

218. Antonescu CR, Zhang L, Shao SY, et al. Frequent PLAG1 gene rearrangements in skin and soft tissue myoepithelioma with ductal differentiation. Genes Chromosomes Cancer 2013;52:675–82.

219. Burke T, Sahin A, Johnson DE, et al. Myoepithelioma of the retroperitoneum. Ultrastruct Pathol 1995;19:269–74.

220. Cibull TL, Gleason BC, O'Malley DP, et al. Malignant cutaneous glomus tumor presenting as a rapidly growing leg mass in a pregnant woman. J Cutan Pathol 2008;35:765–9.

221. Alomari AK, Brown N, Andea AA, et al. Cutaneous syncytial myoepithelioma: a recently described neoplasm which may mimic nevoid melanoma and epithelioid sarcoma. J Cutan Pathol 2017;44:892–7.

222. Stout AP, Gorman JG. Mixed tumors of the skin of the salivary gland type. Cancer 1959;12:537–43.

223. Fernandez-Figueras M-T, Puig L, Trias I, et al. Benign myoepithelioma of the skin. Am J Dermatopathol 1998;20:208–12.

224. Kutzner H, Mentzel T, Kaddu S, et al. Cutaneous myoepithelioma: an under-recognized cutaneous neoplasm composed of myoepithelial cells. Am J Surg Pathol 2001;25:348–55.

225. Michal M, Miettinen M. Myoepitheliomas of the skin and soft tissues. Report of 12 cases. Virchows Arch 1999;434:393–400.

226. Gleason BC, Fletcher CD. Myoepithelial carcinoma of soft tissue in children: an aggressive neoplasm analyzed in a series of 29 cases. Am J Surg Pathol 2007;31:1813–24.

227. Hornick JL, Fletcher CD. Cutaneous myoepithelioma: a clinicopathologic and immunohistochemical study of 14 cases. Hum Pathol 2004;35:14–24.

228. Song W, Flucke U, Suurmeijer AJH. Myoepithelial tumors of bone. Surg Pathol Clin 2017;10:657–74.

229. Flucke U, Palmedo G, Blankenhorn N, et al. EWSR1 gene rearrangement occurs in a subset of cutaneous myoepithelial tumors: a study of 18 cases. Mod Pathol 2011;24:1444–50.

230. Rekhi B, Sable M, Jambhekar NA. Histopathological, immunohistochemical and molecular spectrum of myoepithelial tumours of soft tissues. Virchows Arch 2012;461:687–97.

231. Brandal P, Panagopoulos I, Bjerkehagen B, et al. Detection of a t(1;22)(q23;q12) translocation leading to an EWSR1-PBX1 fusion gene in a myoepithelioma. Genes Chromosomes Cancer 2008;47:558–64.

232. Moller E, Stenman G, Mandahl N, et al. POU5F1, encoding a key regulator of stem cell pluripotency, is fused to EWSR1 in hidradenoma of the skin and mucoepidermoid carcinoma of the salivary glands. J Pathol 2008;215:78–86.

233. Brandal P, Panagopoulos I, Bjerkehagen B, et al. t(19;22)(q13;q12) translocation leading to the novel fusion gene EWSR1-ZNF444 in soft tissue myoepithelial carcinoma. Genes Chromosomes Cancer 2009;48:1051–6.

234. Huang SC, Chen HW, Zhang L, et al. Novel FUS-KLF17 and EWSR1-KLF17 fusions in myoepithelial tumors. Genes Chromosomes Cancer 2015;54:267–75.

235. Folpe AL, Weiss SW. Ossifying fibromyxoid tumor of soft parts: a clinicopathologic study of 70 cases with emphasis on atypical and malignant variants. Am J Surg Pathol 2003;27:421–31.

236. Schneider N, Fisher C, Thway K. Ossifying fibromyxoid tumor: morphology, genetics, and differential diagnosis. Ann Diagn Pathol 2016;20:52–8.

237. Romeo S, Dei Tos AP. Soft tissue tumors associated with EWSR1 translocation. Virchows Arch 2010;456:219–34.

238. Kao YC, Flucke U, Eijkelenboom A, et al. Novel EWSR1-SMAD3 gene fusions in a group of acral fibroblastic spindle cell neoplasms. Am J Surg Pathol 2018;42:522–8.

239. Arbajian E, Magnusson L, Brosjo O, et al. A benign vascular tumor with a new fusion gene: EWSR1-NFATC1 in hemangioma of the bone. Am J Surg Pathol 2013;37:613–6.

240. Panagopoulos I, Thorsen J, Gorunova L, et al. RNA sequencing identifies fusion of the EWSR1 and YY1 genes in mesothelioma with t(14;22)(q32;q12). Genes Chromosomes Cancer 2013;52:733–40.

241. Desmeules P, Joubert P, Zhang L, et al. A subset of malignant mesotheliomas in young adults are associated with recurrent EWSR1/FUS-ATF1 fusions. Am J Surg Pathol 2017;41:980–8.

242. Dashti NK, Wehrs RN, Thomas BC, et al. Spindle cell rhabdomyosarcoma of bone with FUS-TFCP2 fusion: confirmation of a very recently described rhabdomyosarcoma subtype. Histopathology 2018;73:514–52.

Important Recently Characterized Non-Ewing Small Round Cell Tumors

Cody S. Carter, MD[a], Rajiv M. Patel, MD[b,c],*

KEYWORDS

- Round cell sarcoma • Non-Ewing sarcoma • BCOR • CIC • Atypical Ewing sarcoma
- Ewing-like sarcoma • Undifferentiated sarcoma • Sarcoma

Key points

- Ewing-like undifferentiated round cell sarcomas share overlapping morphologic and clinical features with Ewing sarcoma. A subset of Ewing-like sarcomas have oncogenic rearrangements in genes other than *EWSR1* and the *ETS* family of transcription factors.

- Rearrangements in Ewing-like undifferentiated round cell sarcomas most commonly involve *CIC* and *BCOR*. Proposals for these entities to be granted independent classifications have been made based on transcriptome analysis.

- In comparison with Ewing sarcomas, *CIC*-rearranged sarcomas tend to arise in soft tissues rather than bone, exhibit a myxoid component, have prominent nucleoli, and tend to follow a more aggressive clinical course. Before modern molecular diagnostics, these tumors were often previously categorized as atypical Ewing sarcomas.

- *BCOR*-rearranged sarcomas can have variable components of round cell and spindle cell morphology, and most tumors demonstrate nuclear TLE1 expression, features that overlap with poorly differentiated synovial sarcoma.

- Diagnosis of undifferentiated round cell sarcomas is made through the use of morphologic and immunohistochemical features, which guide confirmatory molecular studies.

ABSTRACT

Round cell sarcomas morphologically similar to Ewing sarcoma, but lacking the classic immunohistochemical features, *EWSR-ETS* family fusions, and other signs of differentiation, are classified as Ewing-like sarcomas. Recent molecular advances led to the discovery and characterization of two recurrent oncogenic fusion rearrangements, *CIC-DUX4* and *BCOR-CCNB3*, in a significant subset of Ewing-like sarcomas. Uncovered alternate fusion partners broadened the proposed classification of these tumors to *CIC*-rearranged sarcomas and *BCOR*-rearranged sarcomas. This article summarizes the clinicopathologic and molecular features of these entities, with particular attention paid to those features that overlap with and distinguish these sarcomas from other round cell sarcomas.

OVERVIEW

The prototypical small round cell sarcoma (SRCS) is Ewing sarcoma, a bone and soft tissue sarcoma classically characterized by a proliferation

---

Disclosures: None of the authors have any conflicts of interest to disclose.

[a] Department of Pathology, Michigan Medicine, University of Michigan, 2800 Plymouth Road, Building 35, Ann Arbor, MI 48109, USA; [b] Department of Pathology, Sections of Dermatopathology and Bone and Soft Tissue Pathology, Michigan Medicine, University of Michigan, 2800 Plymouth Road, Building 35, Ann Arbor, MI 48109, USA; [c] Department of Dermatology, Michigan Medicine, University of Michigan, 1500 East Medical Center Drive, Ann Arbor, MI 48109, USA

* Corresponding author. Department of Pathology, Michigan Medicine, University of Michigan, 2800 Plymouth Road, Building 35, Ann Arbor, MI 48109.

E-mail address: rajivpat@med.umich.edu

of uniform small round blue cells with fine chromatin, strong membranous CD99 expression, and recurrent balanced translocations involving the *EWSR1* gene and members of the E26 transformation-specific (*ETS*) gene family, most commonly *FLI1*, followed by *ERG* (and less commonly *ETV1/4*, *FEV*, and *E1A-F*) (**Fig.** 1A, B). A rare subset of these tumors is characterized by rearrangements of *FUS* (rather than *EWSR1*) with select fusion partners including *ERG* and *FEV*, and evolving molecular techniques have demonstrated uncommon tumors characterized by *EWSR1* fusions with non-*ETS* family members (including *NFATc2*, *PATZ1*, *SMARCA5*, and *SP3*).[1–6] These tumors have been collectively called the Ewing sarcoma family of tumors (ESFT).

Nonclassical Ewing sarcoma tumors, that is, tumors that have features other than the classically described cytomorphology and *EWSR1-ETS* fusions, are somewhat bewildering to the uninitiated. Those tumors that have round cell morphology similar to Ewing sarcoma, but

lacking *EWSR1-ETS* rearrangements and any other signs of a specific line of differentiation have been designated as Ewing-like sarcomas in the most recent World Health Organization classification.[7] Historically, a subset of bone and soft tissue sarcomas with round cell morphology were described as having larger, more pleomorphic nuclei with prominent nucleoli, and were characterized as atypical (or less commonly large-cell) Ewing sarcoma (**Fig.** 2A).[8] Although many tumors with these features were found to harbor *EWSR1-ETS* rearrangements, some tumors were found to have fusions between *EWSR1* and non-*ETS* family members, most notably *NFATc2*,[2] and others lacked *EWSR1* fusions all together. Most of these latter tumors lacking *EWSR1* rearrangements were found to have rearrangements in capicua transcriptional repressor (*CIC*). These sarcomas, in combination with round cell sarcomas harboring rearrangements in the Bcl6 corepressor (*BCOR*) gene, comprise the bulk of Ewing-like sarcomas; the remainder are composed of sarcomas with

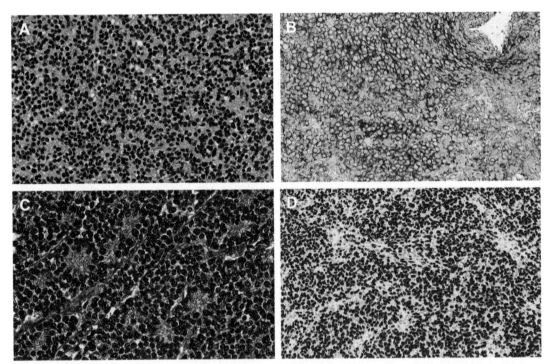

Fig. 1. (*A*) Ewing sarcoma is the prototypical small round blue cell sarcoma. Constituent cells characteristically have uniform round nuclei with fine chromatin and inconspicuous nucleoli (hematoxylin-eosin, original magnification ×400). (*B*) CD99 shows uniform strong membranous expression (original magnification ×200). (*C*) Occasional examples can show neuroectodermal differentiation with Homer Wright rosettes, a feature of tumors that were formerly classified separately as primitive neuroectodermal tumor and not seen in *CIC*- or *BCOR*-rearranged sarcomas (hematoxylin-eosin, original magnification ×400). (*D*) PAX7 nuclear expression is present in nearly all tumors (original magnification ×200). ([*B, D*] *Courtesy of* G. Charville, MD, PhD, Stanford University School of Medicine, Stanford, CA; with permission.)

Fig. 2. (*A*) Atypical Ewing sarcomas have larger nuclei with prominent nucleoli and sometimes a greater degree of nuclear pleomorphism, features that overlap with *CIC*-rearranged sarcomas (hematoxylin-eosin, original magnification ×400). (*B*) Diffuse membranous CD99 expression is still a typical feature of true translocation-defined Ewing sarcomas with atypical features (original magnification ×400).

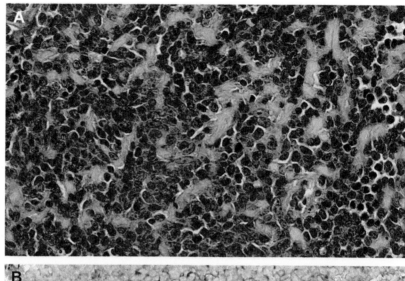

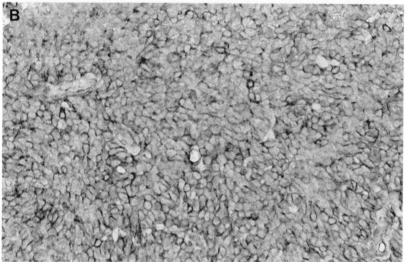

rarely reported, or as-yet unclassified genetic alterations.

Based on a body of emerging molecular evidence, most notably transcriptome analysis by next-generation sequencing (NGS; RNA-seq), many investigators now support classification of tumors harboring *CIC* and *BCOR* rearrangements as entities distinct from Ewing sarcoma. Overall, although there are some overlapping clinical and pathologic features of these tumors with Ewing sarcoma, they also share several features with non-ESFT, which makes accurate classification challenging. However, subtle morphologic features, in combination with the results of a focused immunohistochemical panel, can assist in the diagnosis and guide confirmatory molecular diagnostics.

CAPICUA TRANSCRIPTIONAL REPRESSOR-REARRANGED SMALL ROUND CELL SARCOMAS

INTRODUCTION

The largest subset of Ewing-like undifferentiated SRCSs comprise sarcomas with rearrangements in *CIC*, first characterized in 2006 by Kawamura-Saito and colleagues,[9] accounting for approximately 70% of SRCSs lacking *EWSR* and *FUS* rearrangements.[10–12] *CIC*-rearranged sarcomas affect a wide age range (6–81 years), but most commonly present in young adults (mean age, 30 years), and have a slight male sex predilection.[11,13,14] Nearly 90% of cases arise in soft tissues, split evenly between the extremities and trunk/pelvis, with a minority of cases (approximately 10%) arising in visceral organs. In stark contrast to Ewing sarcoma, of which most arise in bone, less than 5% of *CIC*-rearranged sarcomas arise in bone. There are no known associated risk factors.

GROSS AND RADIOLOGIC FEATURES

There are no specific gross features of *CIC*-rearranged sarcomas. Tumors often show extensive hemorrhage and necrosis, detected grossly and radiologically. By MRI, *CIC*-rearranged sarcomas are typically based in the deep soft tissues of the trunk, pelvis, or proximal extremities and exhibit heterogeneous, but intense postcontrast enhancement.

MICROSCOPIC AND IMMUNOHISTOCHEMICAL FEATURES

Similar to Ewing Sarcoma, *CIC*-rearranged sarcomas are composed of sheets of medium-sized round cells with indistinct cell borders (**Fig. 3**, **Table 1**). However, *CIC*-rearranged sarcomas more often demonstrate lobular growth with dense hyaline bands separating large lobules of tumor cells (**Fig. 4**A).[13–15] An at least focal, distinctive myxoid stroma is a characteristic feature (**Fig. 5**A, B), but this can also be extensive, resembling the stroma seen in extraskeletal myxoid chondrosarcoma, or myoepithelial carcinoma in some cases.[13] Although the tumor cells in *CIC*-rearranged sarcomas most often exhibit a predominantly round or ovoid morphology, they not

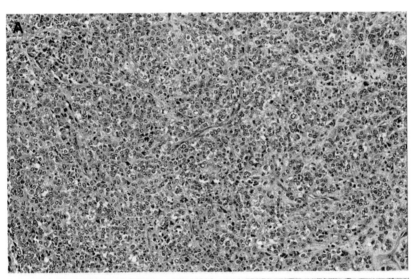

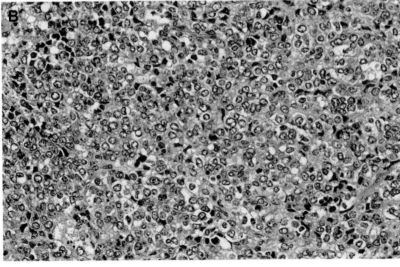

Fig. 3. (*A*, *B*) *CIC*-rearranged sarcomas typically have more vesicular chromatin, prominent nucleoli, and slightly greater nuclear pleomorphism compared with Ewing sarcomas (hematoxylin-eosin, original magnification ×200 [*A*] and ×400 [*B*]).

Table 1
Differential diagnosis of round cell sarcomas

	CIC-Rearranged Sarcoma	BCOR-Rearranged Sarcoma	Ewing Sarcoma	Poorly Differentiated Synovial Sarcoma	DSRCT	ARMS	Mesenchymal Chondrosarcoma	High-Grade Myxoid Liposarcoma
Peak incidence decade (mean age in years)	3rd–4th decade (30)	2nd decade (15)	2nd decade (15)	4th decade (33)	3rd decade (22)	2nd decade	3rd decade	4th decade
Most common anatomic site	Soft tissues of trunk/pelvis and extremities	Pelvic bones and metadiaphysis of long bones of lower extremities	Metadiaphysis of long bones, ribs, pelvis	Soft tissues of extremities	Soft tissues and viscera of abdomen	Soft tissues of extremities	Facial bones, long bones of lower extremities, and pelvic bones	Soft tissues of lower limbs, especially thigh
Cytomorphology	Round cells with moderate eosinophilic cytoplasm	Round cells and spindled cells	Monotonous round cells	At least focal spindling	Monotonous round cells, minimal cytoplasm	Monotonous round cells, rare multinucleated giant cells or striated cells	Round cells and spindled cells	Round cells with rare univacuolated lipoblasts
Nuclear features	Vesicular chromatin, prominent nucleoli, moderate pleomorphism	Fine chromatin, inconspicuous nucleoli	Fine chromatin, inconspicuous nucleoli	Vesicular chromatin, prominent nucleoli	Uniform hyperchromasia, inconspicuous nucleoli, and minimal eosinophilic cytoplasm	Large, fine chromatin, prominent nucleoli	Small, fine chromatin, inconspicuous nucleoli	Vesicular chromatin, prominent nucleoli, moderate pleomorphism
Stroma	Myxoid changes common, subset with dense hyaline bands	Subset with myxoid changes	Scant	Scant	Abundant desmoplastic stroma encasing round cell nests	Fibrotic septae between anastomosing round cells	Geographically variable chondroid matrix	Myxoid changes
Other helpful features	Subset with rhabdoid/plasmacytoid cells	Subset with hemangiopericytoma-like vessels	Focal neural differentiation (Homer Wright rosettes)	Hemangiopericytoma-like vessels	—	—	Hemangiopericytoma-like vessels	Plexiform capillary network, focal hypocellular conventional component
Typical positive immunohistochemical profile	Patchy CD99, ETV4, WT1, can be ERG and FLI1	Patchy CD99, TLE1, BCOR, CCNB3	Diffuse membranous CD99, NKX2-2	TLE1, patchy EMA and keratin	WT1, keratin, EMA, desmin (perinuclear)	Desmin, myogenin, MyoD1	Diffuse membranous CD99, NKX2-2, S100 in chondroid areas	S100
Genetics (in order of incidence)	CIC-DUX4, CIC-DUX4L, CIC-FOXO4	BCOR-CCNB3, BCOR-MAML3, ZC3H7B-BCOR	EWSR1-FLI1, EWSR1-ERG, EWSR1-PATZ1, also FUS-ERG	SS18-SSX1, SS18-SSX2	EWSR1-WT1	PAX3-FOXO1, PAX7-FOXO1	HEY1-NCOA2	FUS-DDIT3 EWSR1-DDIT3

Abbreviations: ARMS, alveolar rhabdomyosarcoma; DSRCT, desmoplastic small round cell tumor; EMA, epithelial membrane antigen.

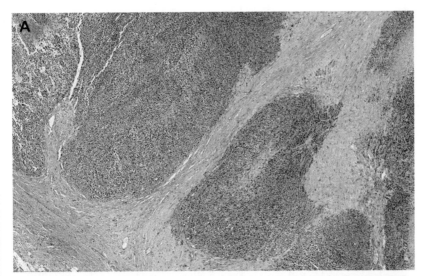

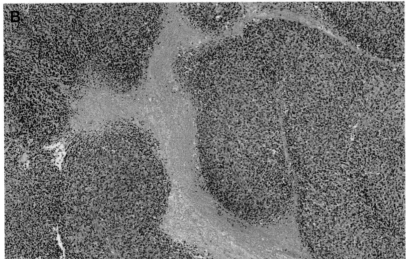

Fig. 4. Fibrous bands (*A*) and geographic necrosis (*B*) are common low-power features of *CIC*-rearranged sarcomas (hematoxylin-eosin, original magnification ×40 [*A*] and ×100 [*B*]).

uncommonly have a minor component of rhabdoid or plasmacytoid morphology (approximately 25%), which rarely may account for most constituent cells (**Fig. 5**C).[14] Less commonly, these tumors exhibit spindle cell morphology (approximately 10%), an important distinction from *BCOR*-rearranged sarcomas detailed later (**Fig. 5**D).[14]

CIC-rearranged sarcomas usually demonstrate more nuclear atypia compared with Ewing sarcoma, displaying vesicular chromatin, prominent nucleoli, and a slightly greater degree of nuclear pleomorphism.[11,13,15,16] In particular, the prominent nucleoli are a useful initial diagnostic clue. These nuclear features have been historically described in the large cell or atypical variant of Ewing sarcoma (**Fig. 2**), and have been seen in ESFTs with *EWSR1-ETS* and *EWSR1*-non-*ETS*

rearrangements, with the strongest correlation being with tumors harboring *EWSR1-NFATc2* translocations.[2,8] Compared with conventional Ewing Sarcoma, *CIC*-rearranged sarcomas also tend to have a greater amount of eosinophilic cytoplasm and occasional clear cell change, and lack any evidence of neuroectodermal differentiation that is seen in Ewing sarcoma, such as Homer Wright rosettes (**Fig. 1**C). Mitotic activity is high, with a mean of approximately 30 mitotic figures (MF) per 10 high-power fields (HPF), with almost all cases having more than 10 MF per 10 HPF.[12,14] Most cases also show geographic coagulative tumor cell necrosis (**Fig. 4**B).

CIC-rearranged sarcomas have a unique immunohistochemical expression pattern from Ewing sarcoma, making immunohistochemistry a useful adjunct (**Table 2**). Although most *CIC*-rearranged

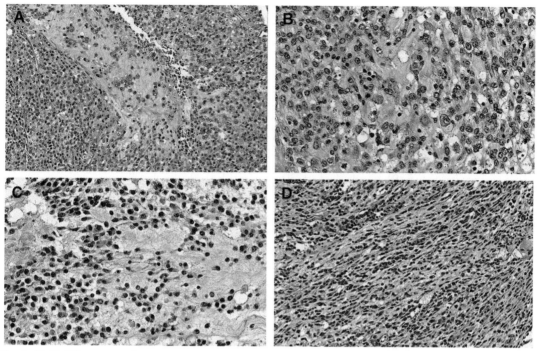

Fig. 5. (*A*, *B*) *CIC*-rearranged sarcomas commonly exhibit prominent myxoid stroma. (*C*) They also often contain a subset of tumor cells with plasmacytoid or rhabdoid morphology. (*D*) Less commonly, they can exhibit areas of prominent spindling, which is usually focal (hematoxylin-eosin, original magnification ×200 [*A*, *D*] and ×400 [*B*, *C*]).

sarcomas exhibit at least focal expression of CD99 (**Fig. 6**A, B), only a small subset demonstrate the diffuse, strong membranous expression seen commonly in Ewing sarcoma, and a large subset are completely negative for this marker.[12,14] Nuclear ETV4 and WT1 expression is seen in more than 90% of *CIC*-rearranged sarcomas (**Fig. 6**C, D),[12,14] whereas Ewing sarcoma, *BCOR*-rearranged sarcoma, and poorly differentiated synovial sarcoma are negative.[17] Importantly, other entities in the morphologic differential diagnosis, namely desmoplastic small round cell tumor (DSRCT) and Wilms tumor, are positive for nuclear WT1 (although DSRCT is only positive for antibodies targeting the carboxyl terminus). *CIC*-rearranged sarcomas are also commonly positive for calretinin, resulting in immunohistochemical overlap with mesothelioma.[12] Focal desmin and cytokeratin AE1/AE3 expression is seen in a small minority of cases (approximately 15% and 4%, respectively).[14] Immunohistochemistry for ERG and FLI1 expression has been reported, an important diagnostic pitfall for differentiating these neoplasms from Ewing sarcoma, especially because previous reports have alleged that FLI1 expression is a specific marker among round cell tumors.[13] In contrast, NKX2-2, a downstream target of EWSR1-FLI1, is expressed in nearly all Ewing

sarcomas, whereas it is negative in almost all *CIC*-rearranged sarcomas.[12,17] Diffuse MYC immunohistochemical expression has been reported in 10 out of 10 cases in a recent series.[13]

MOLECULAR GENETIC FEATURES

The most common genes involved in the oncogenic driver mutations of *CIC*-rearranged sarcomas include the *CIC* gene on chromosome 19q13.1, involved in transcriptional repression of *ETV1*, *ETV4*, and *ETV5*, and either *double homeobox 4* (*DUX4*) gene or *double homeobox4-like* (*DUX4L*) gene, located on 4q35 or chromosome 10q26.3, respectively, which are transcription factors typically expressed in germ cells, but epigenetically silenced by methylation in differentiated cells.[18] These t(4;19)(q35;q13) and t(10;19)(q26;q13) fusions result in upregulated expression of the genes, which the CIC product normally inhibits, namely *polyoma enhancer activator 3* (*PEA3*) family members of *ETS*-related transcription factors *ETV1*, *ETV4*, and *ETV5*.[9,11,19,20] The t(4;19) fusion is slightly more common, and there are no significant clinicopathologic differences between tumors harboring the t(4;19) versus the t(10;19).[14]

Table 2
Extended immunophenotype of round cell sarcomas

	CIC-Rearranged Sarcoma	BCOR-Rearranged Sarcoma	Ewing Sarcoma	Poorly Differentiated Synovial Sarcoma	DSRCT	ARMS	Mesenchymal Chondrosarcoma	High-Grade Myxoid Liposarcoma
Widely available markers								
CD99 (membranous)	±	±	++	±	±	±	±	±
WT1 (nuclear)	++	–	–	–	++[a]	–	–	–
TLE1 (nuclear)	–	++	–	++	–	–	–	±
Keratins/EMA	±	–	±	++	++	–	–	–
Desmin	±	–	–	–	++	++	–	±
Myogenin (nuclear)	–	–	–	–	–	++	–	–
S100	–	–	–	±	–	–	++[b]	++
Less commonly available markers								
ETV4 (nuclear)	++	–	–	–	–	–	–	–
BCOR (nuclear)	–	++	–	–	–	–	–	–
CCNB3 (nuclear)	–	++[c]	–	–	–	–	–	–
NKX2-2 (nuclear)	–	±	++	–	±	–	±	Unknown
PAX7 (nuclear)	–	…	++	±	–	++	±	–

Where not indicated, staining is cytoplasmic.
Abbreviations: ARMS, alveolar rhabdomyosarcoma; DSRCT, desmoplastic small round cell tumor; EMA, epithelial membrane antigen; ++, usually positive (>70%); ±, sometimes positive (10%–70%); –, never or almost never positive (<10%).
[a] WT1 (nuclear) staining by antibodies targeting carboxyl terminal groups on WT1.
[b] In chondroid areas only.
[c] In tumors with BCOR-CCNB3 rearrangements.

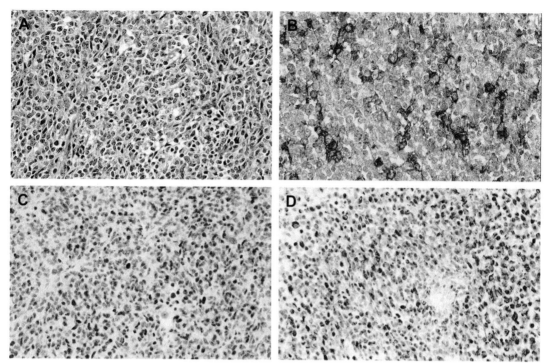

Fig. 6. (*A*) *CIC*-rearranged sarcoma with typical morphology (hematoxylin-eosin, original magnification ×400). (*B*) CD99 is focal or patchy in most tumors, and only rarely shows the diffuse membranous expression seen in Ewing sarcomas (original magnification ×400). (*C*) ETV4 is consistently positive (original magnification ×400). (*D*) Nuclear WT1 is expressed in most cases (original magnification ×400). ([*A, C,* and *D*] *Courtesy of* J. Hornick, MD, PhD, Brigham & Women's Hospital, Boston, MA; with permission.)

SRCSs with alternate fusion partners with *CIC* have also been described, most notably *FOXO4* and *NUT midline carcinoma family member 1* (*NUTM1*), and unknown fusion partners.[6,12,14,21,22] Gene expression profiles of these tumors cluster tightly with *CIC-DUX4* and *CIC-DUX4L* rearranged tumors.[6] Based on this finding, the term "*CIC*-rearranged sarcomas" has been proposed for this class of neoplasms to include alternate fusion partners under the definition of the entity (and thus has been used throughout this article). Furthermore, when comparing tumors with *CIC-DUX4* fusion and other *CIC*-rearranged sarcomas with ESFTs with *EWSR1-ETS* fusions, their transcriptomes show little overlap in differentially expressed genes, providing perhaps the strongest single measure of support for the distinction of these tumors from ESFTs.[16]

In addition to supporting *CIC*-rearranged sarcomas as a distinct entity, transcriptional profiling analysis has been used in the discovery of additional biomarkers, which aid in the diagnosis of round cell sarcomas. RNA in situ hybridization performed on formalin-fixed paraffin embedded sections for detection of *ETV1*, *ETV4*, and *ETV5* transcripts has been proposed as a sensitive and specific ancillary test among SRCSs, which provides an alternative detection method in cases with limited tissue sampling.[23,24] Additionally, *PAX7* was recently identified as one of the genes encoding transcription factors with the highest differential expression between Ewing sarcoma and *CIC*-rearranged sarcoma, and a subsequent immunohistochemical study demonstrated expression of *PAX7* in 102/103 Ewing sarcomas and 0/27 *CIC*-rearranged sarcomas (**Fig. 1**D).[25] Similar to other markers described previously, however, *PAX7* expression has been seen in a high proportion of other round cell sarcomas, most notably *BCOR*-rearranged sarcomas, alveolar rhabdomyosarcoma (ARMS), and poorly differentiated synovial sarcoma[26]; thus it may only be useful as a component of a larger immunohistochemical panel to guide molecular testing.

Apart from the defining translocations involving *CIC*, karyotyping and fluorescence in situ hybridization (FISH) studies have shown recurrent trisomy 8 in *CIC*-rearranged sarcomas, which also show *MYC* amplifications (because of its locus at 8q24).[13,15] Similar chromosome 8 alterations were supported by broad gene panel NGS, which demonstrated recurrent broad copy number

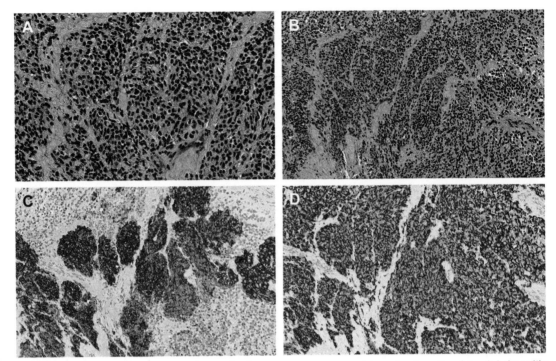

Fig. 7. (*A, B*) Some desmoplastic small round cell tumor cases can consist predominantly of a solid sheet-like component, particularly in limited biopsy samples. These tumors express cytokeratin (*C*) and desmin (in a characteristic perinuclear dot accentuation pattern) (*D*) (hematoxylin-eosin [*A, B*], original magnification ×400 [*A*] and ×200 [*B–D*]).

alterations, most notably gains of chromosome 8 and loss of 1p, in addition to an overall low somatic mutational burden.[27] Although gains of chromosome 8 are also observed in a high proportion of ESFTs, gains of 1q, 12, and loss of 16q are observed in ESFT instead of 1p loss.[28]

DIFFERENTIAL DIAGNOSIS

Ewing sarcoma is obviously the primary entity in the differential diagnosis, particularly atypical variants (see **Figs. 1** and **2**). Clinical factors, such as location, are a helpful diagnostic clue, because *CIC*-rearranged sarcomas rarely arise in bone, where most ESFTs arise. Neuroectodermal differentiation with formation of Homer Wright rosettes (see **Fig. 1**C) is not seen in *CIC*-rearranged sarcomas. Most *CIC*-rearranged sarcomas exhibit at least focal expression of CD99, but rarely demonstrate the diffuse, strong membranous expression seen in Ewing sarcoma (see **Figs. 1**B and **2**B), and many are completely negative for this marker.[12,14] Nuclear WT1 and ETV4 expression are both present in more than 90% of *CIC*-rearranged sarcomas,[12,14] whereas Ewing sarcomas are negative. Conversely, Ewing sarcomas are nearly all positive for NKX2-2 and PAX7, whereas *CIC*-

rearranged sarcomas are negative for these markers.[17,25]

DSRCT can mimic *CIC*-rearranged sarcomas involving the trunk and pelvis, because most DSRCTs are located in the abdominal cavity of young adults with a peak incidence in the late third decade.[29] These tumors are composed of densely cellular nests of uniform small round cells with hyperchromatic nuclei, and minimal eosinophilic cytoplasm.[29,30] Although most DSRCTs show tumor cell nests embedded in a dense, cellular fibrous stroma, a subset of tumors demonstrate predominantly solid growth with little intervening stroma (**Fig. 7**A, B).[31] However, these tumors are unlikely to show the myxoid change that is commonly seen in *CIC*-rearranged sarcomas, and typically have inconspicuous nucleoli. DSRCTs exhibit an overlapping immunoprofile with *CIC*-rearranged sarcomas, because most DSRCTs are WT1 nuclear positive, but are only immunoreactive for antibodies directed toward the carboxyl-terminus of WT1 because of a truncation of the protein (resulting from its pathognomonic gene fusion t[11;22][p13;q12] *EWSR1-WT1* fusion). This is in contrast to *CIC*-rearranged sarcomas, which are positive for antibodies directed against either the C- or N-terminus (**Fig. 7**D).[30,32]

Contrary to other round cell sarcomas, DSRCTs frequently exhibit strong, diffuse expression of cytokeratins (CAM5.2, and AE1/AE3), desmin (in a distinctive perinuclear dot pattern), and epithelial membrane antigen (EMA), and they are negative for myogenin and ETV4 (Fig. 7C, D).[17,33]

Extraskeletal mesenchymal chondrosarcomas with a poorly developed chondroid matrix can mimic the myxoid stroma seen in *CIC*-rearranged sarcomas. Because of the variably prominent foci of cartilaginous differentiation, which can vary markedly throughout a single tumor, these neoplasms can present a pitfall in the context of core needle biopsy when the cartilaginous component is not sampled or minimally present. The cellular component of these tumors is made up of predominantly primitive round cells or slightly spindled cells with fine chromatin, lacking the vesicular chromatin and prominent nucleoli often seen in *CIC*-rearranged sarcomas (Fig. 8). Similar to CIC-rearranged sarcomas, mesenchymal chondrosarcomas most commonly affect teenagers and young adults with a peak incidence in the twenties. Mesenchymal chondrosarcomas originate in the soft tissues approximately 30% of the time, and radiologic correlation is a helpful diagnostic clue, because most tumors exhibit a calcified matrix. Immunophenotypically, only the cells associated with the chondroid matrix are S100 positive, whereas the undifferentiated cells often show diffuse membranous CD99 immunoreactivity, and also often express NKX2-2, but typically lack nuclear WT1 and ETV4 staining.[17] Mesenchymal chondrosarcomas harbor *HEY1-NCOA2* fusions, which can be interrogated by reverse-transcriptase polymerase chain reaction (RT-PCR) or FISH.

ARMS, representing approximately 20% of all rhabdomyosarcomas (the most common soft tissue sarcoma in children), can show significant morphologic overlap with *CIC*-rearranged sarcomas. The classic histology is characterized by a proliferation of small round cells and occasional multinucleated tumor giant cells present in a background fibrotic stroma, with discohesive tumor cells resulting in an artifactual separation of the fibrous septae resembling the alveoli of the lung. However, the percentage of fibrotic stroma varies among tumors, and those cases with less stroma and more cohesive tumor cells result in a solid pattern of ARMS, which is difficult to separate from other round cell tumors based on morphology alone (Fig. 9A, B). As a result, adding myogenin to an immunohistochemical panel is suggested, because it is diffusely positive in ARMS (Fig. 9C).[34] In contrast to *CIC*-rearranged sarcomas, ETV4 is essentially negative in

ARMS.[17,33] When suspected, the characteristic t(2;13) *PAX3-FOXO1A* or t(1;13) *PAX7-FOXO1A* fusions are detected by FISH or RT-PCR.[35]

Although most myxoid liposarcomas contain only a minority of a cellular round cell component, rare tumors are composed predominantly or exclusively of an undifferentiated round cell component and are designated as high-grade myxoid liposarcoma (previously called round cell liposarcoma) (Fig. 10). Although they occur in an older population compared with most round cell sarcomas (with a peak incidence in the fourth decade), there is significant overlap in the affected age range with *CIC*-rearranged sarcomas, which is further confounded by the presence of a prominent myxoid stroma. However, these aggressive round cell–predominant myxoid liposarcomas maintain the characteristic plexiform or chicken-wire vascular pattern seen in conventional myxoid liposarcomas, and harbor the same t(12;16) *FUS-DDIT3* fusions. In contrast to *CIC*-rearranged sarcomas, they express S100 in hypocellular and hypercellular areas, and are negative for WT1 and ETV4.[17]

Although they share a greater morphologic overlap with *BCOR*-rearranged sarcomas, poorly differentiated synovial sarcomas share more clinical features with *CIC*-rearranged sarcomas in that they affect a similar age group (young adults) and often arise in the deep soft tissues of the proximal limbs. These poorly differentiated synovial sarcomas also display round-to-ovoid nuclei with prominent nuclei. In contrast to *CIC*-rearranged sarcomas, they express cytokeratins and/or EMA, and they are negative for WT1 and ETV4.[17,33,36] Unlike *CIC*-rearranged sarcomas, synovial sarcomas also demonstrate a t(X;18) (*SYT-SSX* fusion) detectable by FISH or RT-PCR.

DIAGNOSIS

Making an accurate diagnosis of tumors with round cell morphology on core biopsy is more paramount than ever as the use of minimally invasive image-guided tumor sampling methods expands, in combination with the increasing role of neoadjuvant chemotherapeutic regimens in round cell sarcoma treatment protocols.[37] Most round cell sarcomas with atypical features (ie, tumors other than classical Ewing sarcoma in the anticipated age and location), should be confirmed by molecular methods.

When encountering a core biopsy of a bone or soft tissue mass showing round cell morphology in an adolescent or young adult, a focused immunohistochemical panel should be used, consisting of CD99, desmin, TLE1, S100, WT1, a

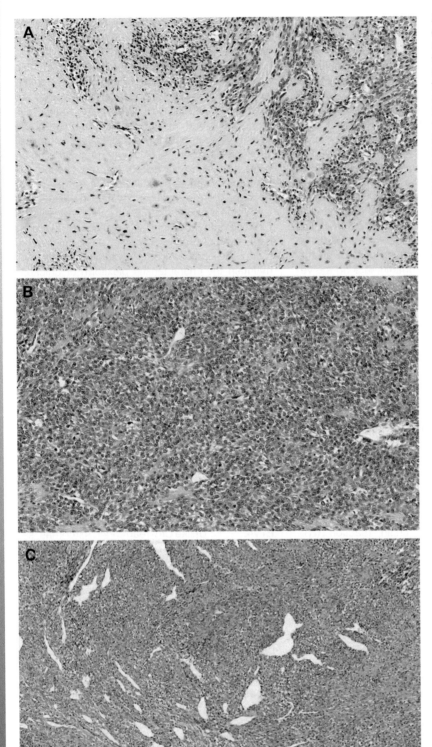

Fig. 8. (*A*) The prominent chondroid matrix in mesenchymal chondrosarcomas can vary markedly throughout the tumor, such that core biopsies may target areas lacking this stroma (hematoxylin-eosin, original magnification ×200). (*B*) Rare tumors can contain little chondroid stroma (hematoxylin-eosin, original magnification ×200). (*C*) Hemangiopericytoma-like vessels are a common feature (hematoxylin-eosin, original magnification ×100).

Fig. 9. (*A*) The solid variant of alveolar rhabdomyosarcoma consists of a solid round cell component in a fibrotic stroma, lacking alveolar morphology (hematoxylin-eosin, original magnification ×100). (*B*) Core biopsy samples can demonstrate a solid pattern with little stroma (hematoxylin-eosin, original magnification ×200). (*C*) Diffuse nuclear myogenin expression is a sensitive and specific marker for alveolar rhabdomyosarcomas, including solid variants (original magnification ×200).

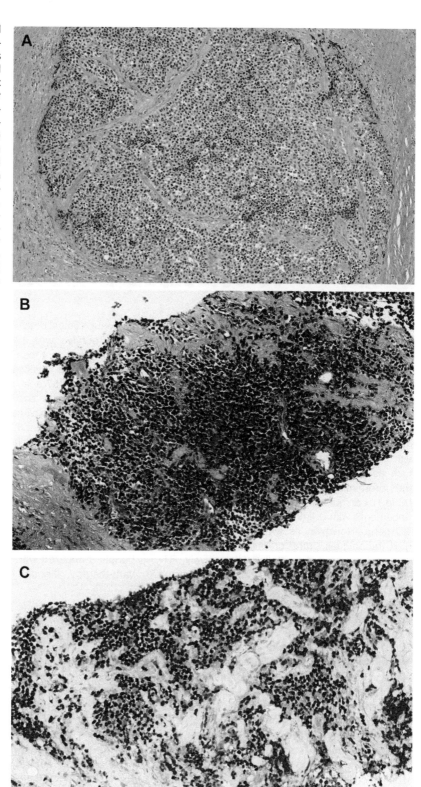

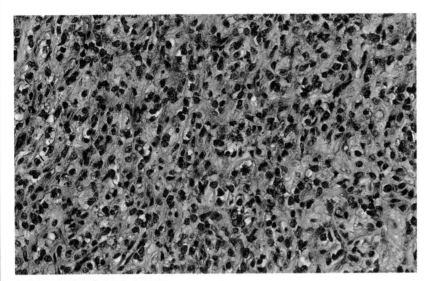

Fig. 10. High-grade myxoid (round cell) liposarcoma may consist of a solid round cell component in rare cases (hematoxylin-eosin, original magnification ×400).

broad-spectrum keratin (eg, AE1/AE3), or EMA, and lymphoid markers, such as CD45, CD3, CD20, and TdT. Although other immunohistochemical stains, such as ETV4, PAX7, NKX2-2, BCOR, and CCNB3 can also be useful, at the time of publication these stains are much less commonly validated and available for clinical use in most laboratories. The previously mentioned immunohistochemical panel, when combined with evaluation of select morphologic features, such as presence of myxoid stroma, necrosis, and prominent nucleoli, among others (see **Table 1**), can guide molecular testing for *CIC*-rearrangements with break-apart FISH probes for the *CIC* gene. However, as with most conventional FISH techniques, rare cryptic rearrangements represent a diagnostic pitfall.[38] Alternatively, RT-PCR is used with probes for the *CIC-DUX4* and *CIC-DUX4L* fusion transcripts. This approach requires further multiplexing to interrogate less common alternate fusion partners, such as *CIC-FOXO4* and *CIC-NUTM1*, but the low variation in breakpoints of the *CIC-DUX4* fusions makes this a viable option.[11] NGS techniques nullify some of these pitfalls, and round cell sarcoma NGS panels will likely become more widely available and reimbursable in the near future. Of note, some fusion callers used with NGS panels filter intronic calls, such as are often present in *CIC*-rearranged sarcoma, and care must be taken to adjust laboratory parameters to take this into account to avoid false-negative calls.

PROGNOSIS AND MANAGEMENT

In the largest published cohort of *CIC*-rearranged sarcomas documenting 115 cases (for which follow-up clinical data were available for 57 cases), 5-year survival was 43% for all cases, and 49% when limited to those presenting with localized disease. This is significantly worse than a comparison cohort of 57 age- and stage-matched Ewing sarcomas, which had 5-year survival rates of 77% and 76% for all cases and localized disease presentation, respectively.[14] These are in line with previously published cohorts.[11–13] Most patients have been treated with a Ewing sarcoma chemotherapy regimen, and initial data show a lower grade III neoadjuvant chemotherapy response rate (defined as <10% residual viable tumor cells) compared with *BCOR*-rearranged sarcoma and Ewing sarcoma.[11,14,39] Thus far, neoadjuvant chemotherapy has not shown a survival benefit compared with surgery followed by adjuvant therapy, although data are limited.[14]

Key Features
OF *CIC*-REARRANGED SARCOMAS

- *CIC*-rearranged sarcomas are SRCS that predominantly arise in the soft tissues of young adults, and often exhibit prominent nucleoli, mild to moderate nuclear pleomorphism, and myxoid stroma.

- Most *CIC*-rearranged sarcomas exhibit nuclear WT1 and ETV4 expression and lack diffuse membranous CD99 expression.

- These tumors seem to have a worse prognosis and response to therapy compared with Ewing sarcoma and *BCOR*-rearranged sarcoma.

Pitfalls
OF *CIC*-REARRANGED SARCOMAS

! Like Ewing sarcoma, *CIC*-rearranged sarcomas commonly express ETS transcription factor family members ERG and FLI1. Immunohistochemistry for CD99 is also commonly expressed; however, only rarely in the form of strong, diffuse membranous expression seen in Ewing sarcoma.

! Myxoid change and rhabdoid or plasmacytoid morphology can each be prominent features in *CIC*-rearranged sarcomas, broadening the morphologic differential diagnosis to include sarcomas with a prominent myxoid matrix and rhabdoid and plasmacytoid features.

! Nuclear WT1 (N- or C-terminal) expression is present in almost all *CIC*-rearranged sarcomas, and is helpful in differentiating these tumors from Ewing sarcoma and *BCOR*-rearranged sarcomas, but is also a feature of DSRCT (C-terminal only). DSRCTs also show at least focal expression of desmin (in a characteristic perinuclear dot pattern) and/or ETV4.

BCL6 COREPRESSOR-REARRANGED ROUND CELL SARCOMAS

INTRODUCTION

First described by Pierron and colleagues,[40] *BCOR*-rearranged undifferentiated round cell sarcomas constitute a much smaller proportion of round cell sarcomas lacking *EWSR1* rearrangements compared with *CIC*-rearranged sarcomas. Overall, the clinical features of *BCOR*-rearranged sarcomas more closely reflect those of classic Ewing sarcoma than *CIC*-rearranged sarcomas. Like Ewing sarcoma, they most commonly present in the second decade, with a median age of 15 years. There is also less age variation, with only a few cases reported beyond the second decade. *BCOR*-rearranged sarcomas arise slightly more commonly in bone (approximately 60% of cases), with the pelvis and long bones of the lower extremities most commonly affected.[39,41–44] By contrast, nearly 85% of Ewing sarcomas arise in bone, and less than 5% of *CIC*-rearranged sarcomas arise in bone.[41] Nearly 85% of *BCOR*-rearranged sarcoma cases occur in males, a much greater sex predilection than either *CIC*-rearranged or Ewing sarcomas.[39,41–45]

GROSS AND RADIOLOGIC FEATURES

Although there are no specific gross features of *BCOR*-rearranged sarcomas, tumors are typically solid and commonly exhibit gross evidence of hemorrhage and necrosis. Similarly, radiologic features are nonspecific, but by MRI, most tumors show a heterogeneously enhancing lytic bone tumor involving the pelvis or metadiaphysis of long bones with cortical destruction and associated infiltration of surrounding soft tissues.[43,46] In tumors of long bones, pathologic facture is common.

MICROSCOPIC AND IMMUNOHISTOCHEMICAL FEATURES

BCOR-rearranged sarcomas demonstrate a greater combination of round cell and spindled morphology compared with Ewing sarcoma and *CIC*-rearranged sarcomas. They range in composition from exclusively medium-sized uniform round cells to a uniform spindled appearance, with most cases showing a mix of round and spindled morphologies (**Fig. 11**).[39,41,43,44] The round cell component is typically present in sheets, whereas the spindled component demonstrates a short fascicular and storiform growth pattern most commonly, with a subset of tumors arranged in longer fascicles with a herringbone pattern. The tumors exhibit a predominantly well-circumscribed border with focal infiltrative edges, and can have a lobular configuration with thick fibrous septa. The chromatin quality is typically smooth to finely stippled, lacking nucleoli (in contrast to the conspicuous nucleoli in *CIC*-rearranged sarcomas), and the cells have scant pale eosinophilic cytoplasm.[41]

Similar to *CIC*-rearranged sarcomas, focal-to-prominent myxoid stroma has been reported, although the incidence of a myxoid component is lower (**Fig. 12**).[42,43] The stroma also contains a rich vascular network of curvilinear thin-walled vessels (see **Fig. 11C**). A subset of reported cases can exhibit dilated hemangiopericytoma-like vessels and thick collagen bundles among the tumor cells, similar to solitary fibrous tumor (SFT) and synovial sarcoma.[44] Brisk mitotic activity is a feature, although lower than in *CIC*-rearranged sarcomas (mean, 12 MF per 10 HPF).[39,41]

Although data are limited, initial reports suggest that a greater degree of nuclear pleomorphism similar to that seen in undifferentiated pleomorphic sarcoma confers a more aggressive behavior, and is more commonly seen in metastases.[41] Focal osteoblastic differentiation with osteoid matrix formation has also been described in a case of lung metastasis.[39] Additional series are required to support this observation, and no grading system

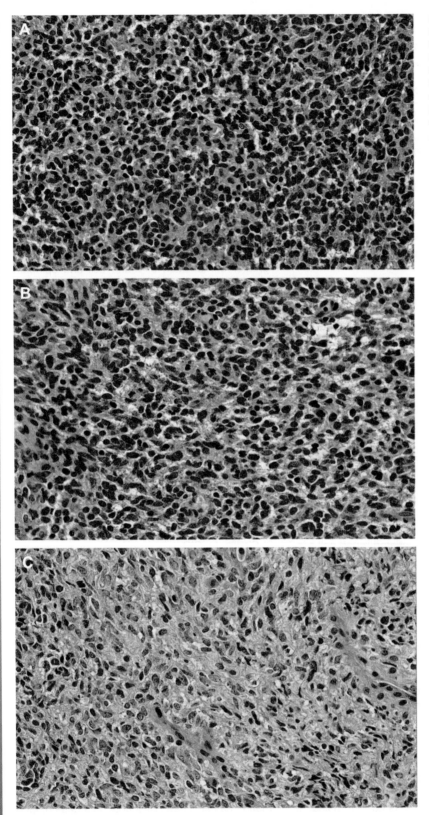

Fig. 11. (A–C) Most *BCOR*-rearranged sarcomas contain a mixture of spindled and round cells. The tumor cell nuclei exhibit fine, evenly dispersed chromatin with inconspicuous nucleoli (hematoxylin-eosin, original magnification ×400).

Fig. 12. (*A*, *B*) Occasionally, *BCOR*-rearranged sarcomas can exhibit myxoid stroma similar to *CIC*-rearranged sarcomas (hematoxylin-eosin, original magnification ×200 [*A*] and ×400 [*B*]).

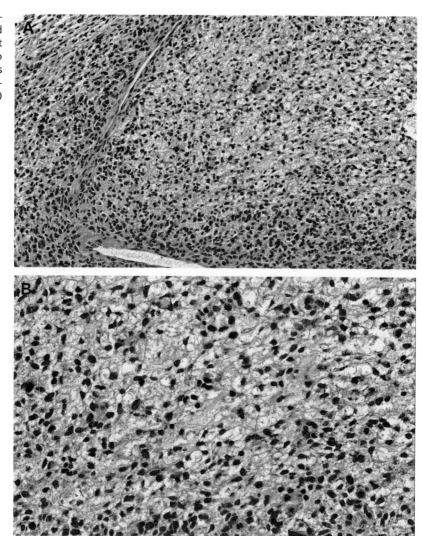

currently exists. Coagulative tumor cell necrosis is present in most cases.[41]

CD99 immunoreactivity is variably reported among cohorts of *BCOR*-rearranged sarcomas, ranging from 0%[42] to 100%.[45] Overall, expression is reported in approximately 40% of cases, but only rarely do tumors show strong membranous staining similar to that seen in typical Ewing sarcoma.[41–45] Strong nuclear CCNB3 expression is present in 95% of tumors, making it the most consistent positive marker, correlating with the most frequent BCOR fusion partner. Similarly, BCOR is strongly and diffusely expressed in 94% of tumors.[42,44] Matsuyama and colleagues[44] stained 412 tumors with small round cell or spindled cell morphologies for CCNB3 and BCOR, and found an expression rate of 1.5% and 4.4%, respectively. Based on these data, the authors concluded that immunohistochemistry

for CCNB3 and BCOR lacked adequate specificity; however, a small number of tumors comprised the group that showed positive staining, including SFTs, synovial sarcoma, Ewing sarcoma, lymphoma, and small cell carcinoma, most of which could be easily discerned by a few additional immunohistochemical stains. The major exception is synovial sarcomas, because the strong TLE1 nuclear expression seen in most synovial sarcomas is also present in a high proportion of *BCOR*-rearranged sarcomas (75%; Fig. 13).[42,44] Combined with morphologic overlap, these features make synovial sarcoma the most significant diagnostic pitfall of *BCOR*-rearranged sarcoma. Additionally, most *BCOR*-rearranged sarcomas express SATB2 (83%); a subset express NKX2-2 (29%); and they are consistently negative for WT1 (nuclear), S100, cytokeratin AE1/AE3, CD34, and desmin.[39,41–44]

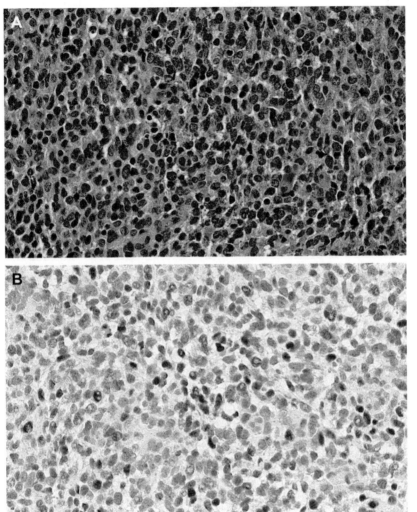

Fig. 13. (*A*) Most *BCOR*-rearranged sarcomas exhibit nuclear expression of TLE1 (*B*), similar to synovial sarcomas (hematoxylin-eosin [*A*], original magnification ×400 [*A, B*]).

MOLECULAR GENETIC FEATURES

BCOR-rearranged sarcomas were discovered through RNA-seq performed on a series of SRCS of bone lacking the typical gene fusions of *EWSR1* and *ETS*. One tumor in the cohort demonstrated fusions between exon 15 of *BCOR* on Xp11.4 and exon 5 of *CCNB3* on Xp11.22, the result of an X-chromosome paracentric inversion.[40] The authors found the same fusion in 23 other tumors with similar morphology, and additionally demonstrated distinct gene expression profiles and copy number alterations compared with classic Ewing sarcoma.

The *BCOR* gene encodes a nuclear corepressor protein that suppresses gene expression of the BCL6 oncoprotein.[47,48] This protein is responsible for epigenetic regulation of mesenchymal stem-cell proliferation and function through histone methylation.[49] *CCNB3* encodes a meiotic cyclin

protein found in spermatocytes, and the resulting BCOR-CCNB3 fusion protein promotes an increased proportion of cells in S-phase in mouse models.[40] Although even more rare, undifferentiated soft tissue and bone sarcomas with *BCOR* alterations other than *BCOR-CCNB3* fusions have subsequently been reported, including *BCOR–MAML3*, *ZC3H7B–BCOR*, *KMT2D-BCOR*, *BCOR* internal tandem duplication (ITD), and unknown fusion partners; thus, the term *BCOR*-rearranged sarcomas has been proposed for this family of neoplasms.[39,50] These tumors with alternate fusions exhibit fairly similar morphology and clinical characteristics, and similarly exhibit clustered transcriptomes.[6] Similar to *CIC*-rearranged sarcomas, *BCOR*-rearranged sarcomas harbor predominantly balanced genomic profiles with occasional recurrent copy number alterations including 10q and 17p deletions, in contrast to the fairly common gains of chromosome 8, 1q, and 12 in ESFT.[28,40] This finding, in concert with the marked difference in gene expression profiling and lack of expression of genes constituent to Ewing sarcoma oncogenesis, supports BCOR-rearranged sarcomas as biologically distinct from ESFT.

Outside of soft tissue–based round cell sarcomas, the BCOR gene is emerging as a recurrent tumor suppressor gene across multiple tissue types. BCOR alterations including ZC3H7B-BCOR and BCOR-ITD have also been described in high-grade uterine sarcomas with myxoid phenotype, proposed to represent high-grade endometrial stromal sarcomas with an alternative gene fusion to the YWHAE-NUTM2A/B.[51] Similarly, mutually exclusive BCOR ITD and YWHAE-NUTM2B/E gene fusions have been found in tumors diagnosed as clear cell sarcomas of the kidney, supporting a phenotypic link between these alterations brought about by activation of distinct signaling pathways.[52–55] BCOR alterations have also been described in ossifying fibromyoid tumors and a small subset of acute myeloid leukemias.[40,56]

DIFFERENTIAL DIAGNOSIS

The differential diagnosis for BCOR-rearranged sarcomas is similar to that of CIC-rearranged sarcomas, with the addition of entities that show a more prominent spindle cell component. Ewing sarcoma remains the foremost entity in the differential diagnosis. Clinical factors including affected ages and involved anatomic sites are much more similar between BCOR-rearranged sarcomas and Ewing sarcoma compared with CIC-rearranged sarcomas. CD99 expression is present in nearly half of BCOR-rearranged sarcomas, but rarely shows strong membranous staining.[41–45] Importantly, a subset of BCOR-rearranged sarcomas express NKX2-2 (~30%), rendering it of low yield in this differential. BCOR and CCNB3 immunohistochemical stains are positive in BCOR-rearranged sarcomas and only rarely so in Ewing sarcoma, making them useful, but unfortunately these stains are currently not widely available.[41–44] An EWSR1-break-apart FISH assay can be used as a screening tool in suspected cases, followed by specific CIC and BCOR molecular testing in negative tumors.

Because of their mixed spindled and round cell morphology and significant immunophenotypic overlap, poorly differentiated synovial sarcoma should always be considered in tandem with BCOR-rearranged sarcomas. Although poorly differentiated (round cell) synovial sarcomas display large ovoid nuclei with prominent nucleoli,

these features are variably prominent throughout a single tumor (Fig. 14). Because diffuse TLE1 nuclear expression is present in a high proportion of both tumors, expression of cytokeratin and/or EMA favors synovial sarcoma.[36] If readily available, a negative assay for the detection of SS18(SYT)-SSX1/2 essentially excludes a poorly differentiated synovial sarcoma, and BCOR molecular testing can be performed in a step-wise fashion.[57]

Because of the spindled nature of many BCOR-rearranged sarcomas and occasional hemangiopericytoma-like vasculature, soft tissue SFT also enters the differential diagnosis. Morphologically, SFTs consist of a syncytial proliferation of bland spindled cells in a haphazard patternless arrangement with stromal hyalinization, but some tumors, particularly malignant SFTs, exhibit cellular sheets of round-to-ovoid cells and can be mitotically active (Fig. 15). Immunohistochemically, most SFTs exhibit diffuse CD34 and STAT6 expression (90% and 97%, respectively).[58] The latter finding is based on a recurrent intrachromasomal rearrangement of 12q resulting in a NAB2-STAT6 fusion, and compared with other mesenchymal tumors, is highly sensitive and specific for SFT.[59–61]

Mesenchymal chondrosarcomas affect overlapping anatomic sites, most notably the pelvis, in addition to its predilection for the jaw, ribs, and vertebrae. The mix of small round and slightly spindle-shaped cells lacking nucleoli is similar to BCOR-rearranged sarcomas in cellular areas, and mesenchymal chondrosarcomas also commonly show branching, thin-walled, ectatic hemangiopericytoma-like vessels (see Fig. 8). Radiologic correlation should typically suggest a component of calcified matrix in cases where core biopsies did not sample the foci of cartilaginous differentiation. Mesenchymal chondrosarcomas are negative for TLE1, BCOR, and CCNB3.[44]

Because most BCOR-rearranged sarcomas arise in bone, small cell osteosarcoma enters the differential diagnosis. This is compounded by the fact that most BCOR-rearranged sarcomas (83%) also express SATB2, a marker of osteoblast differentiation.[39] As a result, bone tumors with SATB2 expression and round cell sarcoma morphology should be tested for BCOR rearrangements.

DIAGNOSIS

The diagnosis is suggested based on a combination of morphologic and immunophenotypic features, but requires molecular testing for confirmation. Overall, a tumor with a mix of round cell and spindled cell morphology lacking high-grade features, such as nucleoli (among other features, see Table 1), with an immunophenotype positive

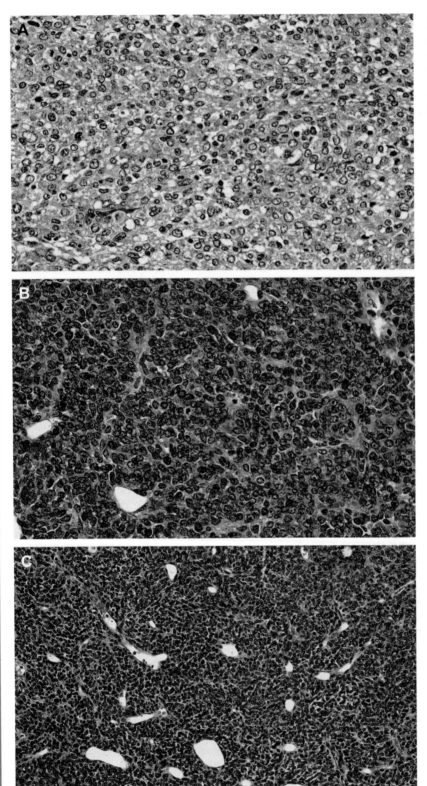

Fig. 14. (*A, B*) In contrast to typical monophasic synovial sarcomas, poorly differentiated synovial sarcomas exhibit more rounded nuclei with prominent nucleoli, and a slightly greater degree of nuclear pleomorphism (hematoxylin-eosin, original magnification ×400). (*C*) They frequently have hemangiopericytoma-like vessels (hematoxylin-eosin, original magnification ×200).

Fig. 15. (*A, B*) SFT, particularly in malignant cases, can show more diffuse round-to-ovoid cell morphology with conspicuous mitotic activity (hematoxylin-eosin, original magnification ×100 [*A*] and ×400 [*B*]). (*C*) STAT-6 nuclear positivity is sensitive and specific for SFTs (original magnification ×400).

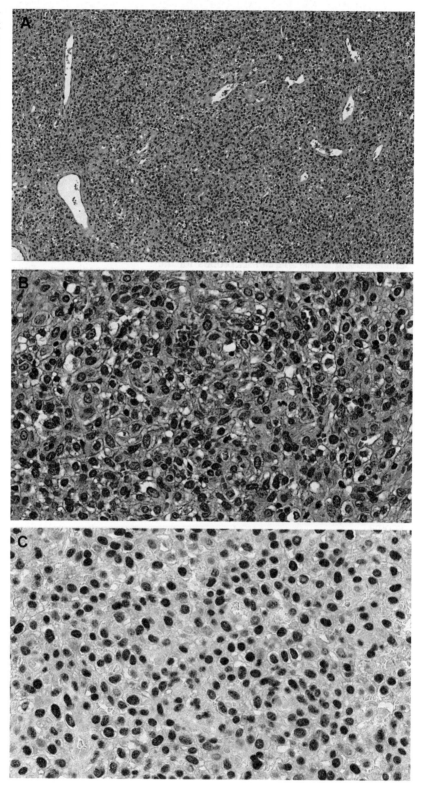

for TLE1 and either CCNB3 or BCOR, negative for WT1 and STAT6, and lacking diffuse membranous CD99 expression, should raise considerable suspicion for a *BCOR*-rearranged sarcoma, which is confirmed by FISH or RT-PCR assays. In laboratories lacking access to CCNB3 and BCOR immunohistochemistry, a tumor with the previously mentioned morphology and strong and diffuse TLE1 expression can be tested for synovial sarcoma fusions (*SS18-SSX1/2*) followed by molecular testing for *BCOR*.

Because of the nature of the *BCOR-CCNB3* fusion (paracentric inversion on the X-chromosome), dual-fusion probes are required for FISH assays targeting the most common rearrangement.[38] The less common rearrangements described previously, *BCOR-MAML3* and *BCOR-ZC3H7B*, are identified using break-apart FISH probes for the *BCOR* gene. RT-PCR is less effective in *BCOR*-rearranged sarcomas compared with *CIC*-rearranged sarcomas, because of a greater variability in breakpoints. This accounts for its more recent discovery requiring RNA-seq techniques.[40]

PROGNOSIS AND MANAGEMENT

The 5-year overall survival for *BCOR*-rearranged sarcomas is approximately 75%, which is similar overall to matched cohorts of Ewing sarcoma.[39,41,43,45] Late recurrences have been published, with one patient dying of disease 157 months after diagnosis.[45] *BCOR*-rearranged sarcomas located in the axial skeleton and soft tissues show a significantly shorter survival, although this finding is similarly seen with Ewing sarcoma.[41,62,63]

BCOR-rearranged sarcomas are most commonly treated with Ewing sarcoma protocols or less commonly rhabdomyosarcoma protocols, with induction chemotherapy followed by surgical resection with chemosensitivity assessment. In the two largest cohorts of *BCOR*-rearranged sarcomas, 10 of 12 tumors treated with neoadjuvant therapy showed less than 10% viable tumor cells after resection, corresponding with a good response based on Ewing sarcoma criteria.[43,64] Unfortunately, few additional conclusions are drawn based on the small number of published cases and heterogeneity of provided treatments, although based on the limited data, prognosis seems to not be significantly worse or better than Ewing sarcoma. Future meta-analysis is required to support these impressions, hopefully with more uniformly applied treatment protocols as oncologists and pathologists become increasingly aware of this entity leading to a higher proportion of prospective diagnoses.

Key Features
OF *BCOR*-REARRANGED SARCOMAS

- *BCOR*-rearranged sarcomas commonly show a mix of round cell and spindle cell morphology with fine chromatin, and can show myxoid stroma and hemangiopericytoma-like vessels.

- The typical immunoprofile includes expression of BCOR, CCNB3, TLE1, and patchy expression of CD99.

- *BCOR*-rearranged sarcoma shows similar clinical features to Ewing sarcoma, most commonly arising in bones of patients in their second decade, and exhibiting similar overall survival rate and response rate to neoadjuvant Ewing sarcoma treatment regimens.

Pitfalls
OF *BCOR*-REARRANGED ROUND CELL SARCOMAS

! *BCOR*-rearranged sarcomas express CD99 in approximately 40% of cases, although typically not in a diffuse, membranous pattern as is seen in Ewing sarcoma. A subset (approximately 30%) can also express NKX2-2.

! There is significant morphologic and immunophenotypic overlap between *BCOR*-rearranged sarcomas and poorly differentiated synovial sarcoma. Most *BCOR*-rearranged sarcomas exhibit diffuse nuclear TLE1 expression, and a component of spindle cell morphology. Furthermore, BCOR is positive in a subset of synovial sarcomas. Mixed round cell and spindled sarcomas with TLE1 expression should be tested in a stepwise fashion for the more common *SS18-SSX1/2* fusions, followed by *BCOR* FISH.

! Although BCOR and CCNB3 are often expressed in *BCOR*-rearranged sarcomas by immunohistochemistry, they can also rarely be expressed by tumors in the morphologic differential, including a subset of Ewing sarcomas and *CIC*-rearranged sarcomas.

! Detection of the X-chromosome paracentric inversion of *BCOR-CCNB3* by FISH testing requires dual fusion probes in addition to a break-apart probe for *BCOR* to detect less common fusion partners.

SUMMARY

Integrated clinical, immunohistochemical, and molecular data, supported by robust transcriptome analysis, support the classification of *CIC*-rearranged sarcomas and *BCOR*-rearranged sarcomas as separate entities from Ewing sarcoma, united under the category of undifferentiated round cell sarcomas. Although these tumors remain rare, prospective recognition and further characterization of these neoplasms promotes a greater understanding of their response to current round cell sarcoma treatment protocols, and hopefully will promote a more optimal treatment regimen and identify new treatment targets in the future. These developments will likely be accelerated as NGS techniques, including RNA-seq, become more widely available, affordable, and reimbursable.

REFERENCES

1. Llombart-Bosch A, Machado I, Navarro S, et al. Histological heterogeneity of Ewing's sarcoma/PNET: an immunohistochemical analysis of 415 genetically confirmed cases with clinical support. Virchows Arch 2009;455(5):397–411.
2. Szuhai K, Ijszenga M, de Jong D, et al. The NFATc2 gene is involved in a novel cloned translocation in a Ewing sarcoma variant that couples its function in immunology to oncology. Clin Cancer Res 2009; 15(7):2259–68.
3. Mastrangelo T, Modena P, Tornielli S, et al. A novel zinc finger gene is fused to EWS in small round cell tumor. Oncogene 2000;19(33):3799–804.
4. Sumegi J, Nishio J, Nelson M, et al. A novel t(4;22)(q31;q12) produces an EWSR1-SMARCA5 fusion in extraskeletal Ewing sarcoma/primitive neuroectodermal tumor. Mod Pathol 2011;24(3):333–42.
5. Wang L, Bhargava R, Zheng T, et al. Undifferentiated small round cell sarcomas with rare EWS gene fusions: identification of a novel EWS-SP3 fusion and of additional cases with the EWS-ETV1 and EWS-FEV fusions. J Mol Diagn 2007;9(4):498–509.
6. Watson S, Perrin V, Guillemot D, et al. Transcriptomic definition of molecular subgroups of small round cell sarcomas. J Pathol 2018;245(1):29–40.
7. Fletcher CD, Hogendoorn PC, Mertens F, et al. WHO classification of tumours of soft tissue and bone. 4th edition. Lyon (France): IARC Press; 2013.
8. Nascimento AGUK, Pritchard DJ, Cooper KL, et al. A clinicopathologic study of 20 cases of large-cell (atypical) Ewing's sarcoma of bone. Am J Surg Pathol 1980;4(1):29–36.
9. Kawamura-Saito M, Yamazaki Y, Kaneko K, et al. Fusion between CIC and DUX4 up-regulates PEA3 family genes in Ewing-like sarcomas with t(4;19)(q35;q13) translocation. Hum Mol Genet 2006;15(13):2125–37.
10. Machado I, Navarro S, Llombart-Bosch A. Ewing sarcoma and the new emerging Ewing-like sarcomas: (CIC and BCOR-rearranged-sarcomas). A systematic review. Histol Histopathol 2016;31(11): 1169–81.
11. Italiano A, Sung YS, Zhang L, et al. High prevalence of CIC fusion with double-homeobox (DUX4) transcription factors in EWSR1-negative undifferentiated small blue round cell sarcomas. Genes Chromosomes Cancer 2012;51(3):207–18.
12. Yoshida A, Goto K, Kodaira M, et al. CIC-rearranged sarcomas: a study of 20 cases and comparisons with Ewing sarcomas. Am J Surg Pathol 2016; 40(3):313–23.
13. Smith SC, Buehler D, Choi EY, et al. CIC-DUX sarcomas demonstrate frequent MYC amplification and ETS-family transcription factor expression. Mod Pathol 2015;28(1):57–68.
14. Antonescu CR, Owosho AA, Zhang L, et al. Sarcomas with CIC-rearrangements are a distinct pathologic entity with aggressive outcome: a clinicopathologic and molecular study of 115 cases. Am J Surg Pathol 2017;41(7):941–9.
15. Choi EY, Thomas DG, McHugh JB, et al. Undifferentiated small round cell sarcoma with t(4;19)(q35;q13.1) CIC-DUX4 fusion: a novel highly aggressive soft tissue tumor with distinctive histopathology. Am J Surg Pathol 2013;37(9):1379–86.
16. Specht K, Sung YS, Zhang L, et al. Distinct transcriptional signature and immunoprofile of CIC-DUX4 fusion-positive round cell tumors compared to EWSR1-rearranged Ewing sarcomas: further evidence toward distinct pathologic entities. Genes Chromosomes Cancer 2014;53(7):622–33.
17. Hung YP, Fletcher CD, Hornick JL. Evaluation of ETV4 and WT1 expression in CIC-rearranged sarcomas and histologic mimics. Mod Pathol 2016; 29(11):1324–34.
18. Krom YD, Thijssen PE, Young JM, et al. Intrinsic epigenetic regulation of the D4Z4 macrosatellite repeat in a transgenic mouse model for FSHD. PLoS Genet 2013;9(4):e1003415.
19. Graham C, Chilton-MacNeill S, Zielenska M, et al. The CIC-DUX4 fusion transcript is present in a subgroup of pediatric primitive round cell sarcomas. Hum Pathol 2012;43(2):180–9.
20. Yoshimoto M, Graham C, Chilton-MacNeill S, et al. Detailed cytogenetic and array analysis of pediatric primitive sarcomas reveals a recurrent CIC-DUX4 fusion gene event. Cancer Genet Cytogenet 2009; 195(1):1–11.
21. Solomon DA, Brohl AS, Khan J, et al. Clinicopathologic features of a second patient with Ewing-like sarcoma harboring CIC-FOXO4 gene fusion. Am J Surg Pathol 2014;38(12):1724–5.

22. Sugita S, Arai Y, Tonooka A, et al. A novel CIC-FOXO4 gene fusion in undifferentiated small round cell sarcoma: a genetically distinct variant of Ewing-like sarcoma. Am J Surg Pathol 2014;38(11):1571–6.

23. Kunju LP, Carskadon S, Siddiqui J, et al. Novel RNA hybridization method for the in situ detection of ETV1, ETV4, and ETV5 gene fusions in prostate cancer. Appl Immunohistochem Mol Morphol 2014;22(8):e32–40.

24. Smith SC, Palanisamy N, Martin E, et al. The utility of ETV1, ETV4 and ETV5 RNA in-situ hybridization in the diagnosis of CIC-DUX sarcomas. Histopathology 2017;70(4):657–63.

25. Charville GW, Wang WL, Ingram DR, et al. EWSR1 fusion proteins mediate PAX7 expression in Ewing sarcoma. Mod Pathol 2017;30(9):1312–20.

26. Toki S, Wakai S, Sekimizu M, et al. PAX7 immunohistochemical evaluation of Ewing sarcoma and other small round cell tumors. Histopathology 2018;73(4):645–52.

27. Lazo de la Vega L, Hovelson DH, Cani AK, et al. Targeted next-generation sequencing of CIC-DUX4 soft tissue sarcomas demonstrates low mutational burden and recurrent chromosome 1p loss. Hum Pathol 2016;58:161–70.

28. Armengol G, Tarkkanen M, Virolainen M, et al. Recurrent gains of 1q, 8 and 12 in the Ewing family of tumours by comparative genomic hybridization. Br J Cancer 1997;75(10):1403–9.

29. Ordonez NG. Desmoplastic small round cell tumor: I: a histopathologic study of 39 cases with emphasis on unusual histological patterns. Am J Surg Pathol 1998;22(11):1303–13.

30. Thway K, Noujaim J, Zaidi S, et al. Desmoplastic small round cell tumor: pathology, genetics, and potential therapeutic strategies. Int J Surg Pathol 2016;24(8):672–84.

31. Rao P, Tamboli P, Fillman EP, et al. Primary intra-renal desmoplastic small round cell tumor: expanding the histologic spectrum, with special emphasis on the differential diagnostic considerations. Pathol Res Pract 2014;210(12):1130–3.

32. Arnold MA, Schoenfield L, Limketkai BN, et al. Diagnostic pitfalls of differentiating desmoplastic small round cell tumor (DSRCT) from Wilms tumor (WT): overlapping morphologic and immunohistochemical features. Am J Surg Pathol 2014;38(9):1220–6.

33. Le Guellec S, Velasco V, Perot G, et al. ETV4 is a useful marker for the diagnosis of CIC-rearranged undifferentiated round-cell sarcomas: a study of 127 cases including mimicking lesions. Mod Pathol 2016;29(12):1523–31.

34. Kumar S, Perlman E, Harris CA, et al. Myogenin is a specific marker for rhabdomyosarcoma: an immunohistochemical study in paraffin-embedded tissues. Mod Pathol 2000;13(9):988–93.

35. Nishio J, Althof PA, Bailey JM, et al. Use of a novel FISH assay on paraffin-embedded tissues as an adjunct to diagnosis of alveolar rhabdomyosarcoma. Lab Invest 2006;86(6):547–56.

36. Miettinen M, Limon J, Niezabitowski A, et al. Patterns of keratin polypeptides in 110 biphasic, monophasic, and poorly differentiated synovial sarcomas. Virchows Arch 2000;437(3):275–83.

37. Gaspar N, Hawkins DS, Dirksen U, et al. Ewing sarcoma: current management and future approaches through collaboration. J Clin Oncol 2015;33(27):3036–46.

38. Le Loarer F, Pissaloux D, Coindre JM, et al. Update on families of round cell sarcomas other than classical Ewing sarcomas. Surg Pathol Clin 2017;10(3):587–620.

39. Kao YC, Owosho AA, Sung YS, et al. BCOR-CCNB3 fusion positive sarcomas: a clinicopathologic and molecular analysis of 36 cases with comparison to morphologic spectrum and clinical behavior of other round cell sarcomas. Am J Surg Pathol 2018;42(5):604–15.

40. Pierron G, Tirode F, Lucchesi C, et al. A new subtype of bone sarcoma defined by BCOR-CCNB3 gene fusion. Nat Genet 2012;44(4):461–6.

41. Puls F, Niblett A, Marland G, et al. BCOR-CCNB3 (Ewing-like) sarcoma: a clinicopathologic analysis of 10 cases, in comparison with conventional Ewing sarcoma. Am J Surg Pathol 2014;38(10):1307–18.

42. Yamada Y, Kuda M, Kohashi K, et al. Histological and immunohistochemical characteristics of undifferentiated small round cell sarcomas associated with CIC-DUX4 and BCOR-CCNB3 fusion genes. Virchows Arch 2017;470(4):373–80.

43. Cohen-Gogo S, Cellier C, Coindre JM, et al. Ewing-like sarcomas with BCOR-CCNB3 fusion transcript: a clinical, radiological and pathological retrospective study from the Societe Francaise des Cancers de L'Enfant. Pediatr Blood Cancer 2014;61(12):2191–8.

44. Matsuyama A, Shiba E, Umekita Y, et al. Clinicopathologic diversity of undifferentiated sarcoma with BCOR-CCNB3 fusion: analysis of 11 cases with a reappraisal of the utility of immunohistochemistry for BCOR and CCNB3. Am J Surg Pathol 2017;41(12):1713–21.

45. Peters TL, Kumar V, Polikepahad S, et al. BCOR-CCNB3 fusions are frequent in undifferentiated sarcomas of male children. Mod Pathol 2015;28(4):575–86.

46. Machado I, Yoshida A, Morales MGN, et al. Review with novel markers facilitates precise categorization of 41 cases of diagnostically challenging, "undifferentiated small round cell tumors." A clinicopathologic, immunophenotypic and molecular analysis. Ann Diagn Pathol 2018;34:1–12.

47. Huynh KD, Fischle W, Verdin E, et al. BCoR, a novel corepressor involved in BCL-6 repression. Genes Dev 2000;14(14):1810–23.

48. Gearhart MD, Corcoran CM, Wamstad JA, et al. Polycomb group and SCF ubiquitin ligases are found in a novel BCOR complex that is recruited to BCL6 targets. Mol Cell Biol 2006;26(18):6880–9.

49. Fan Z, Yamaza T, Lee JS, et al. BCOR regulates mesenchymal stem cell function by epigenetic mechanisms. Nat Cell Biol 2009;11(8):1002–9.

50. Specht K, Zhang L, Sung YS, et al. Novel BCOR-MAML3 and ZC3H7B-BCOR gene fusions in undifferentiated small blue round cell sarcomas. Am J Surg Pathol 2016;40(4):433–42.

51. Marino-Enriquez A, Lauria A, Przybyl J, et al. BCOR internal tandem duplication in high-grade uterine sarcomas. Am J Surg Pathol 2018;42(3):335–41.

52. Kao YC, Sung YS, Zhang L, et al. Recurrent BCOR internal tandem duplication and YWHAE-NUTM2B fusions in soft tissue undifferentiated round cell sarcoma of infancy: overlapping genetic features with clear cell sarcoma of kidney. Am J Surg Pathol 2016;40(8):1009–20.

53. Ueno-Yokohata H, Okita H, Nakasato K, et al. Consistent in-frame internal tandem duplications of BCOR characterize clear cell sarcoma of the kidney. Nat Genet 2015;47(8):861–3.

54. Karlsson J, Valind A, Gisselsson D. BCOR internal tandem duplication and YWHAE-NUTM2B/E fusion are mutually exclusive events in clear cell sarcoma of the kidney. Genes Chromosomes Cancer 2016; 55(2):120–3.

55. Kenny C, Bausenwein S, Lazaro A, et al. Mutually exclusive BCOR internal tandem duplications and YWHAE-NUTM2 fusions in clear cell sarcoma of kidney: not the full story. J Pathol 2016;238(5): 617–20.

56. Grossmann V, Tiacci E, Holmes AB, et al. Whole-exome sequencing identifies somatic mutations of BCOR in acute myeloid leukemia with normal karyotype. Blood 2011;118(23):6153–63.

57. Lewis JT, Oliveira AM, Nascimento AG, et al. Low-grade sinonasal sarcoma with neural and myogenic features: a clinicopathologic analysis of 28 cases. Am J Surg Pathol 2012;36(4):517–25.

58. Huang SC, Ghossein RA, Bishop JA, et al. Novel PAX3-NCOA1 fusions in biphenotypic sinonasal sarcoma with focal rhabdomyoblastic differentiation. Am J Surg Pathol 2016;40(1):51–9.

59. Demicco EG, Harms PW, Patel RM, et al. Extensive survey of STAT6 expression in a large series of mesenchymal tumors. Am J Clin Pathol 2015; 143(5):672–82.

60. Yoshida A, Tsuta K, Ohno M, et al. STAT6 immunohistochemistry is helpful in the diagnosis of solitary fibrous tumors. Am J Surg Pathol 2014;38(4):552–9.

61. Doyle LA, Vivero M, Fletcher CD, et al. Nuclear expression of STAT6 distinguishes solitary fibrous tumor from histologic mimics. Mod Pathol 2014;27(3): 390–5.

62. Bacci G, Ferrari S, Mercuri M, et al. Multimodal therapy for the treatment of nonmetastatic Ewing sarcoma of pelvis. J Pediatr Hematol Oncol 2003; 25(2):118–24.

63. Cotterill SJ, Ahrens S, Paulussen M, et al. Prognostic factors in Ewing's tumor of bone: analysis of 975 patients from the European Intergroup Cooperative Ewing's Sarcoma Study Group. J Clin Oncol 2000; 18(17):3108–14.

64. Oberlin O, Le Deley M, Dirksen U, et al. Randomized comparison of VAC versus VAI chemotherapy (CT) as consolidation for standard risk (SR) Ewing sarcoma tumor (ES): results of the Euro-EWING.99-R1 trial. J Clin Oncol 2011;29(15):2440–8.

Prognostication in Mesenchymal Tumors
Can We Improve?

Wei-Lien Wang, MD

KEYWORDS

- Sarcoma • Prognostic • Biomarker

Key points

- Sarcomas are a diverse group of tumors where histologic appearances are not always predictive of behavior and prognostication challenging.
- Proper classification and grading (generally by the French Federation of Cancer Centers guidelines) remain important prognostic parameters.
- Mutations (translocations, gene mutations) and immune microenvironment show prognostic and therapeutic significance in some sarcomas.
- Prognostic markers that take into account multiple genes/parameters such as gene expression signature (CINSARC, GGI) or nomograms, likely yield the most promise for sarcomas.

ABSTRACT

Prognostication in mesenchymal tumors can be challenging. They exhibit diverse, and sometimes overlapping, histologic features that are not always predictive of their true behavior. This article highlights examples of both traditional and emerging sarcoma biomarkers.

GRADING

Grading is widely recognized as one of the most important prognostic factors to assess aggressive behavior (ie, metastatic potential) in mesenchymal tumors. Although other grading systems exist, the guidelines proposed by the French Federation of Cancer Centers (also abbreviated as FNCLCC) has been adopted by the College of American Pathologists and American Joint Committee on Cancer given its ability to better distinguish tumors into high- or low-grade versus other grading systems.[1] The FNCLCC uses 3 components: tumor differentiation (ie, resemblance to normal mesenchymal counterpart), necrosis, and mitotic rate. A numerical score is assigned to each category, with grade (low, intermediate, or high) determined by the total score. Its simplicity contributes to its reproducibility, and the differentiation score allows it to be applicable to a diverse range of sarcomas.[2–4]

However, these guidelines have limitations. Small biopsies may limit the ability to accurately assess parameters owing to sampling and tumor heterogeneity such as a missed "hot spot" mitotic area or necrosis. Neoadjuvant radiation and/or chemotherapy changes can also make accurate assessment challenging. In addition, not all mesenchymal tumors can be graded by this system. Examples of nongradable tumors include clear cell sarcoma, epithelioid sarcoma, alveolar soft part sarcoma, and Ewing sarcoma. In these tumors, the diagnosis alone confers an expected

---

Disclosure Statement: The author has no financial relationships to disclose.
Departments of Pathology and Translational Molecular Pathology, The University of Texas MD Anderson Cancer Center, 1515 Holcombe Boulevard, Unit 085, Houston, TX 77030, USA
E-mail address: wlwang@mdanderson.org

Surgical Pathology 12 (2019) 217–225
https://doi.org/10.1016/j.path.2018.10.009

high-grade metastatic biological potential. In other tumors, FNCLCC grade fails to predict behavior accurately. These tumors require their own separate guidelines with additional parameters to better assess risk of aggressive behavior. Examples include gastrointestinal stromal tumors, which take into account size, mitotic activity, and site and solitary fibrous tumor; risk models propose the use of size, patient age at primary diagnosis, necrosis, and mitotic activity.[5,6] Similar attempts to integrate clinical and pathologic parameters (such as size, site, and age) and improve the accuracy of prognostication for individual patients have been used in nomograms and show promise as a useful tool.[7–9]

Finally, determining malignant potential in mesenchymal tumors, which lack clear classification (ie, unclassified), can present their own unique challenges. Prior experience in the behavior of similarly appearing tumors and other histologic parameters (like cellularity, pleomorphism, atypia, necrosis, and mitotic activity/proliferative rate) can assist in favoring a malignant potential. Some apply FNCLCC guidelines to unclassified mesenchymal tumors using a differentiation score of 3 owing to undifferentiated/unclassifiable nature. Neither method is always accurate because tumors can deceptively behave worse or better than their histologic appearance. Clinical and radiologic input can provide invaluable information and is one advantage of multidisciplinary treatment centers. For mesenchymal tumors where there is uncertainty, it is reasonable to use the phrase "uncertain malignant potential," particularly in absence of clinical correlation. Additional tools, described elsewhere in this article, may be helpful in assisting pathologists to better grade unclassified tumors.

ROLE OF TRANSLOCATIONS

A growing number of sarcomas harbor recurrent translocations and mutations, which can assist in classification. Because a diagnosis implies a certain behavior, prognosis, and response to therapy, proper classification arguably can be an important prognostic factor. The detection of these recurrent mutations are well-documented (in the appropriate clinical and pathologic context as even vastly different tumors can harbor the same translocations/mutations) to assist in the accurate classification of tumors including in small and suboptimal biopsies. This is especially true in some tumors, which exhibit overlapping morphology. An example of this is small round cells tumors such as Ewing sarcoma, desmoplastic small round cell tumor and undifferentiated Ewing-like round cell sarcomas, which harbor different fusion transcripts, behavior, and prognosis.[10–12]

Although translocations are known to be important to sarcomagenesis, whether variants/types can influence behavior is not entirely certain. Studies have shown that fusion transcript variants (where there are different gene partners) and types (where there is variation in the breakpoints with same gene partners) can sometimes influence phenotypes though not necessarily prognosis. One example is synovial sarcoma and fusion variants SYT-SSX1 and SYT-SSX2. One large study found that biphasic synovial sarcomas were predisposed to harbor the fusion variant SYT-SSX1, whereas monophasic synovial sarcoma were more likely to harbor SYT-SSX2.[13] In this same study, patients with localized tumors at diagnosis with SYT-SSX2 had statistically significant better overall survival using Cox regression analysis. However, this association was not found in another large series.[14] Myoepithelial tumors are another tumor type, which can harbor multiple fusion variants, most often involving EWSR1 and FUS, which seem to be associated with certain histologic phenotypes,[15–24] although the prognostic significance is not known. However, fusion variants may play a role in inflammatory myofibroblastic tumors and alveolar rhabdomyosarcomas. Inflammatory myofibroblastic tumors harbor rearrangements involving ALK and multiple gene partners. Tumors that are ALK negative or have RANBP2 as a fusion partner (often with epithelioid morphology and distinctive perinuclear ALK labeling) can behave more aggressively.[25] The presence of ALK rearrangements also makes these tumors amendable to treatment by ALK inhibitors.[26,27] Prognostic differences are also seen in alveolar rhabdomyosarcoma, where tumors with PAX7-FOXO1A1 fusion variant have a better prognosis than those tumors with PAX3-FOXO1A1 fusion variant.[28,29] Furthermore, those without any FOXO1A1 rearrangements behave more like embryonal rhabdomyosarcoma.[30]

Fusion types may also influence behavior. One example is solitary fibrous tumors. Pleural intrathoracic solitary fibrous tumors have been found to occur in older patients, and are more likely harbor NAB2 exon 4 -STAT6 exon2/4 fusions than solitary fibrous tumors arising at other sites. However, the prognostic significance of fusion types in these tumors remains uncertain. One study found tumors with NAB2ex6-STAT6ex16/17 to have more aggressive behavior, whereas NAB2ex4-STAT6ex2/3 has a better prognosis. However, another series failed to identify disease free survival significance in tumors with NAB2ex4-STAT6

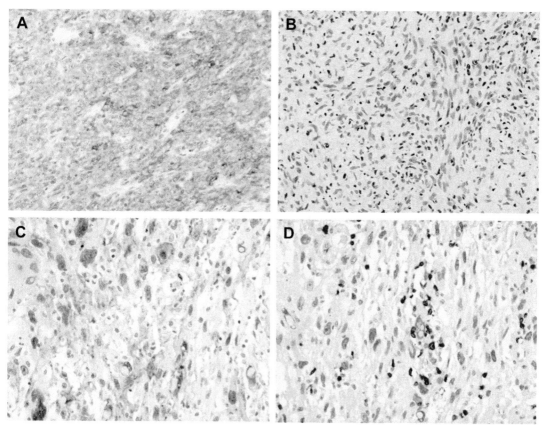

Fig. 1. (*A*). Pan-tropomyosin receptor kinase expression in unclassified sarcomas (Immunohistochemical study, ×100). (*B*). Loss of ATRX in angiosarcomas (Immunohistochemical study, ×100). (*C*). PD-L1 expression (Immunohistochemical study, ×200) (membranous labeling) in undifferentiated pleomorphic sarcoma with concurrent labeling of CD3 lymphocytes (*D*) (Immunohistochemical study, ×200).

ex2/4, although these tumors did have decreased mitotic activity, a known prognostic parameter. The differences may be due to the rarity of these tumors and overall indolent behavior requiring extensive long-term follow-up. Additional validation studies are needed.[31,32]

Some studies have even shown that fusion variants and types can also influence response to therapy. Extraskeletal myxoid chondrosarcoma characteristically harbor rearrangements involving *NR4A3* with various gene partners and with *NR4A3-EWSR1* being the most common fusion variant. One study found that tumors that lack *NR4A3-EWSR1* were more often rhabdoid and of higher grade morphology.[33] However, tumors that have *EWSR1-NR4A3* respond better to sunitinib than tumors harboring other variants.[34] Another example is myxoid liposarcoma, which can have multiple breakpoint points between *FUS* and *CHOP/DDIT3*, resulting in multiple fusion types. Preliminary studies suggest that myxoid liposarcomas with a *FUS* ex 7 - *DDIT3* ex 2 may respond better to trabectedin than those tumors with *FUS* ex 13-*DDIT3* ex 2 fusion variant, although fusion variants have not overall been found to be prognostic by themselves.[35,36]

Interestingly, unclassified sarcomas have recently been found to rarely harbor an actionable fusion involving various genes *NTRK1*, *NTRK2*, and *NTRK3*, which encodes for a family of proteins known as tropomyosin receptor kinase (TRK). Recurrent rearrangements involving *NTRK* have been known to occur in some mesenchymal tumors, including infantile fibrosarcoma and lipofibromatosis-like neural tumor.[37–39] These fusions have also been identified in various tumors, including carcinomas, unclassified sarcomas and wild-type gastrointestinal stromal tumors, where *NTRK* rearrangement results in protein overexpression (**Fig. 1**), and makes affected tumors amendable to therapy with TRK inhibitors, with preliminary evidence of dramatic initial responses.[40,41] These examples highlights that fusions not only play a role in development of sarcomas but some can also influence their appearance, biological behavior, and response to therapies.

> ### Key Features
> OF SARCOMA GENE REARRANGEMENTS
>
> - Fusion variant refers to the presence of alternate gene fusion partners which may be identified in a sarcoma type (eg, *EWSR1-FLI1* or *FUS-FLI1* in Ewing sarcoma)
> - Fusion type refers to the involvement of different exons in fusions of the same genes identified in a sarcoma type (eg, *NAB* exon 4 – *STAT6* exon 2, or *NAB* exon 6 – *STAT6* exon 16 in solitary fibrous tumor)
> - Both gene fusion type and fusion variant may have differential effects on sarcoma histomorphology, behavior, or response to treatment

ROLE OF GENE MUTATIONS

Similar to translocations, recurrent gene mutations are important to both the development and behavior of certain mesenchymal tumors. One example is desmoid-type fibromatosis. The vast majority of sporadic desmoid-type fibromatoses harbor hot spot point mutations in exon 3 *CTNNB1* mutation in 2 codons. These codons predominantly harbor 3 mutation types: T41A (most common), S45F, and S45P. This finding can be useful to confirming the diagnosis in challenging cases (ie, or on small biopsies). In addition, studies now indicate that the behavior of desmoid-type fibromatosis is heterogeneous, with some tumors less locally aggressive than others, and that *CTNNB1* mutation type (S45F) may be associated with more local aggressive course.[42,43] In addition, the absence of a detectable *CTNNB1* mutation in desmoid-type fibromatosis, particularly in young patients, may indicate the tumor is *APC* related, heralding important genetic and familial screening.[44]

Gene mutations can also help to determine whether tumors will respond to therapy. A classic example is the association of *KIT* and *PDGFRA* mutations in gastrointestinal stromal tumors and their response to tyrosine kinase inhibitors. Certain mutations such as those involving *KIT* exon 9 require a high dosage, whereas some mutations such as *PDGFRA* exon 18 D842V are predominantly naïve resistant.[45,46]

Aside from recurrent mutations and translocations, it is important to recognize that multiple pathways are often involved and needed for sarcomagenesis. These pathways include losses of tumor suppressor genes (*TP53*, *RB*, *STAT3*, and *PTEN*) and altered cell signaling pathways, notably PI3K/AKT/mammalian target of rapamycin pathways, some of which have been shown to be prognostic and a potential therapeutic targets in both sarcomas with complex karyotypes and in sarcomas with relatively quiescent karyotypes with translocations.[36,47–51]

GENE EXPRESSION AND DNA METHYLATION PROFILING

Given the complexity of involved pathways in sarcomas,[51] studies have begun to examine the usefulness of using multiple genes to more accurately predict behavior beyond histologic parameters of grading or single recurrent aberration. One example is complexity index in sarcoma (CINSARC), which is a signature of 67 genes involved in mitoses and chromosome management and which was found to predict metastatic outcome better than FNCLCC grading.[52] This signature was subsequently validated with a larger dataset with similar results.[53] Another promising gene signature is genomic grade index (GGI), which uses 108 genes originally derived to predict aggressive behavior in breast cancer and also found applicable to soft tissue sarcomas. The GGI was found to be more predictive of metastases than grading and complementary to CINSARC in sarcomas.[54] With increasing availability of this technology, it may be soon feasible for pathologists to use gene expression profiling to provide additional insights to tumor behavior.

The role of DNA methylation profiling has also been explored in sarcomas for both classification and prognostication. Recently, array-based DNA methylation analysis was found to correctly reclassify undifferentiated round cell sarcomas to other tumors including *CIC* or *BCOR* translocated sarcomas, synovial sarcoma, malignant rhabdoid tumor, and Ewing sarcoma, which was missed by initial molecular testing.[55] Studies have also shown DNA methylation analysis to be useful in discriminating benign and malignant nerve sheath tumors.[56] Finally, differing DNA methylation profiles have been reported in metastasizing versus nonmetastasizing rhabdomyosarcomas, as well as in soft tissue leiomyosarcomas and dedifferentiated liposarcomas with more aggressive behavior, suggesting methylation profiling to be a promising prognostic tool in some sarcomas.[51,57]

Key Features
OF GENE EXPRESSION AND
METHYLATION PROFILING IN SARCOMA

- CINSARC is a 67-gene expression signature that predicts metastatic risk.

- The GGI is a 108-gene expression signature derived to predict aggressive behavior in breast carcinoma, and found applicable to sarcoma.

- DNA methylation array-based analyses can be used to classify undifferentiated round cell sarcomas and peripheral nerve sheath tumors, and may have prognostic value in rhabdomyosarcoma, leiomyosarcomas and dedifferentiated liposarcomas.

Key Features
OF TELOMERE MAINTENANCE
IN SARCOMA

- *TERT* promoter mutations have been reported in atypical fibroxanthoma, pleomorphic dermal sarcoma, myxoid liposarcoma, and solitary fibrous tumor, and may have prognostic significance.

- Alternative lengthening of telomeres is more common in pleomorphic sarcomas with complex karyotypes.

- Loss of ATRX or DAXX correlates with presence of alternative lengthening of telomeres and may be an adverse prognostic feature.

DEFECTS IN TELOMERE MAINTENANCE MECHANISMS

Defects resulting in telomere maintenance have been recognized to be important for promoting cellular survival in many tumors, including in sarcomas. Telomeres are repetitive DNA sequences at chromosomal ends, which can prevent apoptosis and senescence, and tumors use a variety of mechanisms to stabilize them. One of the most common ways is through mutations in the *TERT* promoter region, resulting in constitutive telomerase activation.[58] This predominantly takes the form of 2 recurrent hot spot mutations (C228T and C250T). Aside from epithelial tumors, various sarcomas, including atypical fibroxanthomas/pleomorphic dermal sarcomas, myxoid liposarcomas, and a subset of solitary fibrous tumors, also have been reported to have *TERT* promoter mutations, with some reporting the presence of *TERT* promoter mutations to be prognostic of more aggressive disease.[59–62] Other tumors use a recombination-mediated mechanism known as alternative lengthening of telomeres to avoid telomere shortening[63–68]; this method is more common in sarcomas with complex karyotypes like undifferentiated pleomorphic sarcomas and angiosarcoma. Some studies also show an association (sometimes heterogeneous) between loss of *ATRX* (α-thalassemia/mental retardation X-linked; see **Fig. 1**) and/or *DAXX* (death domain-associated) in these tumors and the formation of alternative lengthening of telomeres[64,69]; loss of these factors can also be an indicator of poor prognosis.

SARCOMA IMMUNE MICROENVIRONMENT

Immunotherapy with immune checkpoint inhibitors, such as PD-1 inhibitors, has become an important oncological treatment modality. Emerging evidence suggests that patients with some types of sarcomas may not only benefit from immunotherapy,[70] but that immune infiltrates including CD3$^+$, CD8$^+$ T cells and CD163/CD68$^+$ macrophages can be prognostic for overall survival in some sarcomas in varying degrees.[51,71] Similar to other tumors types, studies have found PD-1/PD-L1 expression to play a possible role in regulating immune surveillance in some sarcomas and therefore amendable to PD-1 inhibitor. Despite an increase in immune infiltrate in these tumors, PD-L1 expression was found to be poor prognostic factor, indicating that these tumors use negative immune modulator escape mechanisms to persist.[72,73] One reason why certain sarcomas, particularly those with complex karyotypes, are immunogenic is that they can express neoantigens similar to other tumors. These include cancer testes antigens, preferential expressed antigen in melanoma (PRAME), melanoma-associated antigen gene A4 (MAGEA4), and NY-ESO-1/CTAG1, which can be aberrantly overexpressed.[74–77] These neoantigens can also be used as targets to develop cytotoxic T-cell–mediated immune response. PRAME expression was found to negatively correlate with antigen presentation genes in one study, which suggests that some sarcomas have also developed immune surveillance escape mechanisms to compensate for neoantigen expression.[75]

Finally, solid tumors with microsatellite instability have recently been reported to have increased likelihood of response to PD-1 immunotherapy. Loss of microsatellite instability, assessed by loss of mismatch repair proteins (MLH1, MSH2, PMS6, PMS2), by polymerase chain reaction detection or next-generation sequencing detection are theorized to have more complex karyotypes, which potentially makes them more likely to express neoantigens and immunogenic. Microsatellite instability can rarely be seen in sarcomas as a part of the Muir-Torre syndrome and, therefore, its absence may have genetic implications. However, it can also rarely occur in sporadic sarcomas.[78] Whether or not, microsatellite instability in sporadic sarcomas correlates to better response to immunotherapy and prognosis remains to be determined.[79,80]

It is important to recognize that much of the interpretation of immune infiltrates, and even interpretation of PD-L1 (membranous tumoral labeling of >1%; see **Fig. 1**) have been derived from clinical trials in epithelial tumors. There remains uncertainty if results from clinical trials on epithelial tumors can be directly extrapolated to a diverse group of tumors such as sarcomas, and the relationship will likely vary by sarcoma subtype. Similar to gene expression, sarcomas likely use several pathways of immune surveillance and escape, and therefore most likely require assessment of multiple targets rather than a single target to predict response and prognosis.

SUMMARY

With a better understanding and appreciation of the diverse and complex biology of sarcomas and their immune environment, new markers for prognostication and treatment are emerging, although so far, no single marker can accurately predict behavior. Proper classification, subtyping, and grading remains important for prognosis. Increase availability of technologies that can examine multiple pathways or the use of multivariate models such as nomograms can help pathologists to more accurately prognosticate these tumors for clinicians and patients.

REFERENCES

1. AJCC cancer staging manual. New York: Springer Science+Business Media; 2016, pages cm.
2. Guillou L, Coindre JM, Bonichon F, et al. Comparative study of the National Cancer Institute and French Federation of Cancer Centers Sarcoma Group grading systems in a population of 410 adult patients with soft tissue sarcoma. J Clin Oncol 1997;15(1):350–62.
3. Coindre JM. Grading of soft tissue sarcomas: review and update. Arch Pathol Lab Med 2006;130(10):1448–53.
4. Deyrup AT, Weiss SW. Grading of soft tissue sarcomas: the challenge of providing precise information in an imprecise world. Histopathology 2006;48(1):42–50.
5. Demetri GD, von Mehren M, Antonescu CR, et al. NCCN Task Force report: update on the management of patients with gastrointestinal stromal tumors. J Natl Compr Canc Netw 2010;8(Suppl 2):S1–41, [quiz: S42–4].
6. Demicco EG, Wagner MJ, Maki RG, et al. Risk assessment in solitary fibrous tumors: validation and refinement of a risk stratification model. Mod Pathol 2017;30(10):1433–42.
7. Belfiori G, Sartelli M, Cardinali L, et al. Risk stratification systems for surgically treated localized primary Gastrointestinal Stromal Tumors (GIST). Review of literature and comparison of the three prognostic criteria: MSKCC Nomogramm, NIH-Fletcher and AFIP-Miettinen. Ann Ital Chir 2015;86(3):219–27.
8. Tan MC, Brennan MF, Kuk D, et al. Histology-based classification predicts pattern of recurrence and improves risk stratification in primary retroperitoneal sarcoma. Ann Surg 2016;263(3):593–600.
9. Chou YS, Liu CY, Chang YH, et al. Prognostic factors of primary resected retroperitoneal soft tissue sarcoma: analysis from a single Asian tertiary center and external validation of Gronchi's nomogram. J Surg Oncol 2016;113(4):355–60.
10. Li WS, Liao IC, Wen MC, et al. BCOR-CCNB3-positive soft tissue sarcoma with round-cell and spindle-cell histology: a series of four cases highlighting the pitfall of mimicking poorly differentiated synovial sarcoma. Histopathology 2016;69(5):792–801.
11. Ludwig K, Alaggio R, Zin A, et al. BCOR-CCNB3 undifferentiated sarcoma-does immunohistochemistry help in the identification? Pediatr Dev Pathol 2017;20(4):321–9.
12. Yoshida A, Goto K, Kodaira M, et al. CIC-rearranged sarcomas: a study of 20 cases and comparisons with Ewing sarcomas. Am J Surg Pathol 2016;40(3):313–23.
13. Ladanyi M, Antonescu CR, Leung DH, et al. Impact of SYT-SSX fusion type on the clinical behavior of synovial sarcoma: a multi-institutional retrospective study of 243 patients. Cancer Res 2002;62(1):135–40.
14. Guillou L, Benhattar J, Bonichon F, et al. Histologic grade, but not SYT-SSX fusion type, is an important prognostic factor in patients with synovial sarcoma: a multicenter, retrospective analysis. J Clin Oncol 2004;22(20):4040–50.
15. Antonescu CR, Zhang L, Shao SY, et al. Frequent PLAG1 gene rearrangements in skin and soft tissue myoepithelioma with ductal differentiation. Genes Chromosomes Cancer 2013;52(7):675–82.
16. Brandal P, Panagopoulos I, Bjerkehagen B, et al. Detection of a t(1;22)(q23;q12) translocation leading

to an EWSR1-PBX1 fusion gene in a myoepithelioma. Genes Chromosomes Cancer 2008;47(7): 558–64.

17. Brandal P, Panagopoulos I, Bjerkehagen B, et al. t(19;22)(q13;q12) Translocation leading to the novel fusion gene EWSR1-ZNF444 in soft tissue myoepithelial carcinoma. Genes Chromosomes Cancer 2009;48(12):1051–6.

18. Antonescu CR, Zhang L, Chang NE, et al. EWSR1-POU5F1 fusion in soft tissue myoepithelial tumors. A molecular analysis of sixty-six cases, including soft tissue, bone, and visceral lesions, showing common involvement of the EWSR1 gene. Genes Chromosomes Cancer 2010;49(12):1114–24.

19. Flucke U, Palmedo G, Blankenhorn N, et al. EWSR1 gene rearrangement occurs in a subset of cutaneous myoepithelial tumors: a study of 18 cases. Mod Pathol 2011;24(11):1444–50.

20. Matsuyama A, Hisaoka M, Hashimoto H. PLAG1 expression in mesenchymal tumors: an immunohistochemical study with special emphasis on the pathogenetical distinction between soft tissue myoepithelioma and pleomorphic adenoma of the salivary gland. Pathol Int 2012;62(1):1–7.

21. Agaram NP, Chen HW, Zhang L, et al. EWSR1-PBX3: a novel gene fusion in myoepithelial tumors. Genes Chromosomes Cancer 2015;54(2):63–71.

22. Huang SC, Chen HW, Zhang L, et al. Novel FUS-KLF17 and EWSR1-KLF17 fusions in myoepithelial tumors. Genes Chromosomes Cancer 2015;54(5): 267–75.

23. Jo VY, Fletcher CD. Myoepithelial neoplasms of soft tissue: an updated review of the clinicopathologic, immunophenotypic, and genetic features. Head Neck Pathol 2015;9(1):32–8.

24. Verma A, Rekhi B. Myoepithelial tumor of soft tissue and bone: a current perspective. Histol Histopathol 2017;32(9):861–77.

25. Marino-Enriquez A, Wang WL, Roy A, et al. Epithelioid inflammatory myofibroblastic sarcoma: an aggressive intra-abdominal variant of inflammatory myofibroblastic tumor with nuclear membrane or perinuclear ALK. Am J Surg Pathol 2011;35(1): 135–44.

26. Lovly CM, Gupta A, Lipson D, et al. Inflammatory myofibroblastic tumors harbor multiple potentially actionable kinase fusions. Cancer Discov 2014; 4(8):889–95.

27. Lee JC, Li CF, Huang HY, et al. ALK oncoproteins in atypical inflammatory myofibroblastic tumours: novel RRBP1-ALK fusions in epithelioid inflammatory myofibroblastic sarcoma. J Pathol 2017;241(3): 316–23.

28. Harms D. Alveolar rhabdomyosarcoma: a prognostically unfavorable rhabdomyosarcoma type and its necessary distinction from embryonal rhabdomyosarcoma. Curr Top Pathol 1995;89:273–96.

29. Raney RB, Anderson JR, Barr FG, et al. Rhabdomyosarcoma and undifferentiated sarcoma in the first two decades of life: a selective review of intergroup rhabdomyosarcoma study group experience and rationale for Intergroup Rhabdomyosarcoma Study V. J Pediatr Hematol Oncol 2001;23(4): 215–20.

30. Williamson D, Missiaglia E, de Reyniès A, et al. Fusion gene-negative alveolar rhabdomyosarcoma is clinically and molecularly indistinguishable from embryonal rhabdomyosarcoma. J Clin Oncol 2010; 28(13):2151–8.

31. Tai HC, Chuang IC, Chen TC, et al. NAB2-STAT6 fusion types account for clinicopathological variations in solitary fibrous tumors. Mod Pathol 2015; 28(10):1324–35.

32. Barthelmess S, Geddert H, Boltze C, et al. Solitary fibrous tumors/hemangiopericytomas with different variants of the NAB2-STAT6 gene fusion are characterized by specific histomorphology and distinct clinicopathological features. Am J Pathol 2014; 184(4):1209–18.

33. Agaram NP, Zhang L, Sung YS, et al. Extraskeletal myxoid chondrosarcoma with non-EWSR1-NR4A3 variant fusions correlate with rhabdoid phenotype and high-grade morphology. Hum Pathol 2014; 45(5):1084–91.

34. Stacchiotti S, Pantaleo MA, Astolfi A, et al. Activity of sunitinib in extraskeletal myxoid chondrosarcoma. Eur J Cancer 2014;50(9):1657–64.

35. Forni C, Minuzzo M, Virdis E, et al. Trabectedin (ET-743) promotes differentiation in myxoid liposarcoma tumors. Mol Cancer Ther 2009;8(2):449–57.

36. Antonescu CR, Tschernyavsky SJ, Decuseara R, et al. Prognostic impact of P53 status, TLS-CHOP fusion transcript structure, and histological grade in myxoid liposarcoma: a molecular and clinicopathologic study of 82 cases. Clin Cancer Res 2001; 7(12):3977–87.

37. Hung YP, Fletcher CDM, Hornick JL. Evaluation of pan-TRK immunohistochemistry in infantile fibrosarcoma, lipofibromatosis-like neural tumour and histological mimics. Histopathology 2018;73(4):634–44.

38. Nagasubramanian R, Wei J, Gordon P, et al. Infantile fibrosarcoma with NTRK3-ETV6 fusion successfully treated with the tropomyosin-related kinase inhibitor LOXO-101. Pediatr Blood Cancer 2016;63(8): 1468–70.

39. Agaram NP, Zhang L, Sung YS, et al. Recurrent NTRK1 gene fusions define a novel subset of locally aggressive lipofibromatosis-like neural tumors. Am J Surg Pathol 2016;40(10):1407–16.

40. Haller F, Knopf J, Ackermann A, et al. Paediatric and adult soft tissue sarcomas with NTRK1 gene fusions: a subset of spindle cell sarcomas unified by a prominent myopericytic/haemangiopericytic pattern. J Pathol 2016;238(5):700–10.

41. Shi E, Chmielecki J, Tang CM, et al. FGFR1 and NTRK3 actionable alterations in "Wild-Type" gastrointestinal stromal tumors. J Transl Med 2016;14(1):339.

42. Colombo C, Miceli R, Lazar AJ, et al. CTNNB1 45F mutation is a molecular prognosticator of increased postoperative primary desmoid tumor recurrence: an independent, multicenter validation study. Cancer 2013;119(20):3696–702.

43. Lazar AJ, Tuvin D, Hajibashi S, et al. Specific mutations in the beta-catenin gene (CTNNB1) correlate with local recurrence in sporadic desmoid tumors. Am J Pathol 2008;173(5):1518–27.

44. Wang WL, Nero C, Pappo A, et al. CTNNB1 genotyping and APC screening in pediatric desmoid tumors: a proposed algorithm. Pediatr Dev Pathol 2012;15(5):361–7.

45. Wang WL, Conley A, Reynoso D, et al. Mechanisms of resistance to imatinib and sunitinib in gastrointestinal stromal tumor. Cancer Chemother Pharmacol 2011;67(Suppl 1):S15–24.

46. Lasota J, Miettinen M. Clinical significance of oncogenic KIT and PDGFRA mutations in gastrointestinal stromal tumours. Histopathology 2008;53(3):245–66.

47. Lahat G, Tuvin D, Wei C, et al. Molecular prognosticators of complex karyotype soft tissue sarcoma outcome: a tissue microarray-based study. Ann Oncol 2010;21(5):1112–20.

48. Lahat G, Zhang P, Zhu QS, et al. The expression of c-Met pathway components in unclassified pleomorphic sarcoma/malignant fibrous histiocytoma (UPS/MFH): a tissue microarray study. Histopathology 2011;59(3):556–61.

49. Hoffman A, Ghadimi MP, Demicco EG, et al. Localized and metastatic myxoid/round cell liposarcoma: clinical and molecular observations. Cancer 2013;119(10):1868–77.

50. Panse G, Leung CH, Ingram DR, et al. The role of phosphorylated signal transducer and activator of transcription 3 (pSTAT3) in peripheral nerve sheath tumours. Histopathology 2017;70(6):946–53.

51. Cancer Genome Atlas Research Network. Comprehensive and Integrated genomic characterization of adult soft tissue sarcomas. Cell 2017;171(4):950–65.e28.

52. Chibon F, Lagarde P, Salas S, et al. Validated prediction of clinical outcome in sarcomas and multiple types of cancer on the basis of a gene expression signature related to genome complexity. Nat Med 2010;16(7):781–7.

53. Lesluyes T, Delespaul L, Coindre JM, et al. The CINSARC signature as a prognostic marker for clinical outcome in multiple neoplasms. Sci Rep 2017;7(1):5480.

54. Bertucci F, De Nonneville A, Finetti P, et al. The Genomic Grade Index predicts postoperative clinical outcome in patients with soft-tissue sarcoma. Ann Oncol 2018;29(2):459–65.

55. Koelsche C, Hartmann W, Schrimpf D, et al. Array-based DNA-methylation profiling in sarcomas with small blue round cell histology provides valuable diagnostic information. Mod Pathol 2018;31(8):1246–56.

56. Rohrich M, Koelsche C, Schrimpf D, et al. Methylation-based classification of benign and malignant peripheral nerve sheath tumors. Acta Neuropathol 2016;131(6):877–87.

57. Tombolan L, Poli E, Martini P, et al. Global DNA methylation profiling uncovers distinct methylation patterns of protocadherin alpha4 in metastatic and non-metastatic rhabdomyosarcoma. BMC Cancer 2016;16(1):886.

58. Huang FW, Hodis E, Xu MJ, et al. Highly recurrent TERT promoter mutations in human melanoma. Science 2013;339(6122):957–9.

59. Koelsche C, Renner M, Hartmann W, et al. TERT promoter hotspot mutations are recurrent in myxoid liposarcomas but rare in other soft tissue sarcoma entities. J Exp Clin Cancer Res 2014;33:33.

60. Griewank KG, Schilling B, Murali R, et al. TERT promoter mutations are frequent in atypical fibroxanthomas and pleomorphic dermal sarcomas. Mod Pathol 2014;27(4):502–8.

61. Bahrami A, Lee S, Schaefer IM, et al. TERT promoter mutations and prognosis in solitary fibrous tumor. Mod Pathol 2016;29(12):1511–22.

62. Demicco EG, Wani K, Ingram D, et al. TERT promoter mutations in solitary fibrous tumor. Histopathology 2018;73(5):843–51.

63. Heaphy CM, Subhawong AP, Hong SM, et al. Prevalence of the alternative lengthening of telomeres telomere maintenance mechanism in human cancer subtypes. Am J Pathol 2011;179(4):1608–15.

64. Heaphy CM, de Wilde RF, Jiao Y, et al. Altered telomeres in tumors with ATRX and DAXX mutations. Science 2011;333(6041):425.

65. de Wilde RF, Heaphy CM, Maitra A, et al. Loss of ATRX or DAXX expression and concomitant acquisition of the alternative lengthening of telomeres phenotype are late events in a small subset of MEN-1 syndrome pancreatic neuroendocrine tumors. Mod Pathol 2012;25(7):1033–9.

66. Henson JD, Reddel RR. Assaying and investigating Alternative Lengthening of Telomeres activity in human cells and cancers. FEBS Lett 2010;584(17):3800–11.

67. Cesare AJ, Reddel RR. Alternative lengthening of telomeres: models, mechanisms and implications. Nat Rev Genet 2010;11(5):319–30.

68. Panse G, Chrisinger JS, Leung CH, et al. Clinicopathological analysis of ATRX, DAXX and NOTCH receptor expression in angiosarcomas. Histopathology 2018;72(2):239–47.

69. Schwartzentruber J, Korshunov A, Liu XY, et al. Driver mutations in histone H3.3 and chromatin remodelling genes in paediatric glioblastoma. Nature 2012;482(7384):226–31.

70. Topalian SL, Hodi FS, Brahmer JR, et al. Safety, activity, and immune correlates of anti-PD-1 antibody in cancer. N Engl J Med 2012;366(26):2443–54.

71. Gooden MJ, de Bock GH, Leffers N, et al. The prognostic influence of tumour-infiltrating lymphocytes in cancer: a systematic review with meta-analysis. Br J Cancer 2011;105(1):93–103.

72. Guan J, Lim KS, Mekhail T, et al. Programmed death ligand-1 (PD-L1) expression in the programmed death receptor-1 (PD-1)/PD-L1 blockade: a key player against various cancers. Arch Pathol Lab Med 2017;141(6):851–61.

73. Bertucci F, Finetti P, Perrot D, et al. PDL1 expression is a poor-prognosis factor in soft-tissue sarcomas. Oncoimmunology 2017;6(3):e1278100.

74. Ikeda H, Lethé B, Lehmann F, et al. Characterization of an antigen that is recognized on a melanoma showing partial HLA loss by CTL expressing an NK inhibitory receptor. Immunity 1997;6(2):199–208.

75. Roszik J, Wang WL, Livingston JA, et al. Overexpressed PRAME is a potential immunotherapy target in sarcoma subtypes. Clin Sarcoma Res 2017;7:11.

76. Endo M, de Graaff MA, Ingram DR, et al. NY-ESO-1 (CTAG1B) expression in mesenchymal tumors. Mod Pathol 2015;28(4):587–95.

77. Iura K, Kohashi K, Ishii T, et al. MAGEA4 expression in bone and soft tissue tumors: its utility as a target for immunotherapy and diagnostic marker combined with NY-ESO-1. Virchows Arch 2017;471(3):383–92.

78. Lee N, Luthra R, Lopez-Terrada D, et al. Retroperitoneal undifferentiated pleomorphic sarcoma having microsatellite instability associated with Muir-Torre syndrome: case report and review of literature. J Cutan Pathol 2013;40(8):730–3.

79. Davis JL, Grenert JP, Horvai AE. Loss of heterozygosity and microsatellite instability are rare in sporadic dedifferentiated liposarcoma: a study of 43 well-characterized cases. Arch Pathol Lab Med 2014;138(6):823–7.

80. Urso E, Agostini M, Pucciarelli S, et al. Soft tissue sarcoma and the hereditary non-polyposis colorectal cancer (HNPCC) syndrome: formulation of an hypothesis. Mol Biol Rep 2012;39(10):9307–10.

Practical Application of Cytology and Core Biopsy in the Diagnosis of Mesenchymal Tumors

David J. Papke Jr, MD, PhD, Vickie Y. Jo, MD*

KEYWORDS

- Sarcoma • Soft tissue • Core biopsy • Cytology • Fine-needle aspiration

---

Key points

- Minimally invasive biopsy methods of fine-needle aspiration and core biopsy are increasingly used in the diagnosis of soft tissue tumors and are useful in triaging benign and malignant lesions.

- A pattern-based approach in the evaluation of small biopsy specimens is helpful in guiding the formulation of differential diagnoses and application of relevant ancillary testing.

- Detection of tumor-specific immunophenotypes and molecular alterations enables definitive diagnosis for many soft tissue neoplasms in cytologic specimens and core biopsies.

- Diagnostic limitations of small biopsy specimens include overlapping morphologic, immunohistochemical, and molecular features between entities, and judicious interpretation and integration of clinical data are necessary.

- The central goal in small biopsy specimens is to convey biologic behavior to ensure appropriate clinical management, even when definitive classification is not possible.

ABSTRACT

Soft tissue neoplasms are increasingly being sampled by core needle biopsy and fine-needle aspiration (FNA), and these small biopsy specimens pose unique diagnostic challenges. Many advances in ancillary testing enable detection of characteristic immunophenotypes and molecular alterations, allowing accurate classification of soft tissue tumors in these small biopsy samples. This review outlines pattern-based diagnostic approaches to core biopsies and FNAs of soft tissue neoplasms, including formulation of practical differential diagnoses and relevant application of ancillary tests.

OVERVIEW

Minimally invasive biopsy approaches are gaining widespread use, and soft tissue neoplasms are increasingly being sampled by core needle biopsy and fine-needle aspiration (FNA). Although small biopsies pose unique diagnostic challenges, advances in ancillary studies have greatly expanded diagnostic abilities. Core biopsy and FNA are effective in triaging benign and malignant soft tissue neoplasms, which is central to ensuring appropriate clinical management. In many practice centers, core biopsy and FNA are performed concurrently, and FNA has the benefit of allowing rapid on-site evaluation for adequacy, guidance

---

Disclosures: The authors have no relevant disclosures.
Department of Pathology, Brigham and Women's Hospital and Harvard Medical School, 75 Francis Street, Boston, MA 02115, USA
* Corresponding author.
E-mail address: vjo@partners.org

Surgical Pathology 12 (2019) 227–248
https://doi.org/10.1016/j.path.2018.11.002

of core biopsy, and specimen triage (including cell block preparation) for ancillary studies. The detection of specific immunophenotypes and molecular features enables definitive classification of numerous tumor types. This article outlines a pattern-based approach to core biopsies and FNAs of soft tissue tumors, organized broadly into adipocytic, myxoid, spindle cell, epithelioid, round cell, and pleomorphic categories. This discussion is not intended to be comprehensive and focuses on the more commonly encountered soft tissue neoplasms in routine practice, with an emphasis on application of immunohistochemical and molecular tests. Because detailed morphologic and clinical descriptions of many of the entities are provided in other articles of this issue, this discussion focuses on the specific challenges and limitations of small biopsy specimens rather than an overview of typical morphology.

ADIPOCYTIC TUMORS

Although most liposarcoma subtypes have specific cytomorphologic features, adipocytic tumors with well-differentiated fatty components can be diagnostically challenging in core biopsy and cytology specimens. Correlation with clinical history and imaging is important in guiding the differential diagnosis, and discriminating benign tumors from atypical lipomatous tumor/well-differentiated liposarcoma (ALT/WDL).

The diagnosis of benign adipocytic tumors is typically straightforward, especially for superficially located tumors, although it may not be possible to distinguish lipoma subtypes or hibernoma from each other. Smears show discrete lobules of uniformly sized, univacuolated adipocytes with small bland nuclei. ALT/WDL may resemble lipoma in small biopsies when adipocyte size variation and atypical nuclei are not apparent or are sparsely represented (**Figs. 1A, B**). Lipoblasts are not necessary for diagnosis and are actually an infrequent finding.[1] Because biopsies of ALT/WDL may appear deceptively bland, immunohistochemistry for MDM2/CDK4 (positive in 87% and 81% of ALT/WDL, respectively[2,3] [see **Fig. 1C**]) should be performed for any adipocytic tumor greater than 10 cm or arising in a deep-seated or visceral location, because ALT/WDL is more likely in these scenarios. Fat necrosis is common diagnostic pitfall to be aware of in body sites prone to trauma, because it can appear hypercellular and mimic ALT/WDL.[4] Moreover, histiocytes often express MDM2[5]; nevertheless, fat necrosis can be distinguished from true atypia by the presence of foamy histiocytes and multinucleated giant cells. If ALT/WDL is favored, but immunohistochemistry is equivocal or negative, molecular testing (such as fluorescence in situ hybridization [FISH]) should be performed to identify the characteristic amplification of the 12q14-15 region encoding the *MDM2* and *CDK4* genes (see **Fig. 1D**).

On smears, spindle cell/pleomorphic lipomas show fragments of myxoid stroma admixed with mature fat, bland spindle cells, and long collagen strands.[6] Spindle cell lipoma shows CD34 positivity, occasional S100 staining, and loss of expression of retinoblastoma (Rb).[7] Some cases have multinucleated floret-like cells (previously called pleomorphic lipoma) prompting concern for ALT/WDL. Spindle cell lipoma shares morphologic and molecular features with mammary-type myofibroblastoma (MTMF) and cellular angiofibroma. The lack of atypia distinguishes spindle cell lipoma from ALT/WDL and the recently described entity, atypical spindle cell lipomatous tumor (ASCLT).

Key Points
Diagnosis of ALT/WDL in Small Biopsies

- Most cases show variation in adipocytic size and atypical stromal cells, but these findings are often subtle in cytologic smears.

- ALT/WDL should be the first consideration for any retroperitoneal or deep-seated fatty tumor, even if the biopsy is composed of mature adipose tissue with minimal or no atypia.

- MDM2 and CDK4 immunohistochemistry is positive in most cases of ALT/WDL and negative in benign lipoma and ASCLT.

- *MDM2* FISH is more sensitive than MDM2/CDK4 immunohistochemistry and should be considered when immunohistochemical results are equivocal or negative and the diagnosis of ALT/WDL is favored.

- Caution is necessary in interpretation of adipocytic lesions with fat necrosis, because histiocytes may show nuclear MDM2 staining.

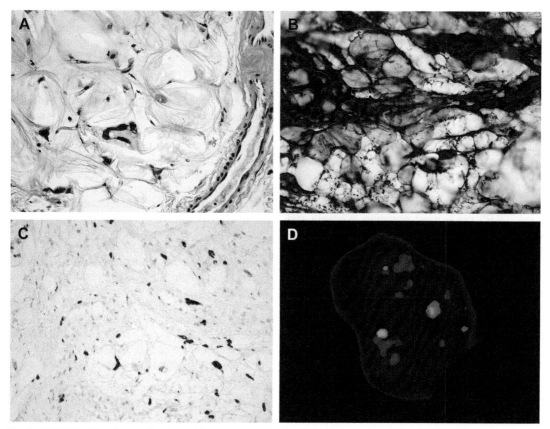

Fig. 1. ALT/WDL. The diagnostic atypical hyperchromatic stromal cells are present in most core biopsies (*A*). Aspirate smears yield large fragments of variably sized adipocytes, a subtle feature that may be overlooked ([*B*] alcohol-fixed, Papanicolaou stain). *MDM2* amplification correlates with nuclear immunoreactivity for MDM2 (*C*) and can be detected by FISH (*D*).

ASCLTs have a broad morphologic and immunophenotypic spectrum which overlaps with spindle cell lipoma and MTMF, with variable expression of CD34 (60%), S100 (40%), and desmin (23%) and loss of Rb expression in 50%. Although nuclear atypia and infiltrative growth are the most helpful morphologic features to discriminate ASCLT from spindle cell lipoma and MTMF, these may not be appreciated in small biopsies. Diffuse desmin positivity favors MTMF,[8] whereas ASCLT is negative for MDM2 and CDK4, thus excluding ALT/WDL.

Dedifferentiated liposarcoma (DDLPS) exhibits a wide range of morphologies and includes cases that mimic other sarcoma types, such as myxofibrosarcoma (MFS), pleomorphic liposarcoma, and myxoid liposarcoma (MLPS).[9,10] Diagnostic areas of residual ALT/WDL are often absent in small biopsies or aspirates. Thus it is important to consider DDLPS in the differential diagnosis of pleomorphic, adipocytic, and spindle cell sarcomas. Testing for *MDM2* amplification should be routinely performed for any retroperitoneal

sarcoma regardless of morphologic appearance. Immunohistochemistry for MDM2 and CDK4 has high diagnostic utility for DDLPS in cytologic samples and small biopsies, with overexpression in approximately 95% and 80%, respectively, of FNAs.[10] Molecular testing should be performed when MDM2/CDK4 immunohistochemistry results are equivocal or negative in cases of suspected DDLPS.

Pleomorphic liposarcoma is a high-grade pleomorphic sarcoma with large, atypical lipoblasts scattered singly or in sheets. Eosinophilic cytoplasmic droplets are a common feature. It is the only type of liposarcoma that requires lipoblasts for diagnosis. Lipoblasts may be only focally present, however, even in resections and are often infrequent in FNA specimens.[11] Pleomorphic liposarcoma can closely resemble DDLPS, undifferentiated pleomorphic sarcoma (UPS), and MFS, whereas the epithelioid variant can mimic carcinoma or melanoma, and 40% show multifocal keratin expression.[12] If diagnostic lipoblasts are not present on biopsy and DDLPS is excluded, then a descriptive diagnosis of high-grade pleomorphic sarcoma is appropriate.

MLPS is characterized by abundant myxoid stroma (sometimes appearing microcystic), delicate branching capillaries, uniform ovoid-to-spindle cells with mild nuclear atypia, and lipoblasts. In smears, myxoid stromal fragments contain delicate branching vessels, tumor cells, and small univacuolated or bivacuolated lipoblasts.[13] Increased cellularity occurs with histologic grade, and high-grade tumors can present as a round cell sarcoma. Although MLPS lacks a specific immunophenotype, *FUS–DDIT3* and *EWSR1–DDIT3* fusions are diagnostic.[14] Lipoblastoma may mimic MLPS but is most common in infants and young children, lacks cytologic atypia, and is positive for PLAG1 secondary to *PLAG1* alterations.[15]

MYXOID TUMORS

Tumors with extensive myxoid stroma encompass a broad spectrum of entities and incorporate challenging differential diagnoses, including several adipocytic tumors discussed previously (**Table 1**). The main goal of small biopsy specimens is to reliably distinguish benign myxoid neoplasms from sarcomas, which is usually straightforward if pleomorphism, high mitotic activity, and necrosis are present. Some sarcomas, however, may appear deceptively bland or uniform, especially in cytologic smears.

Intramuscular myxoma, soft tissue perineurioma, and low-grade fibromyxoid sarcoma (LGFMS), are hypocellular, bland spindle cell tumors with significant cytomorphologic overlap, variable CD34 positivity and epithelial membrane antigen (EMA) positivity, and a predilection for the extremities.[16] Aspirates of both intramuscular myxoma and soft tissue perineurioma tend to be sparsely cellular, with abundant myxoid matrix spread as a background granular film and singly dispersed or clustered bland spindle cells with long, fibrillary cytoplasmic processes and scattered muciphages.[16] Intramuscular myxoma shows copious myxoid stroma with haphazardly distributed bland spindled and stellate cells; infiltration into skeletal muscle is helpful, if present (**Figs. 2**A, B). Soft tissue perineurioma shows storiform architecture of bland spindle cells with long delicate cytoplasmic processes and thin, wavy

Table 1
Differential diagnosis: myxoid soft tissue tumors

Tumor	Useful Immunostains	Molecular Features
Hypocellular neoplasms with bland/minimal atypia		
Intramuscular myxoma	CD34 variable, EMA rare	*GNAS* mutations
Soft tissue perineurioma	CD34, EMA, claudin-1	
LGFMS	MUC4, CD34	*FUS-CREB3L2* (90%)
Lipoblastoma	PLAG1	PLAG1 rearrangement
Adipocytic tumors		
Spindle cell lipoma	CD34, Rb-loss	13q and 16q alterations
Lipoblastoma	PLAG1	PLAG1 rearrangement
MLPS		*FUS-DDIT3*; rare *EWSR1-DDIT3*
Neoplasms with atypia and pleomorphism		
MFS		Complex karyotype
MIFS		*TFGBR3-MGEA5*
Pleomorphic liposarcoma		Complex karyotype
DDLPS	MDM2, CDK4	*MDM2* amplification
Neoplasms with ovoid/epithelioid morphology		
EMC	S100 (50%)	*EWSR1-NR4A3*
OFMT	S100, desmin (50%)	*PHF1* fusions
Myoepithelial neoplasms of soft tissue (myoepithelioma and myoepithelial carcinoma)	Keratin, EMA, S100, SOX10, p63 (50%)	*EWSR1* rearrangements
Chordoma	Brachyury, keratin, EMA, S100	Subset: *T* duplication/amplification SMARCB1 deletions in poorly differentiated tumors

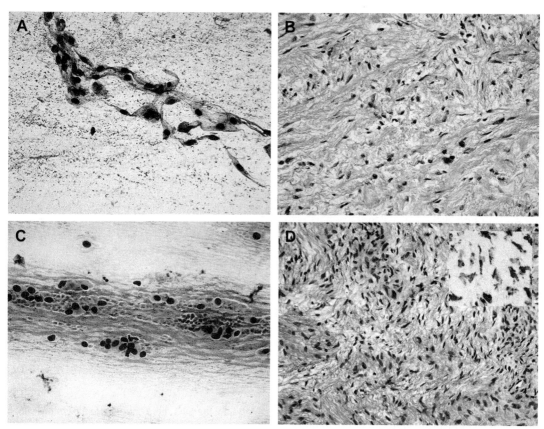

Fig. 2. Overlapping cytomorphologic features of intramuscular myxoma and LGFMS. Smears of intramuscular myxoma show an abundant granular myxoid matrix with bland spindle cells with long, fibrillary cytoplasmic processes ([A] air-dried, Diff-Quik stain). Core biopsies show haphazard distribution of the spindle cells, and cellular examples (as shown) show more collagenous stroma (B). LGFMS appears deceptively bland in smears, appearing as a hypocellular myxoid neoplasm with spindle cells having mild (if any) cytologic atypia ([C] air-dried, Diff-Quik stain). Increased cellularity, mild atypia, and alternating collagenous and myxoid stroma may be appreciated in core biopsies (D), and MUC4 immunoreactivity is diagnostic (*inset*).

nuclei, often with perivascular whorling. Claudin-1 has low sensitivity for soft tissue perineurioma but when positive (30%) it is useful in excluding myxoma, dermatofibrosarcoma protuberans (DFSP), and LGFMS.[17,18] Soft tissue perineurioma is negative for S100 and SOX10, distinguishing it from neurofibroma and schwannoma. Cellular intramuscular myxomas may raise the possibility of low-grade MFS; however, MFS is characterized by pleomorphism and curvilinear vessels. If definitive diagnosis is not possible after exclusion of LGFMS (and other low-grade sarcomas), a diagnosis of benign myxoid spindle cell neoplasm is appropriate.

The diagnosis of LGFMS is challenging on aspirate and core biopsy. Aspirate smears are deceptively bland, appearing hypocellular with clusters of uniform ovoid and spindle cells in a myxoid background[19] (see **Fig.** 2C). There is minimal nuclear atypia, and the characteristic alternating fibrous and myxoid regions with tumor cells arranged in short fascicles and whorls (see **Fig.** 2D) might not be appreciated on small biopsies. Fortunately, MUC4 expression is highly sensitive and specific for LGFMS.[20] Molecular studies may be helpful, because *FUS-CREB3L2* fusions are present in 90% of LGFMS, whereas a small subset has *FUS-CREB3L1* fusions or alternative *EWSR1* rearrangement in lieu of *FUS*.

Extraskeletal myxoid chondrosarcoma (EMC) show a multinodular architecture of myxoid lobules with a reticular arrangement of uniform tumor cells having round-to-ovoid nuclei and eosinophilic cytoplasm. In smears, the tumor cells show a cordlike or beads-on-a-string configuration within myxoid fragments; the matrix appears bright magenta and fibrillary in Romanowsky stain.[21] EMC shows morphologic and immunophenotypic overlap with soft tissue myoepithelial neoplasms, ossifying fibromyxoid tumor (OFMT), and sclerosing epithelioid fibrosarcoma (SEF). S100 is positive in 50% of EMCs, and most cases are negative for EMA and keratin. Myoepithelial neoplasms of soft tissue typically show architectural and cytologic heterogeneity and variable expression of keratin, EMA, S100, and glial fibrillary acidic protein (GFAP). OFMT shows cords and trabeculae of ovoid cells within a fibromyxoid stroma; the peripheral bony shell is often not sampled on biopsy. Most OFMTs are positive for S100 and half are positive for desmin. Molecular testing can be used to detect the characteristic *PHF1* fusions of OFMT,[22] and *EWSR1-NR4A3* fusion of EMC.[23] *NR4A3* rearrangement is specific for EMC, whereas *EWSR1* rearrangements are also present in soft tissue myoepithelial neoplasms and SEF.[24,25]

MFS should be considered for any myxoid neoplasm with cytologic atypia, particularly in superficial tumors of limbs and limb girdles[26] of older adults. The most helpful diagnostic clue on small biopsy is the presence of tumor cells coalesced around curvilinear vessels. Smears typically show variable myxoid matrix, spindled and pleomorphic tumor cells, and long, thin curvilinear vessels.[27] Cellularity increases with histologic grade, and high-grade MFS may show solid growth. MFS has no specific immunophenotype or genomic alterations and may be indistinguishable from pleomorphic liposarcoma and UPS in small biopsies (discussed later). Immunohistochemistry is mainly of use to exclude mimics, such as DDLPS and LGFMS. Myxoinflammatory fibroblastic sarcoma (MIFS) may enter the differential, although most tumors arise in the distal extremities (including digits). MIFS has large pleomorphic cells that have Reed-Sternberg–like vesicular nuclei and inclusion-like nucleoli and no specific immunophenotype, but some cases may be distinguished by *TFGBR3-MGEA5* fusions.[28]

SPINDLE CELL TUMORS

The differential diagnosis of spindle cell neoplasms is broad, and in small biopsies many benign tumors and neoplasms of intermediate biologic grade (locally aggressive or rarely metastasizing) may be difficult to distinguish from spindle cell sarcomas. In aspirate smears, benign tumors often show cohesive fragments and a clean background (**Fig. 3**A) whereas both intermediate-grade spindle cell neoplasms and spindle cell sarcomas tend to yield dense fascicles of spindle cells and a cellular background with singly dispersed tumor cells (see **Fig. 3**B). Pleomorphism, mitotic activity, and necrosis are common in high-grade tumors. Ancillary studies are helpful in resolving most differential diagnoses (**Table 2**). The main goal is to accurately convey biologic potential, and the diagnostic work-up should exclude relevant intermediate-grade neoplasms and sarcomas in the differential even when specific diagnosis is not possible, in which case a descriptive diagnosis conveying grade is recommended.

BENIGN AND INTERMEDIATE-GRADE SPINDLE CELL NEOPLASMS

Nodular fasciitis is a benign, self-limited fibroblastic neoplasm characterized by *USP6* gene rearrangement,[29] and lacking cytologic atypia. Aspirate smears show plump spindle cells with eccentric nuclei and small nucleoli and myxoid stromal fragments.[30] High cellularity and frequent (typical) mitotic figures are common and should not prompt overdiagnosis as a sarcoma. Most cases of nodular fasciitis are positive for smooth muscle actin (SMA) but desmin negative. Immunohistochemistry can exclude other entities in the differential diagnosis, including β-catenin for

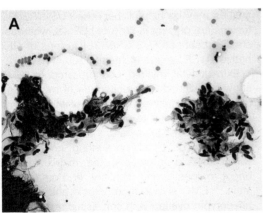
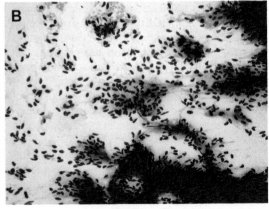

Fig. 3. Comparison of benign and malignant spindle cell neoplasms on FNA. Schwannoma yields large, cohesive fragments and a clean background ([*A*] air-dried, Diff-Quik stain). Smears of synovial sarcoma show alternating dense fascicles and a cellular background with singly dispersed tumor cells ([*B*] air-dried, Diff-Quik stain).

Table 2
Differential diagnosis: spindle cell neoplasms

Tumor	Useful Immunostains	Molecular Features
Benign		
Nodular fasciitis	SMA variable	*USPS-MYH9*
Schwannoma	S100 and SOX10 (both diffuse)	
Neurofibroma	S100 and SOX10 (40%–50% of cells)	
Leiomyoma	SMA, desmin, h-caldesmon	
Intermediate biologic grade		
Desmoid fibromatosis	β-Catenin (80%), SMA variable	*CTNNB1* or *APC* mutations
IMT	SMA, ALK (50%)	*ALK* rearrangements (50%) *ROS1* rearrangements (10%)
GIST	KIT, DOG1	*KIT* mutations (~80%)
DFSP	CD34	*COL1A-PDGFB*
SFT	CD34, STAT6	*NAB2-STAT6*
Sarcomas		
LMS	SMA, desmin, h-caldesmon	Complex karyotype
Spindle cell RMS	Desmin, MyoD1	*MyoD1* mutations
MPNST	Rare S100 and SOX10; H3K27me3 loss	*EED1* and *SUZ12* mutations
Synovial sarcoma	EMA, TLE1	*SS18-SSX*
DDLPS	MDM2, CDK4	*MDM2* amplification

desmoid fibromatosis, S100 for schwannoma, CD34 for DFSP, and MUC4 for LGFMS.

Schwannoma often enters the differential of spindle cell neoplasms. The characteristic capsule and varying hypercellular areas with nuclear palisading (Antoni A) and more sparsely cellular areas with edematous stroma (Antoni B) may not be apparent in small biopsies; however, the presence of thick-walled blood vessels with hyalinized walls and foamy histiocytes are useful diagnostic features, as is the characteristic diffuse nuclear S100 and SOX10 staining.[31] Smears show large, cohesive syncytial fragments of spindled Schwann cells (see **Fig. 3**A). Mimics of schwannoma can be excluded by immunohistochemistry: SMA and desmin (leiomyoma), KIT and DOG1 (gastrointestinal stromal tumor; GIST), STAT6 (solitary fibrous tumor [SFT]), and β-catenin (desmoid fibromatosis). Although cellular schwannoma shows more fascicular growth and may mimic malignant peripheral nerve sheath tumor (MPNST), diffuse S100 and SOX10 staining excludes this entity.

Leiomyomas are frequently encountered on biopsy in the gastrointestinal tract but are rare in somatic sites. In soft tissue (nonuterine) sites, leiomyomas show no cytologic atypia or mitotic activity; the presence of these features is indicative of leiomyosarcoma (LMS). It is important, however, to be aware that core biopsies can underestimate

mitotic activity due to sampling issues. Smears show fascicular fragments of spindle cells and a clean background. Immunoreactivity for SMA, desmin, and h-caldesmon confirms smooth muscle differentiation. h-Caldesmon is most specific for smooth muscle differentiation, although expression may be seen in GIST.[32] Other spindle cell neoplasms can be excluded by immunohistochemistry: schwannoma (S100), GIST (KIT and DOG1), inflammatory myofibroblastic tumor (IMT) (ALK), and desmoid fibromatosis (β-catenin).

Deep (desmoid) fibromatosis is composed of long fascicles of bland spindle cells with tapered nuclei within a collagenous stroma. Smears show fragments of these long fascicles within a clean background[33] (**Fig. 4**A, B). Even in small biopsies, infiltrative growth into adjacent tissue is frequently evident, and entrapped skeletal muscle fibers are often sampled. The differential diagnosis includes schwannoma, leiomyoma, nodular fasciitis, LGFMS, and GIST, which is usually straightforward to resolve with an immunohistochemical panel that includes S100, desmin, MUC4, KIT, and DOG1. Nuclear β-catenin positivity, rare in histologic mimics, is present in 70% to 80% of desmoid fibromatosis (secondary to *CTNNB1* and *APC* mutations) (see **Fig. 4**C).[34]

IMT should be considered in children and young adults with large visceral tumors.[35] In smears,

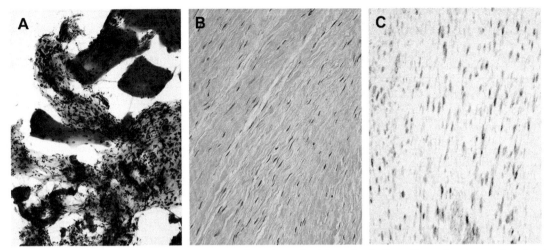

Fig. 4. Desmoid fibromatosis. Aspirate smears show long fascicles of spindle cells, and entrapped skeletal muscle fibers are often sampled ([A] alcohol-fixed, Papanicolaou stain). Histologically, the bland spindle cells are arranged in sweeping fascicles within a collagenized background (B). Most cases show nuclear staining for β-catenin (C).

spindle cells are arranged singly and in loose clusters in a background of lymphocytes and plasma cells.[36] SMA expression is frequent (80%). Nuclear or cytoplasmic immunoreactivity for ALK1 or ROS1 occurs in 50% or 10% of cases, respectively, and correlates with the presence of ALK1 or ROS1 rearrangements.[37,38] ALK-negative IMT poses a diagnostic challenge, with a broad differential that includes reactive processes, nodular fasciitis, desmoid fibromatosis, GIST, and spindle cell sarcomas (including MIFS and inflammatory variants of LMS and DDLPS).

GIST is the most common clinically significant soft tissue tumor of the gastrointestinal tract.[39] Risk stratification (based on primary site, tumor size, and mitotic activity) cannot be assessed on biopsy. Spindle cell morphology predominates, with mixed spindled and epithelioid or purely epithelioid features identified in up to 30%. Paranuclear vacuoles may be present, especially in gastric sites. Smears show uniform spindle cells either singly dispersed or in clusters and fascicles, with wispy cytoplasm and long extensions.[40] KIT and DOG1 are positive in 97%[41]; however, DOG1 is a more robust marker for cytologic specimens fixed in methanol-based solutions.[42] KIT and DOG1 expression is consistently negative in histologic mimics, including leiomyoma, schwannoma, and desmoid fibromatosis.[41,43]

DFSP is a locally aggressive dermal neoplasm characterized by COL1A-PDGFB fusion,[44] most commonly occurring on the trunk and thigh in young adults.[45] In smears, DFSP contains compact, whorled clusters of spindle cells.[46] Conventional DFSP shows strong and diffuse CD34[47]; however, the fibrosarcomatous variant is negative

for CD34 in up to 45%.[48] Mimics include cellular benign fibrous histiocytoma, which is CD34-negative,[49] and SFT, which can be distinguished by STAT6 positivity. Immunohistochemistry is helpful to distinguish fibrosarcomatous DFSP from other spindle cell sarcomas (eg, TLE1 for synovial sarcoma; S100, SOX10, and trimethylation at lysine 27 of histone H3 [H3K27me3] for MPNST).

SFT harbors NAB2-STAT6 fusion, is most common in middle-aged adults, and can arise in at nearly anatomic site.[50] Application of evolving risk stratification schemes is not possible on core biopsy or FNA.[51–53] Smears of SFT show variably interlacing fascicular fragments and numerous isolated single cells (**Fig. 5**A).[54] Core biopsies show considerable histologic variability, resulting in a broad differential diagnosis; however, most cases show stromal collagen and hyalinized staghorn blood vessels (see **Fig. 5**B). Moreover, diffuse nuclear staining for STAT6 is highly sensitive and specific for SFT[55] (see **Fig. 5**C). One pitfall is that a subset (10%–15%) of DDLPS can show nuclear and cytoplasmic STAT6 expression, and MDM2/CDK4 immunohistochemistry should be included when DDLPS is a diagnostic consideration.[56]

HIGH-GRADE SPINDLE CELL SARCOMAS

Soft tissue LMS typically arises in older adults, often in association with large vessels in the retroperitoneum or lower extremity. Smears show highly cellular fascicles and dispersed atypical cells in the background, with frequent mitotic activity and necrosis.[40] Immunoreactivity for SMA, desmin, and h-caldesmon is present in low-

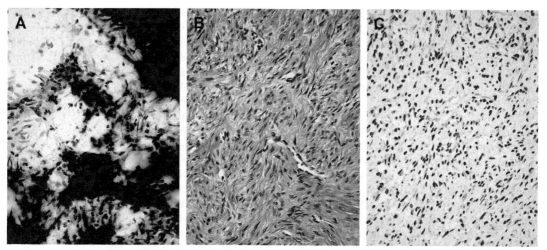

Fig. 5. SFT. Smears tend to be cellular and show interlacing fascicular fragments with isolated tumor cells ([A] alcohol-fixed, Papanicolaou stain). The characteristic patternless pattern may be appear indistinct in core biopsies, although the stromal collagen and hemangiopericytoma-like vessels are helpful (*B*). Nuclear STAT6 positivity identifies SFT (*C*).

grade tumors but is more variable in high-grade tumors.[57] Approximately 40% of cases of LMS show keratin or EMA positivity, which can be a pitfall for sarcomatoid carcinoma.[58] Spindle cell rhabdomyosarcoma (RMS) is also positive for desmin and occasionally for SMA but shows expression of skeletal muscle-specific markers, including diffuse nuclear MyoD1 immunoreactivity, correlating with *MyoD1* mutations.[59]

MPNST is diagnostically challenging without the clinical associations of neurofibromatosis type 1 or prior radiation therapy.[60] Smears show aggregates of atypical spindle cells arranged in large fascicular clusters and singly dispersed, appearing similar to other spindle cell sarcomas (**Fig. 6**A). Histologically, tumors are composed of fascicles of spindle cells with tapered nuclei, often with alternating hypercellular and hypocellular areas (see **Fig. 6**B). S100, SOX10, and GFAP immunohistochemistry has limited diagnostic utility, because only 30% of MPNSTs show focal expression of these markers. Of more utility is the loss of H3K27me3, occurring in half of all cases and detectable by immunohistochemistry[61] (see **Fig. 6**C). High specificity has been confirmed in the setting of FNAs and core biopsies,[62] although loss of H3K27me3 expression can occur in several mimics, including melanoma, synovial sarcoma,

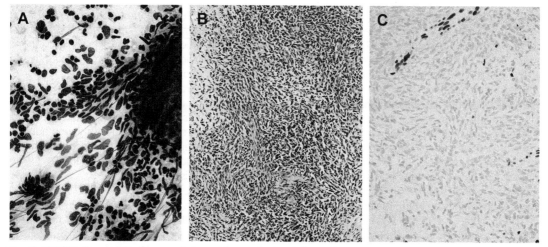

Fig. 6. MPNST. Smears are hypercellular with atypical spindle cells arranged in large fragments and singly dispersed ([A] air-dried, Diff-Quik stain). The characteristic marbling effect of alternating hypercellular and hypocellular areas may be apparent in core biopsies (*B*). Up to half of all cases show immunohistochemical loss of expression for H3K27me3 (*C*).

and DDLPS. Spindle cell melanoma can be distinguished by the more diffuse S100 and SOX10 expression,[63] which is unusual for MPNST. MPNST can show multifocal staining for TLE1 and MDM2, which can be pitfalls for synovial sarcoma and DDLPS and may require additional studies to resolve the differential.

Synovial sarcoma has an overall cytomorphologic appearance resembling MPNST, with alternating tissue fragments and single dispersion of tumor cells.[64] Biphasic tumors show epithelial differentiation with gland or nest formation. TLE1 is a sensitive marker for synovial sarcoma,[65] and although TLE1 may weakly stain mimics, including MPNST,[66] strong and diffuse nuclear expression of TLE1 supports synovial sarcoma.[67] Molecular identification of the characteristic SS18-SSX fusion[68] is diagnostic.

EPITHELIOID TUMORS

Evaluation of many epithelioid soft tissue neoplasms is limited in small biopsies, precluding identification of distinctive histopathologic features and immunophenotypes (Table 3). This section focuses primarily on malignant epithelioid entities, which are characterized by significant cytomorphologic overlap, and all tend to yield cellular aspirate smears with large rounded or polygonal cells in aggregates and singly dispersed. The differential diagnosis also includes epithelioid variants of specific tumor types as well as carcinoma and melanoma. Myxoid neoplasms showing epithelioid morphology are discussed previously.

Epithelioid sarcoma is classified as conventional (distal) and proximal subtypes and is an important differential diagnosis for undifferentiated carcinoma, due to EMA and keratin positivity, and may show overlapping features with several vascular tumors, including epithelioid angiosarcoma, epithelioid hemangioendothelioma (EHE), and pseudomyogenic hemangioendothelioma (PHE). Distal-type epithelioid sarcoma exhibits a nodular growth pattern of epithelioid and spindle cells, with vesicular nuclei and small nucleoli and with frequent central pseudogranulomatous necrosis (Fig. 7A), mimicking deep granuloma annulare and rheumatoid nodules. Proximal-type tumors show nodules of large epithelioid-to-rhabdoid cells with vesicular nuclei and prominent nucleoli.[69] In aspirates, the tumor cells have large round nuclei with prominent nucleoli and frequent binucleation; the cytoplasm is dense with distinct borders, occasional small vacuoles, and perinuclear pale zones (see Fig. 7B). Necroinflammatory debris, granulomata-type structures, and spindle cells may be seen in smears of distal-type epithelioid sarcoma, whereas rhabdoid morphology may

be seen in proximal-type tumors. All epithelioid sarcomas have the distinctive immunophenotype of keratin and EMA positivity, frequent CD34 staining (50%),[70] and consistent loss of INI1 expression[71] (see Fig. 7C, D). Consistent negativity for S100 and SOX10 distinguishes epithelioid sarcoma from melanoma.[31,72] Epithelioid sarcoma is negative for vascular markers CD31 and ERG as well as CAMTA1 and FOSB1, excluding EHE and PHE, respectively. Proximal-type epithelioid sarcoma shows morphologic overlap with myoepithelial carcinoma of soft tissue, epithelioid MPNST, malignant rhabdoid tumor, and poorly differentiated chordoma; these entities are also characterized by loss of INI1 expression[73,74] and require clinical correlation and additional studies to narrow the differential diagnosis.

On cytology, EHE shows dispersed epithelioid cells having mildly atypical nuclei, frequent binucleation, and dense cytoplasm (Fig. 8A). Tumors are composed of cords and strands of uniform epithelioid cells in a myxohyaline stroma (see Fig. 8B). If present, helpful features include the plugging of vessels by tumor cells and the intracytoplasmic vacuoles (blister cells).[75,76] Features specific for EHE in smears are occasional intracytoplasmic vacuoles and tumor cells intermingled with matrix material.[77] Although EHEs show focal keratin staining in 25% of cases, which may be a pitfall for carcinoma and epithelioid sarcoma, EHE is also positive for vascular markers CD31, CD34, and ERG.[76] Nuclear CAMTA1 expression secondary to WWTR1-CAMTA1 fusion is present in 80% to 90% of cases[78,79] (see Fig. 8C) and is nearly 100% specific in distinguishing EHE from other epithelioid and vascular tumors, including epithelioid angiosarcoma.[79] A small subset of vasoformative EHE is characterized by YAP1-TFE3 fusion and shows TFE3 expression.[80] SEF shows cords of epithelioid cells in a hyalinized stroma and may mimic EHE; however, it is negative for CAMTA1 and often positive for MUC4.

Clear cell sarcoma (CCS) of soft tissue is characterized by melanocytic differentiation and commonly arises in aponeuroses and tendon sheaths in the distal extremities of young adults.[81] Smears show epithelioid cells with eccentric nuclei, nuclear pseudoinclusions, and vacuolated cytoplasm with wispy processes.[82] CCS expresses S100, SOX10, HMB-45, and melan-A in most cases, among which HMB-45 staining is usually strongest.[83] Although PEComa is also positive for HMB-45 and melan-A, S100 and SOX10 are negative. Clinical or molecular correlation is often necessary to distinguish CCS from melanoma,[84] because most cases of CCS harbor EWSR1-ATF1 fusions (with EWSR1-CREB1 in approximately 5%).[85]

Table 3
Differential diagnosis: epithelioid soft tissue tumors

Tumor	Specific Morphologic Features	Useful Immunostains	Molecular Features
Epithelioid sarcoma	• Distal type can appear pseudogranulomatous • Proximal type can show rhabdoid morphology	Keratin, EMA, CD34 (50%), INI1 loss	SMARCB1 alterations
EHE	• Intracytoplasmic vacuoles • Myxoid stroma	CD31, CD34, ERG, CAMTA1	WWTR1-CAMTA1; subset YAP1-TFE3
Pseudomyogenic hemangioendothelioma	• Most cells have myoid appearance	AE1/AE3, ERG, CD31, FOSB N.B.: CD34 negative	SERPINE-FOSB
CCS of soft tissue	• Tumor cells have wispy, vacuolated cytoplasm in smears • Multinucleated wreath-like giant cells	S100, SOX10, HMB-45, melan-A	EWSR1-ATF1 (85%); subset EWSRR1-CREB1
ASPS	• Smears show bare nuclei and amorphous granular cytoplasmic contents • Cytoplasmic rhomboid crystals	TFE3	ASPSCR1-TFE3
Granular cell tumor	• Smears show bare nuclei and amorphous granular cytoplasmic contents	S100, SOX10, NKI-C3, TFE3	N.B.: lacks TFE3 fusions
PEComa	• Radial perivascular growth	SMA, desmin, HMB-45, melan-A	Subset with TFE3 fusions
SDH-deficient GIST	• Multinodular growth through gastric wall	KIT, DOG1, SDHB loss; SDHA loss if SDHA mutant	SDHA, SDHB, SDHC, or SDHD mutations
Epithelioid IMT	• Myxoid stroma, delicate capillaries, neutrophils	ALK (nuclear membrane), SMA, desmin, CD30	ALK-RANBP2
Epithelioid MFS	• Curvilinear vessels, myxoid stroma		Complex karyotype
Epithelioid pleomorphic liposarcoma	• Atypical lipoblasts		Complex karyotype

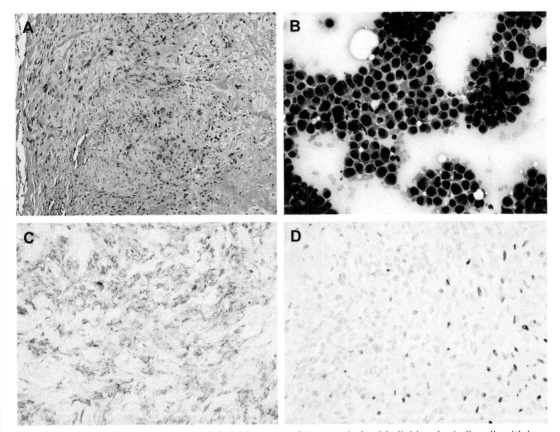

Fig. 7. Epithelioid sarcoma. Distal-type epitheloid sarcoma shows atypical epithelioid and spindle cells with large vesicular nuclei arranged in pseudogranulomatous nodules (*A*). Aspirate smears show polygonal and epithelioid cells with large round nuclei and dense cytoplasm, with occasional binucleation ([*B*] air-dried, Diff-Quik stain). Epithelioid sarcoma shows expression of epithelial markers ([*C*] EMA), frequent CD34 staining, and consistent loss of INI1 expression (*D*).

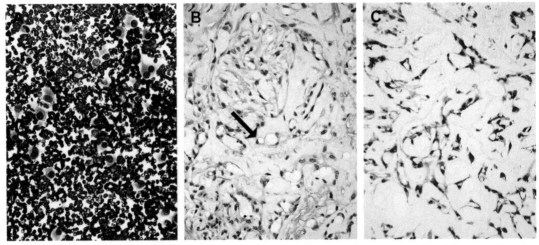

Fig. 8. EHE. Aspirate smears show dispersed epithelioid cells with eccentric round nuclei and frequent binucleation ([*A*] air-dried, Diff-Quik stain). In cores, the tumor cells are arranged in cords and strands within a myxohyaline stroma (*B*), with characteristic blister cells having intracytoplasmic vacuoles (*arrow*). Nuclear CAMTA1 expression is diagnostic (*C*).

Alveolar soft part sarcoma (ASPS) most commonly presents as deep-seated masses in the lower extremities of adolescents and young adults. ASPS shows nests of epithelioid cells with copious eosinophilic cytoplasm that show frequent loss of cohesion; solid growth is common in pediatric cases. In aspirate smears, the fragile tumor cells lyse, yielding bare nuclei dispersed in a background of amorphous granular material.[86] Cytoplasmic rhomboid crystals (which are periodic acid–Schiff positive and diastase resistant) are characteristic but not always present. ASPS is negative for S100 and keratin[87]; desmin expression is variable. Immunohistochemistry can detect nuclear TFE3 overexpression secondary to *ASPSCR1-TFE3* fusion, which is useful for distinguishing ASPS from epithelioid sarcoma, melanoma, and most cases of renal cell carcinoma (RCC) and PEComa. All cases of RCC are positive for EMA and PAX8, and PEComa is positive for HMB-45, unlike ASPS.[88,89] Granular cell tumor is a benign neoplasm that may resemble ASPS, particularly in smears, and shows TFE3 immunoreactivity. Granular cell tumor, however, rarely arises in deep soft tissue and lacks *TFE3* rearrangement[90]; S100, SOX10, and NKI-C3 expression is characteristic.

PEComas are composed of nested growth of epithelioid cells with variably clear and granular-eosinophilic cytoplasm and round nuclei with small nucleoli; some tumors show mixed spindle cell morphology. Radial perivascular growth is common. Unlike other epithelioid neoplasms in the differential, aspirate smears show mixed epithelioid and spindle cells that can appear histiocytoid, sometimes with admixed vessels.[91] Most PEComas are positive for SMA, HMB-45,[88] and melan-A, although staining is more variable for desmin and h-caldesmon. S100 and SOX10 are typically negative,[72] as are keratins and EMA,[92] which is helpful in excluding melanoma and epithelial mimics, including RCC and adrenal cortical carcinoma. CCS is another diagnostic consideration that, unlike PEComa, is almost always positive for S100.[83] A subset of PEComa has *TFE3* gene fusions and shows TFE3 immunoreactivity.[93]

Several tumor types have epithelioid variants with distinctive clinicopathologic features. Succinate dehydrogenase (SDH)–deficient GIST is a distinctive clinicopathologic variant and its accurate diagnosis is important for prognosis and treatment.[94] Tumors arise nearly exclusively in the stomach and show a plexiform, multinodular growth pattern of uniform epithelioid cells. Although wild-type for *KIT*, tumors are positive for KIT and DOG1. SDHB immunohistochemistry is a useful screening tool and loss of expression correlates with SDH deficiency, irrespective of mechanism of SDH dysfunction.[95] The epithelioid variant of IMT is aggressive and commonly presents as an intra-abdominal mass in young adult men. Epithelioid IMT harbors *ALK-RANBP2* fusion and shows a distinctive immunohistochemical ALK immunoreactivity pattern localized to the nuclear membrane.[96]

ROUND CELL TUMORS

Most round cell tumors are high-grade sarcomas and require ancillary testing for definitive classification (**Table 4**). Many diagnostic pitfalls exist, given the frequently overlapping morphologic and

Table 4
Differential diagnosis: round cell sarcomas

Tumor	Useful Immunostains	Molecular Features
Ewing sarcoma	CD99 (diffuse, membranous), FLI1, NKX2.2	*EWSR1-FLI1* (majority); subset *EWSR1-ERGI* and variant *FUS* fusions
Alveolar RMS	Desmin, myogenin, MyoD1	*PAX3-FOXO1A, PAX7-FOXO1A*
DSRCT	CD99 variable, keratin, desmin, NSE, WT1 (C-terminus antibody)	*EWSR1-WT1*
CIC-rearranged sarcoma	WT1, ETV4, CD99 variable	*CIC-DUX4* (majority)
BCOR-rearranged sarcoma	BCOR, SATB2, TLE1, cyclin D1 CD99 variable CCNB3 if *BCOR-CCNB3*	*BCOR-CCNB3* (majority)
High-grade MLPS		*FUS-DDIT3*; rare *EWSR1-DDIT3*
Poorly differentiated synovial sarcoma	EMA, TLE1	*SS18-SSX*
Myoepithelial carcinoma of soft tissue	Keratin, EMA, S100, SOX10, p63 (50%)	*EWSR1* rearrangements (various partners include *POU5F1*, *PBX2*, and *PBX3*)

immunophenotypic features between entities. The initial evaluation of a round cell sarcoma should include a broad immunohistochemical panel that includes CD99 and desmin as well as keratin, S100, and TdT to exclude epithelial mimics, melanoma, and lymphoblastic lymphoma. Immunohistochemistry is helpful to refine the differential diagnosis and direct confirmatory molecular testing.

Most cases of Ewing sarcoma arise in the bone of adolescents and young adults, although some occur in older patients and in extraosseous sites.[97] Ewing sarcoma is composed of sheets of uniform round cells with primitive-appearing round nuclei containing fine chromatin (**Fig. 9**A). Cytoplasmic clearing and pseudorosette formation can sometimes be seen. Aspirate smears show uniform round cells and occasionally a second population of smaller, hyperchromatic cells[98] (see **Fig. 9**B); a tigroid background is common secondary to dispersion of glycogen-rich cytoplasm. Immunohistochemistry shows strong and diffuse membranous CD99 staining, which is specific for Ewing sarcoma (see **Fig. 9**C). Subtotal or cytoplasmic CD99 positivity is nonspecific and can be seen in other tumors

in the differential, including lymphoblastic lymphoma, desmoplastic small round cell tumor (DSRCT), and alveolar RMS.[99] FLI1 is highly sensitive but nonspecific for Ewing sarcoma and can be positive in mimics, in particular lymphoblastic leukemia.[100] In contrast, NKX2.2 is approximately 95% sensitive for Ewing sarcoma (see **Fig. 9**D), although staining occurs in several mimics including mesenchymal chondrosarcoma, neuroblastoma,[101,102] and well-differentiated neuroendocrine tumors, which are an important pitfall to consider, because up to one-third of Ewing sarcomas can aberrantly express keratin, synaptophysin, and chromogranin.[103] A combination of NKX2.2 and CD99 is helpful in most contexts, and when both markers are appropriately positive, the specificity for Ewing sarcoma is 98%.[104] *EWSR1-FLI1* rearrangements are present in 85% of cases, whereas *EWSR1-ERG* rearrangements occur in 10% and correlate with ERG-positivity.[105]

Alveolar RMS arises most commonly in adolescents and young adults in a wide anatomic distribution. Tumors are composed of round cells with large atypical hyperchromatic nuclei and distinct nucleoli,

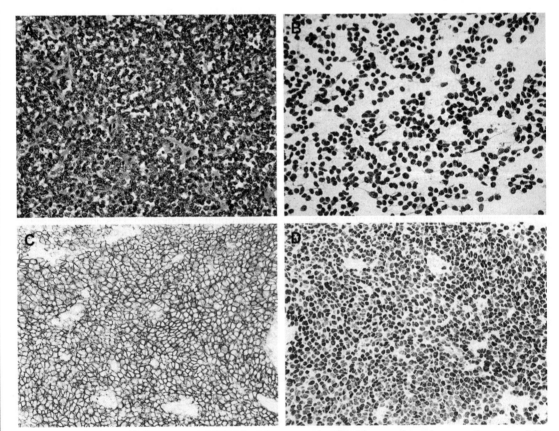

Fig. 9. Ewing sarcoma. Tumors are composed of uniform round cells with smooth nuclear membranes and fine chromatin ([A] core biopsy; [B] alcohol fixed, hematoxylin-eosin stain). Strong membranous CD99 staining is characteristic of Ewing sarcoma (C) and NKX2.2 has high sensitivity (but modest specificity) for Ewing sarcoma (D).

arranged in nests separated by fibrovascular septa. In smears, the nuclear atypia is more apparent. If present, wreath-like multinucleated cells are a helpful feature. Although all RMS subtypes express desmin, myogenin, and MyoD1, alveolar RMS shows diffuse nuclear staining for myogenin and MyoD1 that allows distinction from other RMS subtypes.[106] Keratin and neuroendocrine marker positivity occurs in up to a third of alveolar RMS, presenting a diagnostic pitfall for neuroendocrine carcinoma.[107] Identification of *PAX3-FOXO1A* or *PAX7-FOXO1A* fusions present in 80% of alveolar RMS[108] can confirm the diagnosis.

DSRCT most commonly arises as intra-abdominal masses in young men.[109,110] The characteristic desmoplastic stroma may not be well represented in small biopsies. Irregularly shaped clusters of round cells with nuclear molding at the periphery as well as stromal fragments are seen in smears. DSRCT has a distinctive immunophenotype of keratin, neuron-specific enolase (NSE), and desmin expression.[109] Although nuclear NKX2.2 expression is rare in DSRCT,[101]

DSRCT shows nonspecific CD99 cytoplasmic staining.[104] Nuclear WT1 positivity (using antibodies against the C-terminus) is diagnostic of DSRCT. Although DSRCT harbors *EWSR1-WT1* fusion,[111] sequencing-based methods may be necessary for definitive diagnosis because *EWSR1* rearrangements are present in Ewing sarcoma and other mimics.

CIC-rearranged sarcoma and *BCOR*-rearranged sarcoma both share morphologic features with Ewing sarcoma but tend to show more atypical features apparent in cytologic smears,[112] including cytologic atypia, pleomorphism, more prominent nucleoli, increased cytoplasm, spindled morphology, myxoid stroma, and necrosis (**Fig. 10**). Both *CIC*-rearranged and *BCOR*-rearranged sarcomas have characteristic immunophenotypes; however, currently molecular confirmation is required due to their rarity and novelty. CD99 expression is highly variable, but NKX2.2 staining is rare in both entities.[101] *CIC*-rearranged sarcoma exhibits diffuse nuclear expression of WT1 (see **Fig. 10B**) and ETV4,

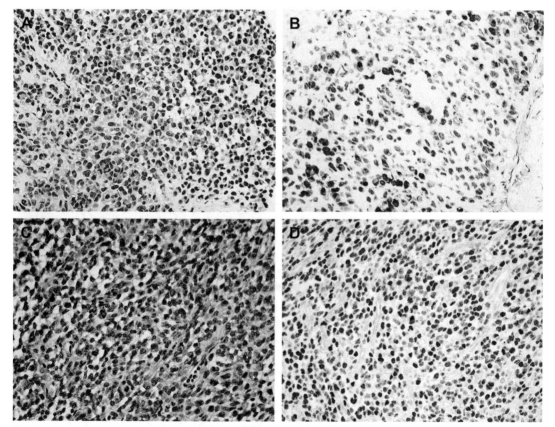

Fig. 10. *CIC*-rearranged sarcoma and *BCOR*-rearranged sarcoma frequently show cytologic atypia, increased cytoplasm, spindled morphology, and myxoid necrosis. *CIC*-rearranged sarcoma (*A*) is characterized by diffuse nuclear staining for WT1 (*B*) and ETV4. *BCOR*-rearranged sarcoma (*C*) shows frequent nuclear expression of staining for *BCOR* (*D*).

both of which are sensitive and specific within the differential, including Ewing sarcoma and *BCOR*-rearranged sarcoma.[113] In contrast, *BCOR*-rearranged sarcoma show nuclear BCOR immunoreactivity (see **Fig. 10D**), which is rare in Ewing sarcoma.[114] Tumors also show frequent staining for SATB2, TLE1, and cyclin D1,[114,115] and CCNB3 is positive in tumors with *BCOR-CCNB3* fusion.[116]

Round cell morphology may be predominant in high-grade MLPS, poorly differentiated synovial sarcoma, and myoepithelial carcinoma of soft tissue (especially in pediatric patients); these tumors may also show nonspecific CD99 staining. Fortunately, these tumors have characteristic molecular alterations (see **Table 4**), which may be identified to confirm the diagnosis.

Pitfalls
ROUND SELL SARCOMAS

! Many round cell sarcomas show nonspecific CD99 expression and should not be interpreted as Ewing sarcoma.

! Aberrant expression of keratin and synaptophysin/chromogranin may be seen in several round cell sarcomas, including Ewing sarcoma and alveolar RMS, which is a pitfall for neuroendocrine neoplasms.

! *EWSR1* and *FUS* rearrangements are present in many tumor types in the differential diagnosis, and interpretation of molecular testing requires correlation with clinical, morphologic, and immunohistochemical features.

PLEOMORPHIC TUMORS

The diagnosis of pleomorphic sarcomas can be challenging on small biopsies or cytology preparations. The differential diagnosis includes DDLPS, high-grade MFS, pleomorphic liposarcoma, pleomorphic LMS, pleomorphic RMS, and UPS. Diagnostic work-up should always include keratin and S100/SOX10 to exclude sarcomatoid carcinoma and melanoma.

DDLPS enters most differential diagnoses, and MDM2 and CDK4 immunohistochemistry should always be included, especially for deep-seated and retroperitoneal tumors. Multifocal MDM2 or CDK4 staining, however, can occur in a small subset of other high-grade sarcomas, including MPNST and MFS,[117] and confirmatory *MDM2* FISH should be performed for equivocal or positive cases.

Immunohistochemistry for desmin is useful to identify pleomorphic RMS (90%)[118] and pleomorphic LMS (85%).[119] Diffuse desmin positivity should prompt further immunohistochemistry for myogenin and MyoD1 to confirm the diagnosis of pleomorphic RMS, and SMA and caldesmon for pleomorphic LMS. Pleomorphic RMS may show multinucleated or polygonal cells with brightly eosinophilic cytoplasm and should be distinguished from tumors showing heterologous rhabdomyoblastic differentiation, such as carcinosarcoma, DDLPS, and MPNST.

MFS, pleomorphic liposarcoma, and UPS all lack specific immunohistochemical features and all have complex karyotypes. Definitive diagnosis of these entities may not be possible on small biopsy specimens if their characteristic features are not present (**Fig. 11**). Many cases are thus

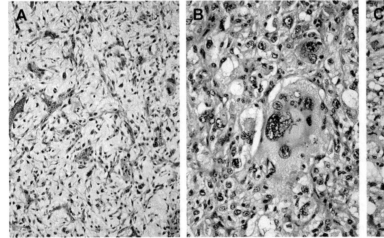

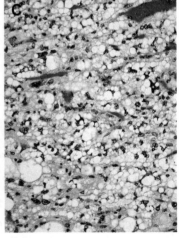

Fig. 11. Pleomorphic liposarcoma. Many cases are indistinguishable from MFS (*A*). Large, bizarre tumor cells are common (*B*), but definitive diagnosis is based on the presence of lipoblasts (*C*), which may be focal in some cases.

assigned a descriptive diagnosis (high-grade pleomorphic sarcoma), with classification deferred to surgical resection. UPS refers to pleomorphic sarcomas showing no recognizable line of differentiation by morphologic, immunohistochemical, and molecular studies and thus is a diagnosis of exclusion that can only rarely be made on small biopsies.

Key Points
DIAGNOSIS OF PLEOMORPHIC SARCOMAS IN SMALL BIOPSIES

- DDLPS should always be considered for small biopsies of pleomorphic sarcomas, especially those located in the retroperitoneum.

- MDM2 and CDK4 coexpression occurs in most cases for DDLPS; although MDM2 expression may be seen in other sarcomas, the diagnosis of DDLPS can be confirmed with *MDM2* FISH.

- The immunohistochemical work-up should also include desmin (for pleomorphic RMS and pleomorphic LMS), keratin (for carcinoma), and S100/SOX10 (for melanoma).

- In core biopsies and smears, MFS, pleomorphic liposarcoma, and UPS are often not distinguishable on cytomorphologic, immunohistochemical, and morphologic grounds.

- The presence of large atypical lipoblasts is consistent with pleomorphic liposarcoma, after exclusion of DDLPS showing homologous dedifferentiation.

- The diagnosis of UPS is rarely made on core biopsy/FNA outside the setting of recurrence or metastasis of known disease.

SUMMARY

A pattern-based approach offers a practical framework for the evaluation of core biopsies and FNAs of soft tissue neoplasms. In most scenarios immunohistochemical panels serve to refine a differential diagnosis and guide confirmatory molecular testing. Immunohistochemical and molecular tests have greatly increased the diagnostic accuracy of small biopsies; however, pitfalls remain given that many tumor types have overlapping morphologic, immunohistochemical, and even molecular features. Accurate classification requires integration of clinical data with morphologic evaluation and ancillary testing results, and

with the goal of triaging lesions based on grade for appropriate clinical management, even if definitive diagnosis is not possible.

REFERENCES

1. Dodd LG. Update on liposarcoma: a review for cytopathologists. Diagn Cytopathol 2012;40: 1122–31.
2. Pilotti S, Della Torre G, Mezzelani A, et al. The expression of MDM2/CDK4 gene product in the differential diagnosis of well differentiated liposarcoma and large deep-seated lipoma. Br J Cancer 2000;82:1271–5.
3. Thway K, Flora R, Shah C, et al. Diagnostic utility of p16, CDK4, and MDM2 as an immunohistochemical panel in distinguishing well-differentiated and dedifferentiated liposarcomas from other adipocytic tumors. Am J Surg Pathol 2012;36:462–9.
4. Miettinen MM, Fetsch JF, Antonescu CR, et al. Cytopathology of soft tissue tumors and tumor-like lesions. AFIP atlas of tumor pathology series 4: tumors of the soft tissues, vol. 20. Washington, DC: American Registry of Pathology; 2014.
5. Stojanov I, Mariño-Enriquez A, Bahri N, et al. Lipomas of the oral cavity: utility of MDM2 and CDK4 in avoiding overdiagnosis as atypical lipomatous tumor. Head Neck Pathol 2018. https://doi.org/10.1007/s12105-018-0928-0.
6. Domanski HA, Carlén B, Jonsson K, et al. Distinct cytologic features of spindle cell lipoma: a cytologic-histologic study with clinical, radiologic, electron microscopic, and cytogenetic correlations. Cancer 2001;93:381–9.
7. Chen BJ, Fletcher CDM, Hornick JL. Loss of retinoblastoma protein expression in spindle cell/pleomorphic lipomas and cytogenetically related tumors: an immunohistochemical study with diagnostic implications. Am J Surg Pathol 2012;36: 1119–28.
8. Howitt BE, Fletcher CDM. Mammary-type myofibroblastoma: clinicopathologic characterization in a series of 143 cases. Am J Surg Pathol 2016;40: 361–7.
9. Sioletic S, Dal Cin P, Fletcher CDM, et al. Well-differentiated and dedifferentiated liposarcomas with prominent myxoid stroma: analysis of 56 cases. Histopathology 2013;62:287–93.
10. Mariño-Enríquez A, Hornick JL, Dal Cin P, et al. Dedifferentiated liposarcoma and pleomorphic liposarcoma. Cancer Cytopathol 2014;122: 128–37.
11. Klijanienko J, Caillaud JM, Lagacé R. Fine-needle aspiration in liposarcoma: cytohistologic correlative

study including well-differentiated, myxoid, and pleomorphic variants. Diagn Cytopathol 2004;30: 307–12.

12. Hornick JL, Bosenberg MW, Mentzel T, et al. Pleomorphic liposarcoma: clinicopothologic analysis of 57 cases. Am J Surg Pathol 2004;28: 1257–67.

13. Qian X. Soft tissue. In: Cibas ES, Ducatman B, editors. Cytology: diagnostic principles and clinical correlates. Saunders/Elsevier Philadelphia; 2014. p. 471–518.

14. Antonescu CR, Elahi A, Humphrey M, et al. Specificity of TLS-CHOP rearrangement for classic myxoid/round cell liposarcoma: absence in predominantly myxoid well-differentiated liposarcomas. J Mol Diagn 2000;2:132–8.

15. Hibbard MK, Kozakewich HP, Dal Cin P, et al. PLAG1 fusion oncogenes in lipoblastoma. Cancer Res 2000;60:4869–72.

16. Yang EJ, Hornick JL, Qian X. Fine-needle aspiration of soft tissue perineurioma: a comparative analysis of cytomorphology and immunohistochemistry with benign and malignant mimics. Cancer Cytopathol 2016;124:651–8.

17. Hornick JL, Fletcher CDM. Soft tissue perineurioma: clinicopathologic analysis of 81 cases including those with atypical histologic features. Am J Surg Pathol 2005;29:845–58.

18. Folpe AL, Billings SD, McKenney JK, et al. Expression of claudin-1, a recently described tight junction-associated protein, distinguishes soft tissue perineurioma from potential mimics. Am J Surg Pathol 2002;26:1620–6.

19. Lindberg G, Maitra A, Gokaslan S, et al. Low grade fibromyxoid sarcoma: fine-needle aspiration cytology with histologic, cytogenetic, immunohistochemical, and ultrastructural correlation. Cancer 1999;87:75–82.

20. Doyle LA, Möller E, Dal Cin P, et al. MUC4 is a highly sensitive and specific marker for low-grade fibromyxoid sarcoma. Am J Surg Pathol 2011;35: 733–41.

21. Jakowski JD, Wakely PE. Cytopathology of extraskeletal myxoid chondrosarcoma: report of 8 cases. Cancer 2007;111:298–305.

22. Gebre-Medhin S, Nord KH, Möller E, et al. Recurrent rearrangement of the PHF1 gene in ossifying fibromyxoid tumors. Am J Pathol 2012;181: 1069–77.

23. Flucke U, Tops BB, Verdijk MA, et al. NR4A3 rearrangement reliably distinguishes between the clinicopathologically overlapping entities myoepithelial carcinoma of soft tissue and cellular extraskeletal myxoid chondrosarcoma. Virchows Arch 2012; 460:621–8.

24. Prieto-Granada C, Zhang L, Chen HW, et al. A genetic dichotomy between pure sclerosing epithelioid fibrosarcoma (SEF) and hybrid SEF/low-grade fibromyxoid sarcoma: a pathologic and molecular study of 18 cases. Genes Chromosomes Cancer 2015;54:28–38.

25. Antonescu CR, Zhang L, Chang NE, et al. EWSR1-POU5F1 fusion in soft tissue myoepithelial tumors. a molecular analysis of 66 cases, including soft tissue, bone and visceral lesions, showing common involvement of the EWSR1 gene. Genes Chromosomes Cancer 2010;49:1114–24.

26. Huang HY, Lal P, Qin J, et al. Low-grade myxofibrosarcoma: a clinicopathologic analysis of 49 cases treated at a single institution with simultaneous assessment of the efficacy of 3-tier and 4-tier grading systems. Hum Pathol 2004;35: 612–21.

27. Olson MT, Ali SZ. Myxofibrosarcoma: cytomorphologic findings and differential diagnosis on fine needle aspiration. Acta Cytol 2012;56:15–24.

28. Antonescu CR, Zhang L, Nielsen GP, et al. Consistent t(1;10) with rearrangements of TGFBR3 and MGEA5 in both myxoinflammatory fibroblastic sarcoma and hemosiderotic fibrolipomatous tumor. Genes Chromosomes Cancer 2011;50:757–64.

29. Erickson-Johnson MR, Chou MM, Evers BR, et al. Nodular fasciitis: a novel model of transient neoplasia induced by MYH9-USP6 gene fusion. Lab Invest 2011;91:1427–33.

30. Allison DB, Wakely PE, Siddiqui MT, et al. Nodular fasciitis: a frequent diagnostic pitfall on fine-needle aspiration. Cancer Cytopathol 2017; 125:20–9.

31. Karamchandani JR, Nielsen TO, Van De Rijn M, et al. Sox10 and s100 in the diagnosis of soft-tissue neoplasms. Appl Immunohistochem Mol Morphol 2012;20:445–50.

32. Miettinen M, Sarlomo-Rikala M, Lasota J. Gastrointestinal stromal tumors: recent advances in understanding of their biology. Hum Pathol 1999;30: 1213–20.

33. Owens CL, Sharma R, Ali SZ. Deep fibromatosis (desmoid tumor): cytopathologic characteristics, clinicoradiologic features, and immunohistochemical findings on fine-needle aspiration. Cancer 2007;111:166–72.

34. Carlson JW, Fletcher CDM. Immunohistochemistry for β-catenin in the differential diagnosis of spindle cell lesions: analysis of a series and review of the literature. Histopathology 2007;51:509–14.

35. Coffin CM, Watterson J, Priest JR, et al. Extrapulmonary inflammatory myofibroblastic tumor (inflammatory pseudotumor). Am J Surg Pathol 1995;19: 859–72.

36. Stoll LM, Li QK. Cytology of fine-needle aspiration of inflammatory myofibroblastic tumor. Diagn Cytopathol 1983;329:663–72.

37. Gleason BC, Hornick JL. Inflammatory myofibro-blastic tumours: where are we now? J Clin Pathol 2008;61:428–37.

38. Antonescu CR, Suurmeijer AJ, Zhang L, et al. Molecular characterization of inflammatory myofibro-blastic tumors with frequent ALK and ROS1 fusions and rare novel RET gene rearrangement. Am J Surg Pathol 2015;39:957–67.

39. Doyle LA, Hornick JL. Gastrointestinal stromal tu-mours: from KIT to succinate dehydrogenase. His-topathology 2014;64:53–67.

40. Wieczorek TJ, Faquin WC, Rubin BP, et al. Cyto-logic diagnosis of gastrointestinal stromal tumor with emphasis on the differential diagnosis with leiomyosarcoma. Cancer 2001;93:276–87.

41. Miettinen M, Wang ZF, Lasota J. DOG1 antibody in the differential diagnosis of gastrointestinal stromal tumors: a study of 1840 cases. Am J Surg Pathol 2009;33:1401–8.

42. Hwang DG, Qian X, Hornick JL. DOG1 antibody is a highly sensitive and specific marker for gastroin-testinal stromal tumors in cytology cell blocks. Am J Clin Pathol 2011;135:448–53.

43. Hornick JL, Fletcher CDM. Immunohistochemical staining for KIT (CD117) in soft tissue sarcomas is very limited in distribution. Am J Clin Pathol 2002; 117:188–93.

44. Sirvent N, Maire G, Pedeutour F. Genetics of der-matofibrosarcoma protuberans family of tumors: from ring chromosomes to tyrosine kinase inhibitor treatment. Genes Chromosomes Cancer 2003;37: 1–19.

45. Fletcher CD, Evans BJ, MacArtney JC, et al. Dermatofibrosarcoma protuberans: a clinicopath-ological and immunohistochemical study with a review of the literature. Histopathology 1985;9: 921–38.

46. Domanski HA, Gustafson P. Cytologic features of primary, recurrent, and metastatic dermatofi-brosarcoma protuberans. Cancer 2002;96: 351–61.

47. Kutzner H. Expression of the human progenitor cell antigen CD34 (HPCA-1) distinguishes dermatofi-brosarcoma protuberans from fibrous histiocytoma in formalin-fixed, paraffin-embedded tissue. J Am Acad Dermatol 1993;28:613–7.

48. Mentzel T, Beham A, Katenkamp D, et al. Fibrosar-comatous ('high-grade') dermatofibrosarcoma protu-berans: clinicopathologic and immunohistochemical study of a series of 41 cases with emphasis on prog-nostic significance. Am J Surg Pathol 1998;22: 576–87.

49. Calonje E, Mentzel T, Fletcher CDM. Cellular benign fibrous histiocytoma: clinicopathologic analysis of 74 cases of a distinctive variant of cuta-neous fibrous histiocytoma with frequent recur-rence. Am J Surg Pathol 1994;18:668–76.

50. Fletcher CDM. Tumors of soft tissue. In: Fletcher CDM, editor. Diagnostic histopathology of tumours, vol. 2. New York: Elsevier Inc.; 2013. p. 1796–870.

51. Demicco EG, Wagner MJ, Maki RG, et al. Risk assessment in solitary fibrous tumors: validation and refinement of a risk stratification model. Mod Pathol 2017;30:1433–42.

52. Gold JS, Antonescu CR, Hajdu C, et al. Clinico-pathologic correlates of solitary fibrous tumors. Cancer 2002;94:1057–68.

53. Gholami S, Cassidy MR, Kirane A, et al. Size and location are the most important risk factors for ma-lignant behavior in resected solitary fibrous tumors. Ann Surg Oncol 2017;24:3865–71.

54. Tani E, Wejde J, Åström K, et al. FNA cytology of solitary fibrous tumors and the diagnostic value of STAT6 immunocytochemistry. Cancer Cytopathol 2018;126:36–43.

55. Doyle LA, Vivero M, Fletcher CDM, et al. Nuclear expression of STAT6 distinguishes solitary fibrous tumor from histologic mimics. Mod Pathol 2014; 27:390–5.

56. Doyle LA, Tao D, Mariño-Enríquez A. STAT6 is amplified in a subset of dedifferentiated liposar-coma. Mod Pathol 2014;27:1231–7.

57. Demicco EG, Boland GM, Brewer Savannah KJ, et al. Progressive loss of myogenic differentiation in leiomyosarcoma has prognostic value. Histopa-thology 2015;66:627–38.

58. Iwata J, Fletcher CDM. Immunohistochemical detection of cytokeratin and epithelial membrane antigen in leiomyosarcoma: a systematic study of 100 cases. Pathol Int 2000;50:7–14.

59. Agaram N, Chen CL, Zhang L, et al. Recurrent MYOD1 mutations in pediatric and adult sclerosing and spindle cell rhabdomyosarcomas: evidence for a common pathogenesis. Genes Chromosomes Cancer 2014;53:779–87.

60. Antonescu CR, Scheithauer B, Woodruff J. Malig-nant tumors of the peripheral nerves. In: AFIP atlas of tumor pathology series 4: tumors of the peripheral nervous system, vol. 19. Washington, DC: American Registry of Pathology; 2013. p. 381–5.

61. Schaefer IM, Fletcher CDM, Hornick JL. Loss of H3K27 trimethylation distinguishes malignant pe-ripheral nerve sheath tumors from histologic mimics. Mod Pathol 2016;29:4–13.

62. Mito JK, Qian X, Doyle LA, et al. Role of histone H3K27 trimethylation loss as a marker for malignant peripheral nerve sheath tumor in fine-needle aspi-ration and small biopsy specimens. Am J Clin Pathol 2017;148:179–89.

63. Nonaka D, Chiriboga L, Rubin BP. Sox10: a Pan-Schwannian and melanocytic marker. Am J Surg Pathol 2008;32:1291–8.

64. Åkerman M, Ryd W, Skytting B. Fine-needle aspiration of synovial sarcoma: criteria for diagnosis: retrospective reexamination of 37 cases, including ancillary diagnostics. A Scandinavian sarcoma group study. Diagn Cytopathol 2003;28:232–8.

65. Terry J, Saito T, Subramanian S, et al. TLE1 as a diagnostic immunohistochemical marker for synovial sarcoma emerging from gene expression profiling studies. Am J Surg Pathol 2007;31:240–6.

66. Kosemehmetoglu K, Vrana JA, Folpe AL. TLE1 expression is not specific for synovial sarcoma: a whole section study of 163 soft tissue and bone neoplasms. Mod Pathol 2009;22:872–8.

67. Foo W, Cruise M, Wick M, et al. Immunohistochemical staining for TLE1 distinguishes synovial sarcoma from histologic mimics. Am J Clin Pathol 2011;135:839–44.

68. Clark J, Rocques PJ, Crew AJ, et al. Identification of novel genes, SYT and SSX, involved in the t(X;18)(p11.2;q11.2) translocation found in human synovial sarcoma. Nature 1994;8:340–4.

69. Hasegawa T, Matsuno Y, Shimoda T, et al. Proximal-type epithelioid sarcoma: a clinicopathologic study of 20 cases. Mod Pathol 2001;14:655–63.

70. Miettinen M, Fanburg-Smith JC, Virolainen M, et al. Epithelioid sarcoma: an immunohistochemical analysis of 112 classical and variant cases and a discussion of the differential diagnosis. Hum Pathol 1999;30:934–42.

71. Hornick JL, Dal Cin P, Fletcher CDM. Loss of INI1 expression is characteristic of both conventional and proximal-type epithelioid sarcoma. Am J Surg Pathol 2009;33:542–50.

72. Miettinen M, McCue PA, Sarlomo-Rikala M, et al. Sox10 – A marker for not only Schwannian and melanocytic neoplasms but also myoepithelial cell tumors of soft tissue. A systematic analysis of 5134 tumors. Am J Surg Pathol 2015;39:826–35.

73. Sigauke E, Rakheja D, Maddox DL, et al. Absence of expression of SMARCB1/INI1 in malignant rhabdoid tumors of the central nervous system, kidneys and soft tissue: an immunohistochemical study with implications for diagnosis. Mod Pathol 2006;19:717–25.

74. Shih AR, Cote GM, Chebib I, et al. Clinicopathologic characteristics of poorly differentiated chordoma. Mod Pathol 2018;1–9. https://doi.org/10.1038/s41379-018-0002-1.

75. Weiss SW, Enzinger FM. Epithelioid hemangioendothelioma a vascular tumor often mistaken for a carcinoma. Cancer 1982;50:970–81.

76. Mentzel T, Beham A, Calonje E, et al. Epithelioid hemangioendothelioma of skin and soft tissues: clinicopathologic and immunohistochemical study of 30 cases. Am J Surg Pathol 1997;21:363–74.

77. VandenBussche CJ, Wakely PE, Siddiqui MT, et al. Cytopathologic characteristics of epithelioid vascular malignancies. Acta Cytol 2014;58:356–66.

78. Tanas MR, Sboner A, Oliveira AM, et al. Identification of a disease-defining gene fusion in epithelioid hemangioendothelioma. Sci Transl Med 2011;3:98ra82.

79. Doyle LA, Fletcher CDM, Hornick JL. Nuclear expression of CAMTA1 distinguishes epithelioid hemangioendothelioma from histologic mimics. Am J Surg Pathol 2016;40:94–102.

80. Antonescu C, Le Loarer F, Mosquera JM, et al. Novel YAP1-TFE3 fusion defines a distinct subset of epithelioid hemangioendothelioma. Genes Chromosomes Cancer 2013;52:775–84.

81. Enzinger M. Clear-cell sarcoma of tendons and aponeuroses a n analysis of 21 cases. Cancer 1965;18:1163–74.

82. Creager AJ, Pitman MB, Geisinger KR. Cytologic features of clear cell sarcoma (malignant melanoma) of soft parts: a study of fine-needle aspirates and exfoliative specimens. Am J Clin Pathol 2002;117:217–24.

83. Hisaoka M, Ishida T, Kuo TT, et al. Clear cell sarcoma of soft tissue: a clinicopathologic, immunohistochemical, and molecular analysis of 33 cases. Am J Surg Pathol 2008;32:452–60.

84. Doyle LA. Non-mesenchymal mimics of sarcoma. Surg Pathol Clin 2015;8:493–513.

85. Wang WL, Mayordomo E, Zhang W, et al. Detection and characterization of EWSR1/ATF1 and EWSR1/CREB1 chimeric transcripts in clear cell sarcoma (melanoma of soft parts). Mod Pathol 2009;22:1201–9.

86. Wakely PE, McDermott JE, Ali SZ. Cytopathology of alveolar soft part sarcoma. Cancer Cytopathol 2009;117:500–7.

87. Folpe AL, Deyrup AT. Alveolar soft-part sarcoma: a review and update. J Clin Pathol 2006;59:1127–32.

88. Folpe AL, Mentzel T, Lehr HA, et al. Perivascular epithelioid cell neoplasms of soft tissue and gynecologic origin: a clinicopathologic study of 26 cases and review of the literature. Am J Surg Pathol 2005;29:1558–75.

89. Cho HY, Chung DH, Khurana H, et al. The role of TFE3 in PEComa. Histopathology 2008;53:236–9.

90. Schoolmeester JK, Lastra RR. Granular cell tumors overexpress TFE3 without corollary gene rearrangement. Hum Pathol 2015;46:1242–3.

91. Zhou H, Guo M, Gong Y. Challenge of FNA diagnosis of angiomyolipoma: a study of 33 cases. Cancer Cytopathol 2017;125:257–66.

92. Doyle L a, Hornick JL, Fletcher CDM. PEComa of the gastrointestinal tract: clinicopathologic study of 35 cases with evaluation of prognostic parameters. Am J Surg Pathol 2013;37:1769–82.

93. Argani P, Aulmann S, Illei PB, et al. A distinctive subset of PEComas harbors TFE3 gene fusions. Am J Surg Pathol 2010;34:1395–406.

94. Miettinen M, Wang ZF, Sarlomo-Rikala M, et al. Succinate dehydrogenase deficient gists – a clinicopathologic, immunohistochemical, and molecular genetic study of 66 gastric gists with predilection to young age. Am J Surg Pathol 2011;35:1712–21.

95. Janeway KA, Kim SY, Lodish M, et al. Defects in succinate dehydrogenase in gastrointestinal stromal tumors lacking KIT and PDGFRA mutations. Proc Natl Acad Sci U S A 2011;108:314–8.

96. Mariño-Enríquez A, Wang WL, Roy A, et al. Epithelioid inflammatory myofibroblastic sarcoma: an aggressive intra-abdominal variant of inflammatory myofibroblastic tumor with nuclear membrane or perinuclear ALK. Am J Surg Pathol 2011;35:135–44.

97. Cash T, McIlvaine E, Krailo MD, et al. Comparison of clinical features and outcomes in patients with extraskeletal versus skeletal localized ewing sarcoma: a report from the Children's Oncology Group Thomas. 2016;63:1771–9.

98. Klijanienko J, Couturier J, Bourdeaut F, et al. Fine-needle aspiration as a diagnostic technique in 50 cases of primary ewing sarcoma/peripheral neuroectodermal tumor. Institut Curie's Experience. Diagn Cytopathol 2010;40:19–25.

99. Yoshida A, Goto K, Kodaira M, et al. CIC-rearranged sarcomas: a study of 20 cases and comparisons with Ewing sarcomas. Am J Surg Pathol 2016;40:313–23.

100. Lin O, Filippa DA, Teruya-Feldstein J. Immunohistochemical evaluation of FLI-1 in acute lymphoblastic lymphoma (ALL): a potential diagnostic pitfall. Appl Immunohistochem Mol Morphol 2009;17:409–12.

101. Hung YP, Fletcher CDM, Hornick JL. Evaluation of NKX2-2 expression in round cell sarcomas and other tumors with EWSR1 rearrangement: imperfect specificity for Ewing sarcoma. Mod Pathol 2016;29:370–80.

102. Russell-Goldman E, Hornick JL, Qian X, et al. NKX2.2 immunohistochemistry in the distinction of ewing sarcoma from cytomorphologic mimics: diagnostic utility and pitfalls. Cancer Cytopathol 2018;1–8. https://doi.org/10.1002/cncy.22056.

103. Doyle LA, Wong KK, Bueno R, et al. Ewing sarcoma mimicking atypical carcinoid tumor: detection of unexpected genomic alterations demonstrates the use of next generation sequencing as a diagnostic tool. Cancer Genet 2014;207:335–9.

104. Shibuya R, Matsuyama A, Nakamoto M, et al. The combination of CD99 and NKX2.2, a transcriptional target of EWSR1-FLI1, is highly specific for the diagnosis of Ewing sarcoma. Virchows Arch 2014;465:599–605.

105. de Alava E, Lessnick S, Sorensen P. Ewing sarcoma. In: Fletcher CDM, Bridge JA, Hogendoorn PCW, et al, editors. WHO classification of tumours of soft tissue and bone. Lyon (France): International Agency for Research on Cancer; 2013. p. 306–9.

106. Wang NP, Marx J, McNutt MA, et al. Expression of myogenic regulatory proteins (myogenin and MyoD1) in small blue round cell tumors of childhood. Am J Pathol 1995;147:1799–810.

107. Bahrami A, Gown AM, Baird GS, et al. Aberrant expression of epithelial and neuroendocrine markers in alveolar rhabdomyosarcoma: a potentially serious diagnostic pitfall. Mod Pathol 2008;21:795–806.

108. Nishio J, Althof PA, Bailey JM, et al. Use of a novel FISH assay on paraffin-embedded tissues as an adjunct to diagnosis of alveolar rhabdomyosarcoma. Lab Invest 2006;86:547–56.

109. Gerald WL, Ladanyi M, de Alava E, et al. Clinical, pathologic, and molecular spectrum of tumors associated with t(11;22)(p13;q12): desmoplastic small round-cell tumor and its variants. J Clin Oncol 1998;16:3028–36.

110. Gerald WL, Miller HK, Battifora H, et al. Intra-abdominal desmoplastic small round-cell tumor. Report of 19 cases of a distinctive type of high-grade polyphenotypic malignancy affecting young individuals. Am J Surg Pathol 1991;15:499–513.

111. Lae ME, Roche PC, Jin L, et al. Desmoplastic small round cell tumor: a clinicopathologic, immunohistochemical, and molecular study of 32 tumors. Am J Surg Pathol 2002;26:823–35.

112. Chebib I, Jo VY. Round cell sarcoma with CIC-DUX4 gene fusion: discussion of the distinctive cytomorphologic, immunohistochemical, and molecular features in the differential diagnosis of round cell tumors. Cancer Cytopathol 2016;124:350–61.

113. Hung YP, Fletcher CDM, Hornick JL. Evaluation of ETV4 and WT1 expression in CIC-rearranged sarcomas and histologic mimics. Mod Pathol 2016;29:1324–34.

114. Matsuyama A, Shiba E, Umekita Y, et al. Clinicopathologic diversity of undifferentiated sarcoma with BCOR-CCNB3 fusion: analysis of 11 cases with a reappraisal of the utility of immunohistochemistry for BCOR and CCNB3. Am J Surg Pathol 2017;41:1713–21.

115. Kao YC, Owosho AA, Sung YS, et al. BCOR - CCNB3 fusion positive sarcomas: a clinicopathologic and molecular analysis of 36 cases with comparison to morphologic spectrum and clinical behavior of other round cell sarcomas. Am J Surg Pathol 2018;42:604–15.

116. Shibayama T, Okamoto T, Nakashima Y, et al. Screening of BCOR-CCNB3 sarcoma using immunohistochemistry for CCNB3: a clinicopathological

report of three pediatric cases. Pathol Int 2015;65: 410–4.

117. Binh MBN, Sastre-Garau X, Guillou L, et al. MDM2 and CDK4 immunostainings are useful adjuncts in diagnosing well-differentiated and dedifferentiated liposarcoma subtypes: a comparative analysis of 559 soft tissue neoplasms with genetic data. Am J Surg Pathol 2005;29:1340–7.

118. Gaffney EF, Dervan PA, Fletcher CD. Pleomorphic rhabdomyosarcoma in adulthood. Analysis of 11 cases with definition of diagnostic criteria. Am J Surg Pathol 1993;17:601–9.

119. Nicolas MM, Tamboli P, Gomez JA, et al. Pleomorphic and dedifferentiated leiomyosarcoma: clinicopathologic and immunohistochemical study of 41 cases. Hum Pathol 2010;41:663–71.

Moving?

Make sure your subscription moves with you!

To notify us of your new address, find your **Clinics Account Number** (located on your mailing label above your name), and contact customer service at:

Email: journalscustomerservice-usa@elsevier.com

800-654-2452 (subscribers in the U.S. & Canada)
314-447-8871 (subscribers outside of the U.S. & Canada)

Fax number: 314-447-8029

Elsevier Health Sciences Division
Subscription Customer Service
3251 Riverport Lane
Maryland Heights, MO 63043

*To ensure uninterrupted delivery of your subscription, please notify us at least 4 weeks in advance of move.

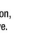

ELSEVIER